World Animal Science, B7

CATTLE GENETIC RESOURCES

World Animal Science

Editors-in-Chief:
Professor A. Neimann-Sørensen
Royal Veterinary & Agricultural University
Institute of Animal Production & Health
23 Rolighedsvej
1958 Frederiksberg C
Denmark

Emeritus Professor D.E. Tribe
Executive Director
Crawford Fund for International Agricultural Research
Hilda Stevenson House
1 Leonard Street
Parkville, Victoria 3052
Australia

Volumes in the Series

Subseries A: Basic information
Domestication, conservation and use of animal resources (ISBN 0-444-42068-1) - A 1
Development of animal production systems (ISBN 0-444-42050-9) - A 2
Dynamic biochemistry of animal production (ISBN 0-444-42052-5) - A 3
General and quantitative genetics (ISBN 0-444-42203-X) - A 4
Ethology of farm animals (ISBN 0-444-42359-1) - A 5
Microbiology of animals and animal products (ISBN 0-444-43010-5) - A 6
Anatomical basis of animal production
Basic physiological systems
Physioloy of production

Subseries B: Disciplinary approach
Grazing animals (ISBN 0-444-41835-0) - B 1
Parasites, pests and predators (ISBN 0-444-42175-0) - B 2
Meat science, milk science and technology (ISBN 0-444-42578-0) - B 3
Feed science (ISBN 0-444-42662-0) - B 4
Bioclimatology and the adaptation of livestock (ISBN 0-444-42690-6) - B 5
Animal production and environmental health (ISBN 0-444-42731-7) - B 6
Cattle genetic resources (ISBN 0-444-88638-9) - B 7
Genetic resources of pig, sheep and goat (ISBN 0-444-88279-0) - B 8
Animal reproduction
Animal housing and accommodation
Health management and preventive veterinary medicine
Animal feeding and nutrition

Subseries C: Production-system approach
Sheep and goat production (ISBN 0-444-41989-6) - C 1
Laboratory animals (ISBN 0-444-42464-4) - C 2
Dairy-cattle production (ISBN 0-444-42680-9) - C 3
Production of aquatic animals (Crustaceans, Molluscs, Amphibians and Reptiles) - C 4
Production of aquatic animals (Fishes)
Beef-cattle production
Pig production
Horse breeding and management
Buffalo production
Production of other domesticated mammals
Furred-animal production
Poultry production
Concluding volume (and cumulative index)

World Animal Science, B7

CATTLE GENETIC RESOURCES

Edited by

C.G. HICKMAN

Resources Management Services,
Box 6246, Station J, Ottawa,
Ont. K2A 0A0, Canada

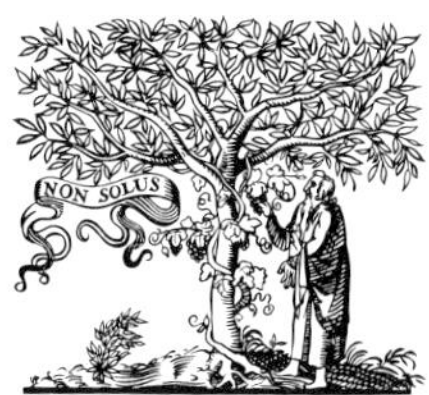

ELSEVIER SCIENCE PUBLISHERS B.V.

Amsterdam – Oxford – New York – Tokyo 1991

ELSEVIER SCIENCE PUBLISHERS B.V.
Sara Burgerhartstraat 25
P.O. Box 211, 1000 AE Amsterdam, The Netherlands

Distributors for the United States and Canada:

ELSEVIER SCIENCE PUBLISHERS COMPANY INC.
655, Avenue of the Americas
New York, NY 10017, U.S.A.

ISBN 0-444-88638-9

This book has been printed on acid-free paper.

Printed in The Netherlands

General Preface

Several factors make it desirable at this time to collect and integrate existing knowledge in Animal Science in its widest sense.

Millions of people in the world are today suffering from starvation or malnutrition and the number will increase with the inevitable rise in the world population. This poses an inexorable challenge to all scientists involved in problems underlying the production of food for man. Yet the development of livestock industries does not only aim to improve the nutritional standards of the human population, important though that is. From man's point of view animals are multipurpose and their use can have different objectives: economic, social and ecological. In addition to being important as sources of food, clothing and certain forms of power, animals can also represent forms of wealth, recreation, means of employing labour, aesthetic enjoyment, and determinants of landscape.

Animal production must increasingly compete with other forms of production for resources, especially energy, but also for land, water, finance and labour. This creates a greater need than ever to develop systems which maximize efficiency. At the same time, these systems need also to meet other requirements. They must be environmentally beneficial, ethically defensible, socially acceptable, and relevant to the particular aims, needs and resources of the community they are designed to serve.

Rapid advances in knowledge within practically all areas of the animal sciences are now being made. Solutions to many of the problems which face the livestock producer, whether he is working in, say, a cattle feedlot in the U.S.A. or in a traditional system of village goat production in West Africa, are now resulting from the research being carried out in the various disciplines of Animal Sciences. However, too often the results of this research remain confined to the specialized journals of different scientific disciplines when, increasingly, the approach of those working in animal production needs to be interdisciplinary and global. Furthermore, Animal Science has attained a new dimension in recent years. Whatever form it takes, animal production constantly influences and interacts with the other components of the total ecosystem within which it operates. New disciplines, like ecology, ethology and conservation have become important; new forms of production, such as aquaculture and the use of non-conventional feed resources are receiving increasing attention.

The scientists and planners in animal production have to work within the framework of these developments. Extensive inquiries among such specialists in many parts of the world have revealed the need for a comprehensive and up-to-date review of the Animal Science literature covering the entire range of technical knowledge that is now required in animal production and development. Therefore, Elsevier Science Publishers has initiated this major work of reference under the title 'World Animal Science'. Inevitably such a task must cover many volumes and involve the collaboration of a great number of editors and authors. Through an elaborate preparatory phase and with continuous editorial guidance from the Chief Editors and the Editorial Advisory Board, including scientists from all parts of the world, the aim has been to produce an integrated series of volumes which, although not encyclopaedic and not intended to be exhaustive in each branch of knowledge, does give appropriate emphasis to coherence and applicability. With this in mind the series has been divided into three parts: the volumes in subseries A provide information on the anatomical, genetical, biochemical, behavioural, physiological and microbiological bases of animal production; those in subseries B are each devoted to a particular discipline important to animal production, e.g. reproduction, breeding, feed science, bioclimatology and adaptation; and finally, in subseries C, production systems are described on a species basis, covering beef and dairy cattle, sheep, pigs, horses, buffaloes, poultry and some newly or partially domesticated mammals.

Emphasis is laid throughout on the careful reviewing and integration of significant knowledge in the total field of animal production with the aim of reporting not only what is known but also of drawing attention to important gaps in our knowledge. Account is taken of current trends in thinking and development and controversial topics are also dealt with, e.g. ethical aspects of animal use. Traditional farm animals, i.e. cattle, horses, sheep, goats and pigs, are given major emphasis and their production systems are treated in special volumes. There are also separate volumes on the conservation and use of their genetic resources. Other forms of animal production, such as poultry and fur production, are given less attention in the early volumes but still have their special volumes dealing with production systems. Other topics of less over-all importance, or about which less is known, are treated in separate chapters within volumes. Because of the increasing importance of animal production in less developed areas of the world, attention is paid to domesticated mammals such as buffalo, camel, llama, alpaca, yak, reindeer and elephant, and to such newly or partially domesticated mammals as the eland, oryx, red deer and musk-ox. The series deals with both intensive and extensive animal production systems. In this way an attempt has been made to set the whole world animal production into an appropriate and contemporary perspective.

Although, by editorial concept and by cross-referencing between volumes, the series functions as a single entity, each volume is nevertheless constituted as an independent unit, suitable for separate use. To achieve this and still avoid undue overlap, each volume only summarizes those essential elements of topics which are treated in detail in other volumes. Thus each volume aims to approach the breadth of World Animal Science from its own particular point of view, with supporting references to details in other volumes.

The series is written primarily for use by people who have a specialist interest in animal production as students, teachers, extension officers and consultants, policy-makers, and research scientists. The volumes are planned for world-wide use, which implies that the information presented covers systems and principles of more than local or national interest.

Preface to Volume B7

This volume has a paramount relevance to the food yield problems of the many vital food production systems that include cattle or buffalo. About 75% of the world's agricultural land produces forages of one kind or another that can be utilized only by ruminants. The cattle and buffalo population, projected to be approximately 2 billion by year 2000 are now maintained for the most part under conditions where modern husbandry does not exist. The present population has a very low percentage of productivity. Prospects for correcting this low level of production in time to offset the world's increasing need for food supplies depend largely on a greater understanding of the technology of present production conditions including the genetic adaption of present breeds to the environment.

The first four chapters give an overview of administrative, organizational and other features of present and past genetic resource activity and technology at the national and international level. They show that our knowledge of livestock and its origins are very extensive but also indicate serious gaps in our understanding of how best to avoid dangers for future generations resulting from inadequate genetic variability.

Chapter 1, by Phillips, reveals the official functions and the interrelationships of the organizations involved in aspects of animal genetic resources. Many of the major projects which have been carried out in different parts of the world are used as examples to present a very clear picture of the interplay between local, national, and international activities involving the two species dealt with in this volume.

Chapter 2, by Turton, deals with the subject of animal genetics as required in modern times and the related conditions of livestock breeding and production. This is an exhaustive treatment of the subject of genetic variability as it exists presently and of how best to maintain it. This chapter should have a major influence on the design of genetic resource programmes. The need for such programmes is increasingly urgent because of the ever decreasing genetic variability among livestock populations in the face of the reality that genetic variability, once diminished, can never be recovered.

Chapter 3, by Payne, reviews the origins and the history of domestication of cattle and buffalo. It vividly presents the distribution of these species around the world and their transition into breeds throughout the history of animal agriculture. This presentation of the introduction of animals from the Old World to the New will be of great interest to the students of the subject of animal migration. In addition, the geneology of species by scientific name will make this chapter of value to an understanding of the evolution of domesticated animals.

The next five chapters describe livestock industries in major livestock-producing areas of the world. These cases illustrate the importance of adapted breeds. In North America, it is obvious that modern genetic techniques have developed an adaptation to intensive production environments. There, modern breeds are developed for maximizing level of production with economic justification based on minimizing capital cost inputs per unit of output. In other examples, an entirely different method of production is presented which is non-specialized and dependent upon optimum inputs for optimum outputs which apparently maximizes economic benefits. The only major livestock production system that is not present in this volume is that of pastoral dry-land management. The basic genetic resource requirements are similar between this and the migratory breeds that are presented in Chapter 4 on Cattle Genetic Resources of West Africa. All together these presentations instil a sense of urgency with regard to maintenance of genetic resources.

Other major livestock producing areas dealt with here are Latin America, Chapter 5, West and Central Africa, Chapter 4 and the most productive livestock populations in Chapters 6 and 7 for the Northern Hemisphere.

The last three chapters of the volume deal with critical technical subjects associated with animal genetic resources. Chapter 8, by Starkey, on Draught Animals is of special importance mainly because of the neglect that has occurred over the decade of this extremely valuable source of power for agriculture. The treatment of the subject of draught animals is extremely thorough, presenting many aspects not available elsewhere. In its original presentation, the chapter included a section on nutrition and feeding which was eliminated due to the necessary limits on the size of this volume and the need to maintain the focus on genetic resource subjects. It is also important to note that this chapter indicates promising possibilities for the future in improving the use of draught animals in a wide range of agricultural needs. In general it highlights something that is also evident in most other chapters, that is, the need for more careful consideration in designing projects for developing countries and the need for a greater appreciation and understanding by industrialized countries of livestock development possibilities.

Chapter 9, on official methods of breed management, is another example of the need for more recognition of native breeds. It outlines the procedures used for breed management in advanced livestock industries. Here it appears obvious that modern methods of husbandry should be introduced for at least the most important native breeds in developing countries. Presented here is an up-to-date picture of modern methods of genetic resource management. It conveys an important premise that genetic resource management is not only a subject for control by governments or government organizations but can be operated successfully by the private sector.

The last chapter serves to present information related to the importance of gene libraries. The vast amount of information on gene identification that is presented here makes up the largest chapter of the volume. It also includes valuable records of the disappearance of breeds and of situations that did harm to important genetic resource material. The chapter points out the need for greater knowledge of facts related to gene identification and genetic engineering. As a final presentation this chapter appropriately highlights the important genetic abilities of many breeds that are now extinct or almost extinct. It can be concluded from this chapter that improved communication between all those interested in the subject of genetic resource is badly needed. This and related volumes will stimulate a demand for a regular exchange of current information of the subject of animal genetic resources.

If there is a single theme for this volume it cannot be better expressed than by the father of modern animal breeding who stated (Jay L. Lush, 1949): The only kind of a world in which concentrating on only one breed is to be encouraged, other than for immediate economic advantage in costs and convenience, is one in which all genes combine their effects additively and it is known that standards of what is desirable are not going to change. The costs of maintaining living museums in which all breeds and strains would be preserved forever seem so high, however, that animal breeding seems unable to go as far in this direction as plant breeding can. That is for the future to determine. Here we can only mention the genetic desirability of encouraging those who are willing to maintain and improve the rare breeds.

CHARLES G. HICKMAN
Ottawa, Canada

Contents

Chapter 1

International Administration and Coordination of Efforts to Conserve and Utilize Effectively Cattle and Water Buffalo Genetic Resources

RALPH W. PHILLIPS

1. MAN'S DEPENCENCE UPON THE GENETIC RESOURCES OF DOMESTICATED PLANTS AND ANIMALS

1.1. Overall importance of genetic resource management

Man has domesticated many plants, and a substantially smaller number of animals. These plants and animals provide man with most of his food and fibre. Without their products man could not have moved from the status of a hunter, dependent upon what he could find or kill, to the status of a settled farmer and, as his numbers increased, to a situation in which millions upon millions live in cities where they have no food and fibre production capacity of their own. Without the domesticated plants and animals that serve him, man could not possibly exist in his present numbers, much less in the substantially larger numbers that are projected for the next century and beyond.

Given man's near total dependence upon the products of domesticated plants and animals, it is essential to understand the present status of the development of these resources, the needs that may be projected for future development, and the dangers that lie ahead if the genetic resources now available are not safeguarded, so that man's future needs may — hopefully — be met. Although the focus in this volume is upon cattle and water buffalo resources, there are important lessons to be learned from the plant field, lessons that should be taken into account as we consider how to cope with the problems of evaluating, conserving and effectively utilizing animal genetic resources, and in particular the cattle and water buffalo genetic resources, that are now available.

The plants and animals that man has domesticated have evolved over many millennia. In recent times man has done much to shape their evolution into more productive types. As man himself evolved, and began to develop the various aspects of science, he began to study the inheritance of different traits, particularly in plants, then in animals. As the science of genetics emerged, it is not surprising that plant geneticists came into prominence ahead of animal geneticists. For, apart from the biologists who worked with such small insects as *Drosophila,* the plant geneticists generally utilized breeding materials that could be maintained at substantially less expense, could be managed more easily, and in which generations could be turned over more rapidly than was possible with larger domesticated animals. Also, the traits of concern to the animal geneticist tended to be inherited in a more complex manner than many of those the plant geneticist sought to understand and control. So, in terms of human generations, the first major 'crop' of plant geneticists emerged at least a generation ahead of the time when substantial numbers of animal geneticists began to appear.

Chapter 1 references, p. 18

The fact that plant breeders were able to make relatively rapid progress, coupled with the fact that the results of their successes could in most cases be quickly transported to other parts of the world, brought them face to face with the problem of conservation of genetic resources at an earlier stage than has occurred with farm animals. As Harlan (1961) pointed out, the geographic centres of diversity upon which plant breeders in the advanced countries had depended so much for their sources of genetic materials were in danger of extinction. Modern agriculture and modern technology were spreading rapidly around the world. New, uniform varieties were replacing the old, mixed populations. The old centres of diversity were disappearing. As a consequence, Harlan urged that adequate and thorough exploration be undertaken before it was too late. He also emphasized that world collections should be preserved with great care, lest the breeding materials be lost, and could never be replaced.

The maintenance of stocks of plant genetic resources is, fortunately, a relatively inexpensive matter, compared with comparable programmes for large domesticated animals. This fact, coupled with the more advanced stage to which plant genetics has progressed, and the more general recognition of the problem among plant geneticists and others concerned with agriculture, led to effective action on a number of fronts. A few examples of the institutions or programmes that have been established as a result of this recognition illustrate the point:

(1) The Crop Genetic Resources Center, that functioned as a part of FAO's Plant Production and Protection Division, in Rome, Italy, under the supervision of the International Board for Plant Genetic Resources, and which is sponsored by the Consultative Group on International Agricultural Research (CGIAR).

(2) The International Potato Center, near Lima, Peru, where a world collection of potato genetic materials is maintained. This centre is also sponsored by the CGIAR.

(3) The National Seed Storage Laboratory, at Ft Collins, Colorado, U.S.A., that is maintained by the U.S. Department of Agriculture, and where extensive collections of seeds are maintained as part of a national collection of plant genetic resources.

(4) The International Rice Research Institute, at Los Banos, near Manila, in the Philippines, where a bank of genetic stocks of rice is maintained. This institute is also sponsored by the CGIAR.

Other examples could be cited, but these will be sufficient to indicate that the need for conserving plant genetic stocks has been recognized by the world agricultural community, and that some important substantive actions have been taken. Symptomatic of the relative lack of such recognition in relation to genetic stocks of domestic animals is that, when efforts were made following the establishment of the Crop Genetic Resources Center mentioned above, to develop a similar programme for animal genetic resources, those in control of possible financial resources showed no interest in such an undertaking.

Although developments do not occur as rapidly in the field of animal breeding as they do in plant breeding, the time has already arrived when many types and breeds of animals that have potential value for use in future animal breeding programmes are being diluted and are in danger of being lost, while some have been lost already.

In a world that has problems in meeting the food and nutritional needs of its present population of some 5 billion people, there is urgent need to safeguard the genetic resources that will be needed in producing the food for the much larger populations of the future. Present projections are that – given the current growth rate – the world's population will double to 10 billion by the year 2050. Since both plants and animals are essential in providing the link between what the earth can produce and what man consumes, it is necessary, if such vast populations are to be fed, to have available the best animal genetic resources as well as the essential plant genetic resources for use in breeding programmes.

In many respects the identification, conservation and effective use of genetic resources is a national or even a local problem. However, because of the increasing interdependence of countries, and because of the importance of ensuring an adequate food supply for all of mankind, now and in the future, it is a peculiarly international problem.

1.2. Special nature and importance of cattle and water buffalo genetic resources

Among the animals that man has domesticated, and which he now maintains in his service, cattle and water buffaloes are, as a group, certainly the most important. In terms of numbers, and using FAO (1982) data for 1981, there were approximately 1331 million cattle and water buffaloes, or approximately three-tenths of an animal for each person in the world, on the average. Leaving chickens aside, their nearest rivals among the domestic animals were sheep, of which there were some 1130 million head.

Cattle and water buffaloes produced about 46.9 million tonnes of beef, veal and buffalo meat in 1981. This amounted to about 10.6 kg of meat per person, for the year, on the average.

Hides are important by-products of the slaughter of cattle and water buffaloes, since they provide the raw materials for shoes, belts, purses and many other useful products made from leather. The 1981 annual production of hides from cattle and water buffaloes amounted to 6.5 million tonnes. Thus, about 1.45 kg of hides were available per person, on the average.

Pigs produced somewhat more meat than cattle and water buffaloes combined, i.e., about 55 million tonnes. However, in terms of total food production, cattle and water buffaloes produced more since, in addition to 46.9 million tonnes of meat, they produced over 456 million tonnes of milk. This amounted to about 103.4 kg of milk for each person, on average, in 1981.

Many cattle and water buffaloes are used for draft, and the power they produce is essential for the tilling of the soil on large numbers of the world's farms. The power they produce is also important for the lifting of water, for the threshing and grinding of grain, and for transport of agricultural products and requisites on and off the farms. Although there are no accurate statistical measures or estimates of the amount of power these animals produce, it is certainly enormous.

Here it should also be recalled that some 68.2% of the world's agricultural land consists of permanent pasture and range land. Cattle, water buffaloes and other ruminants provide the primary mechanism, and in many areas the only mechanism, through which forage can be harvested from these vast areas and converted into products usable by man. In addition, much of the volume of the product of the 31.8% of the agricultural land that is arable or in tree crops, such as straw or fodder from which grain has been harvested, cannot be utilized directly by man, and he is dependent upon cattle, water buffaloes and other animals to convert such materials into products he can consume, or otherwise utilize.

If one considers the meat, milk, skins and draft power cattle and water buffaloes produce, together with the manure, tankage, glands from which hormones are extracted, and other products utilized by man, it is evident that these animals contribute much to man's well-being.

This global overview of the contributions of cattle and water buffaloes underlines the significance not only of their current value to man, but also the

Chapter 1 references, p. 18

very great importance that must be attached to ensuring that their contributions will be available, in greatly increased volume, to meet the needs of substantially larger numbers of people in future generations.

2. NEED FOR EFFECTIVE ANIMAL GENETIC RESOURCE MANAGEMENT AT THE LOCAL, NATIONAL AND INTERNATIONAL LEVELS

2.1. Historical developments and present situation

The available evidence regarding the domestication of sheep, goats, pigs and cattle indicates that the centre of their domestication was in southwestern Asia, and adjacent Greece (for cattle), according to Reed (1980). By at least 6800 BP (before the present) all these four classes of animals were being moved by herders and farmers up the Danube valley into central Europe. Although evidence is lacking about such early domestication in other areas, the Near East is not necessarily the only area in which domestication took place. The ancestors of domestic cattle were found in Europe, North Africa, and in Asia from northern India and southern China northward. So the idea of domestication may have travelled faster than the movement of animals, or people in other areas could well have settled into villages and could have been domesticating cattle and other animals, thus achieving independently what the people of the Near East had already done. In any event, domesticated cattle spread over the European, Asian and African land masses, and were eventually taken by man to other continents.

Water buffaloes were probably domesticated in northern India before 2500 BC (about 4500 BP), according to Reed (1980). From there domesticated water buffaloes spread over the land masses of the Near East, southeastern Europe, southern Asia, the islands of the south Pacific, Egypt, south central Africa, and eventually were taken to northern Australia, and to portions of South America.

Two basic types of cattle emerged, the humpless cattle of Europe and northern Asia (*Bos taurus*), and the humped Zebu cattle (*Bos indicus*). There are many distinctive breeds in each of these two basic types, and there are also many breeds and local groups that are intermediate in type. The broad distribution of the *B. taurus, B. Indicus* and intermediate types has been mapped by Phillips (1961b). The *B. taurus* types are found throughout Europe, northern Asia, Australia, New Zealand, portions of northwestern Africa, and the temperate portions of North and South America. Zebu cattle predominate in India, Pakistan, southeastern Asia, northern Australia, most of central Africa, the Gulf Coast of the United States, the Caribbean, and east central South America. Intermediate types are found in the eastern and western portions of southern Asia, and in southern Africa. Phillips (1961b) lists and maps the points of origin of some 195 recognized breeds of cattle, and many of the minor types and breeds are not included in that listing. Many of the world's breeds of cattle are described in references cited elsewhere in this chapter (Joshi and Phillips, 1953; Joshi et al., 1957; Phillips, 1944, 1963; French et al., 1966). In addition, Rouse (1970/73), in his three-volume work on 'World Cattle', and in his volume on 'The Criollo' (Rouse, 1977), has provided much information on the many diverse breeds throughout the world. Also, Felius (1985) has provided a beautifully illustrated description of the cattle breeds of the world.

Three basic types of water buffaloes evolved, the river breeds, the Mediterranean types, and the swamp types and breeds. According to the mapping of the distribution of these types (Ross Cockrill, 1974), all three types appear to have spread rather widely throughout the tropics and parts of the subtropics, but river breeds predominate in the Indian subcontinent and in central Africa, swamp breeds in the remainder of southern Asia and the islands of the Pacific, Mediterranean types predominate in southeastern Europe and the Near East, and all three types appear to have found some limited place in parts of Latin America. The many breeds that are recognized within these three types are described by Ross Cockrill (1974).

Against this brief and quite general background as to how cattle and water buffaloes evolved and are now distributed around the world, several points should be noted that have a bearing upon the problem of how to evaluate, conserve and most effectively use the available genetic resources of these important groups of domestic animals:

(1) Many types and breeds of cattle have remained quite local in character. They may occupy small geographic areas, and in many cases be quite limited in numbers.

(2) Although these local types may be well-adapted to the environment in which they are maintained, and may have potential value elsewhere, they may be under pressure of encroachment from animals from neighbouring areas, or from animals imported from more distant areas, and in consequence may be in danger of dilution, or of extinction, as distinct types or breeds.

(3) Other types and breeds have, for various reasons, spread over larger and sometimes vast areas, and exist in large numbers. Beef breeds like the Hereford and Angus, and dairy breeds like the Holstein, were taken by settlers to North America, Australia and New Zealand, for example. Spanish cattle were taken by Spanish settlers to Latin America. The Simmental spread overland from Switzerland to eastern Europe and into the U.S.S.R., where it found wide acceptance. So many of the more productive and better known breeds are well-established in various areas, and there is no immediate problem of conserving genetic stocks of such breeds.

(4) On the other hand, the cattle that settlers took with them to new lands were generally those to which they were accustomed in their homelands, and were not necessarily the breeds that would have been most productive in the new situations. This aspect of the problem is discussed in some detail elsewhere (Phillips, 1961a, 1963). Here it is worth noting that during the last two to two-and-a-half decades breed names such as Charolais, Chiana and Simmental have found their way into the vocabularies of North American cattle breeders who, at the beginning of that period, hardly knew of their existence. However, this process of testing out breeds in areas to which they are new is yet only in its beginning.

(5) The situation with water buffaloes is similar to that with cattle, but differs in three important respects. First, since the water buffalo is basically a tropical animal, it has spread over a relatively small area, compared with the worldwide distribution of cattle. Secondly, the recognized types and breeds are generally more local in character, i.e., more of them are limited to specific geographic areas, and only a few, like the Murrah which is especially regarded for its capacity as a milk producer, have been moved to other areas in recent times for breeding purposes. Thirdly, the water buffalo has been a largely neglected animal since, in terms of genetic, nutritional and management research, it has received little attention compared with cattle. This is reflected in the fact that the volume edited by Ross Cockrill (1974) was the first comprehensive compilation of information regarding the husbandry and health of the domestic water buffalo.

(6) In some areas, for example in southern China and in Indonesia, the water buffalo serves primarily as a draft animal, and practically no effort has been made to develop measures of draft-power capacity in these animals that would make possible objective comparisons with draft water buffaloes in other areas or countries.

Chapter 1 references, p. 18

2.2. Approaches needed to cope with the problem

As was pointed out earlier, the evaluation, conservation and effective use of cattle and water buffalo genetic resources is a local and a national problem, and — given the importance of the contributions of these animals to human welfare, now and in the future — it is also a matter of major international importance and concern. Thus, there is need to approach the problem at all three levels.

At the local level, the approach to the problem is necessarily very different in areas where cattle production is well-developed and highly productive breeds are maintained, than in areas where production methods are not well-developed, and breeding, feeding and management problems have been given little or no attention.

In areas where production methods are well-developed, and animals of the established and widely distributed breeds are maintained, there are generally no immediately urgent problems regarding the maintenance of genetic stocks. Nevertheless, there is need for attention to certain points in most such areas. These include:

(1) Continuing attention to methods of measuring performance, particularly in types used for beef and for work, since much remains to be done to develop practical methods of measuring such performance, and in the application of such measures in breeding programmes.

(2) Continuing attention to the possible experimental testing of new types, or types or breeds that have not been tested in the particular local circumstances but for which there is reason to believe that their productive performance might exceed that of the type or types presently used.

(3) Exercising restraint, in those areas from which animals may be exported to developing areas, to be reasonably certain that through such exports, the breeders in the developing areas are not being supplied with ill-adapted stock, and that their indigenous animals are not being diluted in an inappropriate way. This is perhaps a utopian hope, but if such restraint had been exercised in the past, many disappointing animal introductions might have been avoided.

In areas where animal production methods are not well-developed, and where modern methods of animal breeding are not generally applied, yet where local types of animals have evolved that survive and perform reasonably well under local circumstances, somewhat different approaches are needed, including:

(1) Developing an appreciation among animal owners of the merits of their animals, and of the importance of selecting and conserving the most productive animals for use in future breeding programmes.

(2) Collecting information on the true productive capacity of the local animals.

(3) Where it is deemed appropriate, experimental testing of animals from other areas that give promise of being more productive, and which may be adapted to the local environment.

(4) Encouraging the maintenance of nuclear herds of local types or breeds until such time as it may be clearly demonstrated that they are no longer needed in long-range breeding programmes.

In between the areas where animal production is highly developed, and areas where conditions of production are primitive, there are many gradations, and the approaches that are needed must, of course, be adapted to the skills and economic circumstances of the owners of cattle and water buffaloes.

At the national and local level, it is important that the Ministry of Agriculture and/or any other arm of government that is concerned with the productivity of the national herd of cattle and/or water buffaloes, and with that herd's contribution to the national welfare, should be well aware of problems related to genetic resources, and that it should:

(1) take the lead in ensuring that any potentially important types or breeds that have not been evaluated are adequately studied to assess their productivity, and their present and potential usefulness to the country;
(2) identify problem areas, where important types are in danger of dilution or extinction, and take the necessary steps to ensure that valuable genetic resources are not lost;
(3) exercise effective guidance and control over the importation of breeding stock, to ensure that such stock is used widely in breeding programmes, and that it is not allowed to dilute or replace local genetic stocks that may be useful in the long-term breeding programmes of the country; and
(4) conversely, cooperate and consult with countries desiring to import cattle or water buffalo breeding stock, to ensure that stock exported to other countries is to be tested or used in areas to which it may reasonably be expected to be adapted.

The above comments regarding the movements of animals between countries apply equally to inter-country movements of semen and ova. Also, it goes without saying, appropriate steps should be taken in connection with all inter-country movements of animals or of breeding materials to prevent the spread of diseases across national borders.

Needs at the international level naturally reflect the needs at the local and national levels. Thus, whether it be at a world or a regional level, any organization that is concerned with animal agriculture should:

(1) recognize that continuing and increasing productivity by cattle and water buffaloes is essential to man's welfare;
(2) recognize also that if these contributions are to be assured over the centuries ahead, the essential genetic resources must be identified and preserved;
(3) bring the problem, and the specific problem areas, to the attention of the countries concerned and, as appropriate, provide assistance to those countries in dealing with the problems;
(4) facilitate cooperation among countries in the safe exchange of breeding animals and materials, and in their use in experimental testing and in improvement programmes; and
(5) make pertinent information and technical personnel available to countries for improving cattle and water buffalo genetic resources, presenting the results of tests of types and breeds in new environments, and promoting potentially useful approaches to breeding improvement programmes and to more effective means of identifying and conserving the genetic resources needed in carrying out such breeding programmes over the long term.

This broad outline of the needs at the local, national and international levels appears deceptively simple. However, given the vast areas of land and numbers of animals involved, the great diversity in the animals and in the conditions under which they are maintained, and the vast complex of local and national jurisdictions within which the animals are located and under which efforts to achieve progress must be carried out, the meeting of these needs is a complex matter indeed. There is no practical possibility of meeting all of them. One can only hope that there will be some possibility of meeting a reasonable portion of such a complex set of needs.

In the subsequent sections of this chapter, attention is given to ways in which some of the existing national, regional and international institutions may contribute to the meeting of these needs.

Chapter 1 references, p. 18

3. ROLES OF EDUCATIONAL AND RESEARCH INSTITUTIONS

In this generalized discussion of the roles of educational and research institutions, the two types of institutions are treated together since, more often than not, such institutions undertake both education and research, and in many instances carry out extension activities as well. Also the discussion refers to the roles of both private and public institutions, and the roles of divisions of Ministries of Agriculture and other comparable departments of governments and to research and/or educational institutions maintained by them. Consequently, every point does not apply to every institution that may be concerned in one way or another with the evaluation, conservation and effective use of cattle and/or water buffalo genetic resources. Neither do all such institutions fit neatly into the education and research categories. Given the broad range of institutions to which this section refers, the discussion of their roles is necessarily quite generalized in nature.

3.1. Roles of educational and research institutions at the national level

National educational and research institutions that are concerned with various aspects of animal production are in key positions to contribute to the identification, conservation and effective use of cattle and/or water buffalo genetic resources. These include:

(1) taking the lead in developing an understanding, at the local and national levels, of the importance of these genetic resources and of coping effectively with problems relating to them;
(2) training the manpower that is needed to deal with the various aspects of evaluating, conserving and utilizing important genetic resources;
(3) assisting in the identification and evaluation of local types and breeds that have not been studied adequately, or not studied at all;
(4) assisting in the identification of problem areas in which valuable or potentially valuable genetic stocks of cattle or water buffaloes are in danger of being diluted, or of becoming extinct.
(5) participating in the planning and carrying out of experimental breeding programmes to test the adaptability and productivity of imported types under local conditions;
(6) utilizing some portion of the physical facilities that are usually available in educational and research institutions for the maintaining of important types or breeds, as parts of overall programmes to ensure the continuing availability of such genetic resources; and
(7) participating, through extension programmes or through other means, in the development of local and/or national programmes, in cooperation with cattle and/or water buffalo breeders and others concerned, to help ensure effective action in the evaluation, conservation and effective use of their respective countries' genetic resources.

Institutions of the types mentioned above are making contributions along the lines recommended in a number of countries. FAO (1981) brought together information on some such efforts, in a Technical Consultation organized jointly with UNEP in Rome in 1980. Some examples are summarized below to illustrate both the extent of the problem and the kinds of actions being taken to cope with it.

United Kingdom. Alderson (1981) points out that a 'rare breed' movement began in the U.K. only in 1964, with a view to maintaining distinct breeds of livestock. He also points out that six breeds of cattle have become extint during the 20th century. A Rare Breeds Survival Trust is the most important organization concerned with genetic resource conservation in the U.K. It is a charitable company, administered by an elected Council, and its policy is implemented by a technical consultant.

Alderson also notes that there are 55 rare or endangered breeds of large animals (cattle, sheep, pigs, horses) in the U.K., 45 of which are presently recognized by the Rare Breeds Survival Trust, on the basis of two criteria, numerical status and genetic value. Among the 55 rare breeds, 15 are cattle. Ten of these 15 rare breeds of cattle appeared to be considered worthy of attention by the Rare Breeds Survival Trust. The most important methods used by the Trust are: (a) preventing rare breeds from becoming extinct; (b) long-term storage of frozen embryos and semen; (c) creation of new breeding units, either as independent units, or as units within larger commercial units; (d) increasing the numerical status of each rare breed; (e) improving the management of rare breeds; (f) evaluation of rare breeds; and (g) promotion and utilization of rare breeds.

Bulgaria. Hinkovski and Alexiev (1981) point out that in Bulgaria the intensification of animal production in recent decades has resulted in decreasing numbers of animals in the breeds used as the basic means of production. Consequently, an attempt is being made, by direct subsidies to breeders, to conserve all the breeds that are in danger of extinction. These include three indigenous breeds of cattle, one of water buffalo, and some recently developed crossbred types of cattle and water buffaloes. Subsidies to the owners of breeds that are being conserved are paid annually by the National Agricultural–Industrial Union.

India. Bhat (1981) points out that there is very little real awareness of the animal resources India possesses, but that the need for conservation of animal genetic resources has now become clear. Consequently, a National Bureau of Animal Genetic Resources has been sanctioned. This Bureau will basically be a centre for information regarding the animal genetic resources of the country, and will serve as a link between Indian Council of Agricultural Research Institutes, Agricultural Universities, Government or private agencies, and national and international organizations concerned with livestock. It will provide support to such agencies for the maintenance of rare species and breeds that are in danger of extinction. The functions envisioned for the Bureau include attention to most of those listed at the beginning of this section, together with some extensions and refinements. Since cattle and water buffaloes are both very numerous and very important in India, it follows that the genetic resources of these two groups of animals will receive major attention.

France. Devillard et al. (1981) indicate that in France almost half the 80 existing breeds of asses, horses, cattle, sheep, goats and pigs are threatened with extinction, since they number no more than a few thousand head and in some cases far less. These endangered breeds include 12 breeds of cattle, while the numbers of some other breeds of cattle are decreasing at a rate sufficiently rapid to cause concern. Up until 1965 the Merino de Rambouillet breed of sheep was the only breed for which a preservation programme had been established, through a flock of 100–200 ewes kept in a closed breeding system at the Ecole Nationale d'Enseignement Ovin (National Sheep Training School). Conservation measures, supported by the Ministry of Agriculture, were initiated in 1968–69 for the preservation of Aubrac and Bazadaise cattle, and Solognote sheep. Little more was done until 1976, when the number of programmes began to increase rapidly, and by 1980 some 15 programmes were in place, of which nine were either management programmes or more modest programmes relating to cattle.

Chapter 1 references, p. 18

Devillard et al. (1981) indicate further that support had been given to the various activities in France through national agencies or public service agencies such as the Institut National de la Recherche Agronomique (National Agricultural Research Institute), higher education institutions, and professional associations. The experience in France shows that success in such efforts depends upon the existence of a local body to act as leader, the presence of an active worker, and a wish to conserve a breed on the part of the farmers who use it.

The foregoing examples from four countries in which breeds, conditions of livestock management, and other factors vary widely indicate some of the approaches being made. Evidence that the problem is being taken seriously or is at least recognized in other countries is obtained in the summaries of actions presented at the FAO/UNEP Technical Consultation on Animal Genetic Resources Conservation and Management (FAO, 1981), for Africa as a whole, and for Argentina, Botswana, Brazil, Canada, Colombia, Egypt, Ethiopia, Federal Republic of Germany, Hungary, Indonesia, Italy, Libya, Morocco, the Netherlands, Niger, Nigeria, Pakistan, Rwanda, Scandinavia (including Finland, Denmark, Iceland, Norway and Sweden), Spain, Sri Lanka, Thailand and Turkey. These summaries reflect varying degrees of awareness of the problem, and great variations in the kinds and levels of action being taken. A few examples of effective action will serve to indicate further what is being done:

(1) In Colombia, the selection and conservation of six criollo breeds of cattle is being undertaken by the Instituto Colombiano Agropecuario.

(2) In Hungary, six herds, numbering 850 cows, of the Hungarian breed of cattle are being maintained on state or cooperative farms.

(3) In Italy a 'Defense of Animal Genetic Resources' project was started in 1976 by the National Research Council, to promote and coordinate research on breed populations, mainly in the marginal land areas of the country.

(4) In the Netherlands the Dutch Rare Breed Foundation carried out a survey in 1977–78, and classified five domestic breeds of cattle as very rare, one as rare, and two as rather rare. Subsequently, a number of activities were undertaken by the Foundation to encourage the preservation of these rare breeds.

(5) In 1973 the Finnish Academy set up a working group to map threatened genetic resources of farm animals, and in 1975 the Finnish Animal Breeders' Association made an agreement with five state agricultural schools on maintaining their Finncattle herds until the time when the results of a breed comparison trial become available.

(6) In 1971 semen banks were established in Denmark for the three most important breeds of cattle.

3.2. Potential contributions of educational and research institutions at the inter-country and international levels

One such contribution was mentioned in the previous section, i.e., the evaluation of types or breeds of cattle from other countries. In addition, educational and research institutions are in position to make contributions at the inter-country and international levels in a number of other ways, including:

(1) Cooperating with institutions in other countries in the evaluation and conservation of cattle and/or water buffalo genetic resources in which the host countries of the cooperating institutions have mutual interests.

(2) Cooperating with institutions in other countries in the testing of types and breeds already known to be highly productive in their home countries, to determine if they are adapted to and can be useful in new locations.

(3) Supplying information to other countries, either directly or through in-

ternational organizations, on types and breeds evaluated as noted in points 1 and 2.

(4) Training and otherwise serving as a source of supply of competent manpower for international organizations, and for international programmes and projects relating to the evaluation, conservation and effective use of cattle and/or water buffalo genetic resources.

Activities of these various types are not as easy to carry out as are activities at the strictly national level. However, each time an institution imports breeding animals (or frozen ova or semen), tests them out either in pure form or in crossbreeding experiments, and publishes or otherwise makes the results available to other countries, it makes a contribution at the inter-country or international level to the evaluation of genetic resources and to how such resources may best be utilized in breeding practice.

Professionally trained workers who are active in the conduct of breeding research in their own countries, and who develop interest in the international aspects of the identification, conservation and effective utilization of cattle and water buffalo genetic resources, constitute the most likely source of talent to advise on or conduct genetic resource projects in other countries, or to provide leadership for such work in international organizations.

Experience in Canada provides an unusual example of how one country can contribute significantly in this field (FAO, 1981). In 1965 the Government of Canada established quarantine facilities to permit the importation of large domestic animals from outside the North American continent, and following that, animals of about two dozen breeds of beef cattle were imported. This brought the combined number of beef and dairy cattle breeds to nearly 60. Purebred herds of each of the imported breeds were established, and they were also used in crossbreeding. Some breeds were used more extensively than others. For example, in 1978 it was estimated that 16 484 cows were bred artifically with Simmental semen, 3591 with Limousin semen, 166 with Chianina semen, 88 with Tarentaise semen, and 4 with Parthenay semen. Additional cows were bred in natural matings by imported bulls. Since some of the breeds imported into Canada are on the decline in their countries of origin, Canada may also play a role in conserving the genetic resources of these breeds.

4. ROLES OF INTERNATIONAL ORGANIZATIONS

The term 'international organizations' is interpreted rather broadly in this section to include international companies or corporations that conduct business across national boundaries, non-governmental organizations that are regional or international in scope, and inter-governmental organizations that are regional or international in their memberships. This latter group is also interpreted to include international institutes that operate under the sponsorship of inter-governmental organizations, but which are not themselves inter-governmental organizations.

4.1. Essential contributions of international organizations

For reasons outlined at the beginning of this chapter, the identification, conservation and effective utilization of valuable genetic resources of cattle are matters of importance to all countries. This is also true in regard to water buffaloes in all tropical and subtropical countries where they are maintained. Also, there are advantages for many countries in being able to tap the cattle and/or water buffalo genetic resources of other countries. Consequently, attention to the identification of valuable stocks of these animals, and to their effec-

Chapter 1 references, p. 18

tive conservation and use, are matters uniquely suited to inclusion in the programmes of international and regional organizations whose objectives include attention to animal agriculture.

Translated into specific programme objectives, these considerations mean that organizations composed of nations, and institutions sponsored by such organizations, can help meet the needs of the countries they serve by:

(1) Alerting countries to the importance of identifying, conserving and effectively utilizing their valuable genetic resources of all types and, in particular, to the special significance of their cattle and/or water buffalo genetic resources.

(2) Assembling, publishing and distributing information on cattle and water buffalo genetic resources, and on national programmes wherein such resources have been conserved and utilized to the advantage of their member nations or, in the case of international or regional institutions, to the advantage of the countries they serve.

(3) Providing assistance to countries, where needed and upon request, to ensure that their cattle and/or water buffalo resources are accurately assessed, and that the more valuable of these resources are wisely conserved and used in constructive breeding programmes.

(4) Facilitating the exchange between and among countries of cattle and/or water buffalo genetic resources that give promise of being useful outside their countries of origin.

(5) Encouraging, facilitating and, where appropriate, providing for the training of personnel, in numbers adequate to ensure that the valuable genetic resources of cattle and/or water buffaloes in the respective countries are identified, and that appropriate steps are taken where needed for their conservation; Also that effective breeding programmes for their use are designed and carried out.

Institutes that operate in the international sphere may also contribute to national efforts through some or all of the above programme objectives. In addition, such institutes may utilize their own land and laboratory facilitates to maintain selected genetic stocks, and may distribute breeding animals or breeding materials to the countries that they serve.

4.2. Respective roles of various kinds of international organizations

In relation to the foregoing general list of the ways international organizations may contribute to the identification, conservation and effective utilization of cattle and water buffalo genetic resources, the following sections contain examples of ways in which the various kinds of organization have and/or may carry out their roles.

4.2.1. Role of FAO

The Food and Agriculture Organization of the United Nations (FAO), with headquarters in Rome, Italy (Fig. 1.1), is the primary international intergovernmental organization in the agricultural field. As such, its programme of work covers the whole range of agriculture, including animal agriculture. Consequently, FAO is in position to contribute through activities aimed at meeting all the objectives set out in the preceding section. In fact, because it is the pre-eminent international agricultural organization, FAO to a considerable degree holds the key to effective worldwide understanding and cooperative action in dealing with the problems of evaluation, conservation and use of valuable cattle and water buffalo genetic resources.

Attention was given to animal genetic resources even before the Organization formally initiated its work in agriculture. At the time of the Second Ses-

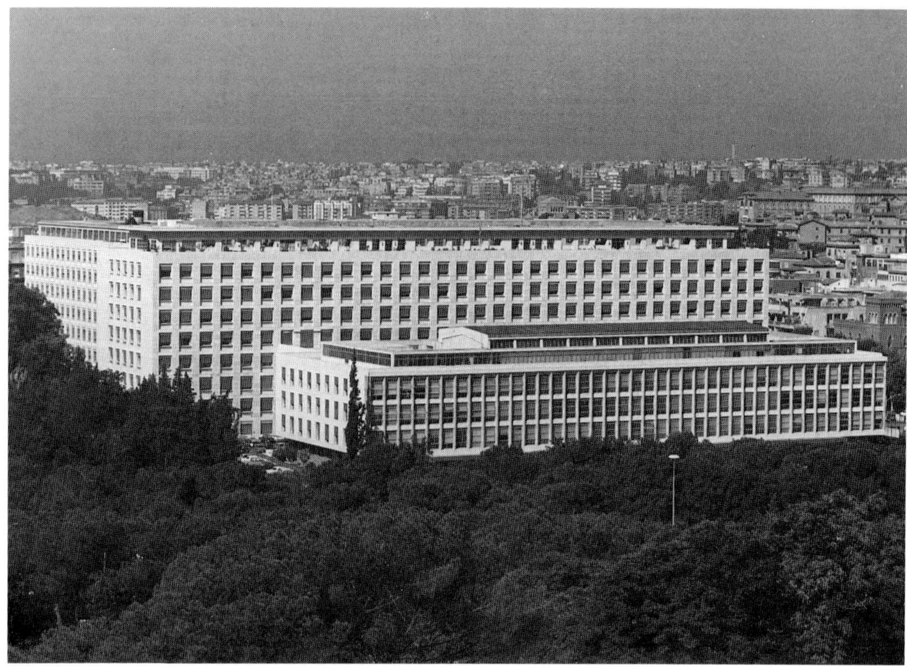

Fig. 1.1. Headquarters of the Food and Agriculture Organization of the United Nations, Rome.

sion of FAO Conference in the summer of 1946 the Director General convened a session of a Standing Committee on Agriculture. The main function of that session was to tender advice on the work of the yet to be formed Agriculture Division (which was eventually transformed into the present Agriculture Department). One of the recommendations of the Committee was that FAO should undertake work on the cataloguing of animal genetic stocks (Phillips, 1981). Among the publications prepared as a consequence of that recommendation were: 'Zebu cattle of India and Pakistan' (Joshi and Phillips, 1953); 'Types and breeds of African cattle' (Joshi et al., 1957); and, 'European breeds of cattle', Vols I and II (French, et al., 1966).

Another early FAO publication, entitled 'Breeding livestock adapted to unfavorable environments' (Phillips, 1948), also stressed the importance of some of the lesser known breeds of cattle, and of water buffaloes, in the more difficult environments of the tropics and subtropics. Subsequently, in a volume on *The Husbandry and Health of the Domestic Buffalo,* edited by Ross Cockrill (1974), all the important types and breeds of water buffaloes were described.

Volumes such as those mentioned above not only constituted solid contributions to the cataloguing of genetic stocks; they also served to focus attention upon the importance of identifying and conserving valuable genetic resources of cattle and water buffaloes.

During the first three decades of its existence FAO carried out many other activities aimed at stimulating interest in animal genetic resources and in the taking of effective action to identify and conserve the most valuable of those resources. Only a few of those activities can be mentioned here, as examples. They included:

(1) The holding of many meetings in various parts of the world, to focus attention upon the problem, to assemble information, and to stimulate action. As examples, the first such meeting, held in Lucknow, India, dealt with improving livestock, including cattle and water buffaloes, under tropical and subtropical conditions (Phillips, 1950a); the second with livestock production in the Americas (Phillips, 1950b).

Chapter 1 references, p. 18

(2) Preparing papers for presentation at international gatherings, and for publication in leading journals, on various aspects of the problem. Two early examples were a paper on the cataloguing and perpetuating of genetic stocks, presented to the Eighth International Genetics Congress (Phillips, 1948), and a paper on methods of assessing adaptability of animals to climatic stress (Lee and Phillips, 1948).

(3) Holding a series of four consultations on animal genetic resources, from 1966 through 1973, one of which involved an overall examination of the problem (in 1966), and one of which dealt specifically with the problem in cattle (in 1968).

In 1974 a series of activities was launched, in cooperation with the United Nations Environmental Program (UNEP), and these activities continued through 1980 (Mason, 1981). Here also, only some examples can be given, as follows:

(1) A survey of the cattle breeds of Europe, which revealed that of 149 indigenous breeds in this region, only 33 were holding their own, and the others were declining in numbers.

(2) A meeting, held in 1977, on the utilization of Mediterranean cattle (and sheep), in six countries of southern Europe and western Turkey.

(3) A study of the trypanotolerant cattle of West Africa, conducted in cooperation with the International Livestock Center for Africa (ILCA) (Trail, 1981).

(4) An expert consultation on dairy cattle breeding in the humid tropics, held in Hissar, India in February 1978.

(5) Preparation of a draft inventory (including cattle and water buffaloes) of conservation herds of rare breeds, feral populations formed from domestic animals, herds and flocks of domestic animals in zoological gardens, and experimental and selection strains developed in research stations.

(6) Preparation of a bibliography on the criollo cattle of the Americas, by B. Müller-Haye, in 1977.

(7) An expert consultation on the evaluation and conservation of animal genetic resources in Latin America, held in Bogata, Colombia in 1978, in which major attention was given to criollo cattle.

(8) A Technical Consultation on Animal Genetic Resources Conservation and Management, held at FAO Headquarters in Rome, Italy in 1980 (FAO, 1981). This was the culmination of the series of cooperative activities initiated by FAO and UNEP in 1974.

One further example of FAO's efforts should be cited. Under its Constitution FAO has formed numerous subsidiary bodies to deal with specific subjects and problems. One of these is the Animal Production and Health Commission for Asia, the Far East and South-West Pacific (APHCA), that was established in December 1975 under Article XIV of FAO's Constitution. Among the projects the Commission approved for early implementation, and which related to problems of animal genetic resources, was one on Buffalo Research and Development (Barker, 1981).

4.2.2. Roles of other intergovernmental organizations

In addition to FAO, other inter-governmental organizations of various types have undertaken work on cattle and/or water buffalo genetic resources. Three examples of such organization are mentioned below; a body of the United Nations, a regional inter-American organization, and an international agricultural research laboratory.

Reference has already been made to the United Nations Environmental Program (UNEP), and to cooperation between it and FAO. UNEP was established as a body of the United Nations, following the United Nations Conference on the Environment held in Stockholm, Sweden in 1972. Its headquarters are in Nairobi, Kenya. While it is concerned with all aspects of the environment, UNEP numbers among its specific objectives in the field of agriculture the following, according to Mason (1981):

(1) To promote the production and conservation of plants and animals, especially rare or endangered species.

(2) To initiate the preparation of a comprehensive catalogue of threatened species and varieties of crop plants, fish, domestic animals and micro-organisms, and to cooperate with FAO in its programmes for genetic resource conservation.

(3) To support regional and national institutions in developing countries for promoting the collection, evaluation and conservation of gene pools of plants and animals for maintaining genetic diversity for the future use of mankind.

From 1974 to 1980 FAO and UNEP carried out a series of cooperative activities on the conservation of animal genetic resources. These activities related to various classes of animals, and some key examples of the activities related to cattle and water buffaloes are given in the previous section, hence they are not repeated here.

The Inter-American Institute for Cooperation on Agriculture (IICA), formerly known as the Inter-American Institute for Agricultural Sciences, with headquarters in San Jose, Costa Rica, is the agricultural arm of the Organization of American States. It carried out useful work with criollo cattle and did much to focus attention upon the importance of evaluating and conserving these animals, during the several decades when the Institute maintained its headquarters and a central laboratory at Turrialba, Costa Rica. A herd of criollo milking cattle was assembled from various countries in the area, and used in breeding research and on the physiological aspects of adaptability to the tropical environment. The central laboratory that was formerly maintained by IICA is now the Centro Agronomico Tropical de Investigacion y Ensenanza (Tropical Agricultural Institute for Research and Training). It continues to be located in Turrialba, Costa Rica, works cooperatively with IICA, and continues to give some attention to criollo cattle.

Among the some dozen international agricultural institutes and centres operating under the sponsorship of a Consultative Group on International Agricultural Research (CGIAR), the International Livestock Center for Africa (ILCA) provides an example of how such an institute or centre can contribute to the evaluation and conservation of cattle genetic resources.

The CGIAR is a Group that was organized by FAO, the International Bank for Reconstruction and Development (World Bank), and UNDP to sponsor and finance international agricultural research (Saouma et al., 1976). Most of the institutes and centres that operate under the sponsorship of CGIAR do research on plants, but several work on various aspects of animal production and health. ILCA, which has its headquarters in Addis Ababa, Ethiopia does research aimed at improving systems of production and marketing, and has carried out one activity on trypanotolerant livestock in cooperation with FAO and UNEP, and one on the potential of Sahiwal cattle to contribute to milk and beef production programmes in Africa.

The basic aims of the project on trypanotolerant livestock were to survey the present status, appraise existing information on animal productivity, and present comparisons between trypanotolerant and non-trypanotolerant livestock maintained under comparable conditions (Trail, 1981). This work included attention to the two main trypanotolerant cattle groups, N'Dama and West African Shorthorn, as well as trypanotolerant sheep and goats. The data assembled, and their comparison with data from other breeds in Africa, suggested that the productivity of trypanotolerant livestock relative to other indigenous types may be much higher than was previously assumed. In the

Chapter 1 references, p. 18

follow-up of this cooperative activity, ILCA, with the limited resources at its disposal, is taking steps to establish a network of trypanotolerant herds, to help coordinate research and project work already in progress, in order to ensure a flow of reliable data on the biological and economic productivity of various breeds under different environmental conditions and levels of trypanosomiasis challenge.

The work with Sahiwal cattle involved the examination of purebred Sahiwal, Sahiwal crosses with various percentages and combinations of *Bos taurus* cattle, purebred Ayrshire, Boran and East African Zebu, in five environments in Kenya, ranging from sea level to 2200 m, and with annual precipitation of from 610 to 1043 mm. The production units varied considerably in production potential, goals and objectives in regard to emphasis on milk production relative to beef production (Trail, 1981). The results indicate that the Sahiwal has the potential to contribute increased milk and beef production in major ecological zones in Africa when used in combination with breeds of *B. taurus* cattle that have a high response capability for milk and beef production, but lack in adaptability. Trail (1981) also concluded that the formation of composite breeds is one logical approach to achieving and maintaining the optimum contribution by appropriate *B. indicus* and *B. taurus* breeds of cattle.

4.2.3. Roles of non-governmental organizations

The Society for the Advancement of Breeding Researches in Asia and Oceania (SABRAO) is an international scientific society whose members are interested in plant and animal breeding (Barker, 1981). Its members are not representatives of their respective countries. Following the Third Congress of SABRAO in 1977, an Expert Committee on Animal Genetic Resources was set up to investigate the collection and collation of data on the breeds, strains and varieties of the economically important domestic animals in the SABRAO region. The Expert Committee recognized that the complete study of animal genetic resources involved documentation, evaluation, conservation and utilization, but chose to emphasize documentation, i.e., to collect and collate information on various types of animals, including cattle and water buffaloes, in readily available form, in order to:

(1) identify gaps in knowledge, and areas where research should be maximized:
(2) fully document productivity and assess adaptability of local or native strains:
(3) ensure that local or native strains are not displaced by so-called improved breeds before their present or potential value is known;
(4) allow research workers to know the extent of information in their areas of interest; and
(5) allow planners and administrators to make rational decisions with regard to national and international development programmes.

SABRAO is, therefore, a good example of how scientists can band together to contribute to national and international efforts in relation to the identification, conservation and effective utilization of cattle and water buffalo genetic resources.

Some of the private foundations have also supported international efforts in the conquest of hunger, including the giving of support to work on genetic resources. The Rockefeller Foundation and the Ford Foundation are two such foundations and, while their interests have been more in the plant field, they have contributed in various ways to international research in the animal field, including, for example, support for the institutes and centres sponsored by CGIAR, of which one, ILCA, is cited above as having done important work on cattle genetic resources.

Private companies and corporations are also often in position to contribute to the evaluation, conservation and/or effective use of genetic resources. Private breeders have, over the centuries, been largely responsible for the selection and perpetuation of the many breeds of cattle and water buffaloes that exist today. In some cases, large farmers or farming companies have been responsible for the establishment of breeds. The Santa Gertrudis, developed on the King Ranch in southern Texas, U.S.A., is an example of such a breed. In other cases a single breeder may have had a predominant although not the sole influence in the development of a breed. One example is the Kangayam, of which one of the most notable herds was developed on the estate of the Pattagar of Palayakottai, in Madras State in India (Phillips, 1944; Joshi and Phillips, 1953).

Private breeders, companies and corporations have long served as sources of breeding stock for those who wished to import stock for use in their breeding programmes. With the advent of artificial insemination, and more recently with the development of techniques for the transport of fertilized ova, breeding materials from sources specializing in the use of these techniques have entered into international trade.

The contributions of such private breeders, companies and corporations have often been positive, sometimes negative. When the breeding materials used have been keyed to the needs of the importers, taking account of the environmental and other circumstances under which the offspring will be used, the contributions have generally been positive. On the other hand, when interests in making sales have dominated the transactions, importations often have resulted in offspring ill-adapted to the situations in which they were to be maintained, with negative results. If such breeders, companies and corporations are to make maximum, positive contributions to the conservation and distribution of superior genetic resources, it is essential that, in the conduct of their business, they practise enlightened selfishness, with a view not only to their own profits but also to the long-term benefits to the breeding programmes in areas to which their breeding stock and/or breeding materials may be exported.

5. SUMMARY AND CONCLUSIONS

Man is almost totally dependent upon his domesticated plants and animals for the food and fibre he needs to maintain his present numbers and way of life. He will be even more dependent as his numbers reach higher levels. Among the domesticated animals, cattle and water buffaloes as a group are most important. Through their meat, milk, skins, draft power and other products, they contribute greatly to man's welfare. Also, together with other ruminants, they make possible the utilization of vast areas of grassland that otherwise would produce little of use to man, and they also convert much of the residue from crop production into products usable by man.

In the 6800 or more years since cattle were first domesticated, and the some 4500 years since water buffaloes were domesticated, many useful types and breeds have evolved; types and breeds that are highly variable in their capacities to produce meat, milk and/or draft power, and in their adaptability to the many environments and conditions of production under which man has found it to his advantage to use these animals. Consequently, man possesses in them a highly valuable genetic resource; a resource to which he should be giving much greater attention at the local, national and international levels if he is to be reasonably assured that his needs for meat, milk, draft power, skins and other products will be met over the decades and centuries ahead.

The identification of valuable genetic resources, and their effective conser-

Chapter 1 references, p. 18

vation and use, are problems that must be attacked at the local and national levels. But they are matters of such great concern to all mankind that they deserve special attention at the inter-country and international levels as well. The varied approaches that are needed at these several levels, together with some examples of achievements, are presented in broad outline in the preceding sections, including approaches needed through national educational and research institutions, companies and corporations that trade in breeding stock and materials across national borders, non-governmental regional and international organizations, and inter-governmental organizations that are regional and international in scope. The role of FAO is particularly emphasized since, as the pre-eminent international agricultural organization, it has the key place in ensuring an adequate understanding of the problem, and effective action at the international level in seeking solutions; also in stimulating national action and in providing support to it where needed.

The evaluation, conservation and effective use of genetic resources, be they plant or animal, are matters of serious import to all peoples. There has been greater recognition of the importance of action in these areas in regard to plants than in regard to animals, in part because progress in plant breeding evolved at an earlier time and at a faster pace than in animal breeding. But, with the advent of modern techniques and rapid transportation, and the spread of the better known breeds, the time has arrived when effective action is essential to prevent the loss of valuable or potentially valuable genetic resources of both cattle and water buffaloes. In fact, that time has already passed since, for example, as Alderson (1981) points out, six British breeds of cattle have become extinct during the 20th century.

So, as man strives for even greater productivity in agriculture, it is essential that he makes the necessary effort and devotes the necessary resources to ensuring that he has at hand the essential tools with which to work. For cattle and water buffaloes, this means identifying and conserving the valuable genetic resources that are available to him in these useful animals. Thus, the effective administration and coordination of national and international efforts to identify, conserve and utilize these resources, deserve a place high on man's list of priorities.

6. REFERENCES

Alderson, G.L.H., 1981. The conservation of animal genetic resources in the United Kingdom. In: Animal Genetic Resources Conservation and Management. FAO Animal Production and Health Paper 24, Food and Agriculture Organization, Rome, pp. 53–76.

Barker, J.S.F., 1981. Work by SABRAO on conservation of animal genetic resources. In: Animal Genetic Resources Conservation and Management. FAO Animal Production and Health Paper 24, Food and Agriculture Organization, Rome, pp. 42–52.

Bhat, P.N., 1981. Conservation of animal genetic resources in India. In: Animal Genetic Resources Conservation and Management. FAO Animal Production and Health Paper 24, Food and Agriculture Organization, Rome, pp. 86–95.

Devillard, J.M., Bougler, J. and Duplan J.M., 1981. La politique Francaise de conservation des races domestiques en peril. In: Animal Genetic Resources Conservation and Management. FAO Animal Production and Health Paper 24, Food and Agriculture Organization, Rome, pp. 96–120.

FAO, 1981. Animal Genetic Resources Conservation and Management. FAO Animal Production and Health Paper 24, Food and Agriculture Organization, Rome, 338 pp.

FAO, 1982. 1981 FAO Production Yearbook. Food and Agriculture Organization, Rome, 306 pp.

Felius, Marleen, 1985. Genus *Bos*: Cattle Breeds of the World. Merck and Co. Rahway, NJ, U.S.A., 234 pp.

French, M.H., Johansson, I., Joshi, R.N. and McLaughlin, E.A., 1966. European Breeds of Cattle, Vols I and II. Agricultural Study 67, Food and Agriculture Organization, Rome, 389 and 421 pp.

Harlan, Jack R., 1961. Geographic origin of plants useful to agriculture. In: Ralph E. Hodgson (Editor), Germ Plasm Resources. AAAS Publication 66, American Association for the Advancement of Science, Washington, DC., pp. 3–19.

Hinkovski, Tz. and Alexiev, A., 1981. Conservation of animal genetic resources in Bulgaria. In: Animal Genetic Resources Conservation and Management. FAO Animal Production and Health Paper 24, Food and Agriculture Organization, Rome, pp. 77–85.
Joshi, N.R. and Phillips, Ralph W., 1953. Zebu Cattle of India and Pakistan. Agricultural Study 19, Food and Agriculture Organization, Rome, 256 pp.
Joshi, N.R., McLaughlin, E.A. and Phillips, Ralph W., 1957. Types and Breeds of African Cattle. Agricultural Study 37, Food and Agriculture Organization, Rome, 297 pp.
Lauvergne, J.J., 1981. L'Organisation de la conservation et de la gestion des stock genetiques pour les gros animaux de ferme. In: Animal Genetic Resources Conservation and Management. FAO Animal Production and Health Paper 24, Food and Agriculture Organization, Rome, pp. 318–334.
Lee, Douglas H.K. and Phillips., Ralph W., 1948. Assessment of the adaptability of livestock to climatic stress. J. Animal Science, 7: 391–425.
Mason, I.L., 1981. Cooperative work by FAO and UNEP on the conservation of animal genetic resources. In: Animal Genetic Resources Conservation and Management. FAO Animal Production and Health Paper 24, Food and Agriculture Organization, Rome, pp. 15–28.
Phillips, Ralph, W., 1944. The cattle of India. J. Heredity, 35: 273–288.
Phillips, Ralph W., 1948. Breeding Livestock Adapted to Unfavorable Environments. Agricultural Study 1, Food and Agriculture Organization, Rome, 182 pp.
Phillips, Ralph W. (Editor), 1950a. Improving Livestock Under Tropical and Sub-Tropical Conditions. Agricultural Development Paper 6, Food and Agriculture Organization, Rome, 55 pp.
Phillips, Ralph W. (Editor), 1950b. Report of the Inter-American Meeting on Animal Production. Agricultural Development Paper 8, Food and Agriculture Organization, Rome, 95 pp.
Phillips, Ralph W., 1961a. Untapped sources of animal germ plasm. In: Ralph E. Hodgson (Editor), Germ Plasm Resources. AAAS Publication 66, American Association for the Advancement of Science, Washington, DC, pp. 43–75.
Phillips, Ralph W., 1961b. World distribution of the major types of cattle. J. Heredity, 52: 207–213.
Phillips, Ralph W., 1963. Beef cattle in various areas of the world. In: T.J. Cunha, M. Koger and A.C. Warnick (Editors), Crossbreeding Beef Cattle. University of Florida Press, Gainesville, pp. 3–32.
Phillips, Ralph W., 1981. The identification, conservation and effective use of valuable animal genetic resources. In: Animal Genetic Resources Conservation and Management. FAO Animal Production and Health Paper 24, Food and Agriculture Organization, Rome, pp 1–5.
Reed, Charles A., 1980. The beginnings of animal domestication. In: H.H. Cole and W.N. Garrett (Editors), Animal Agriculture: The Biology, Husbandry and Use of Domestic Animals, W.H. Freeman and Company, San Francisco, pp. 3–20.
Ross Cockrill, W. (Editor), 1974. The Husbandry and Health of the Domestic Buffalo. Food and Agriculture Organization, Rome, 993 pp.
Rouse, John E., 1970/73. World Cattle, Vols I, II and III. University of Oklahoma Press, Norman, Oklahoma. 1046 and 650 pp.
Rouse, John E., 1977. The Criollo: Spanish Cattle in the Americas. University of Oklahoma Press, Norman, Oklahoma, 303 pp.
Saouma, Edouard, McNamara, Robert S. and Morse, Bradford, 1976. CGIAR — Consultative Group on International Agricultural Research. United Nations Development Program, United Nations, New York, 67 pp.
Trail, J.C.M., 1981. Work on Conservation of animal genetic resources by the International Livestock Center for Africa (ILCA). In: Animal Genetic Resources Conservation and Management. FAO Animal Production and Health Paper 24, Food and Agriculture Organization, Rome, pp. 29–41.

Chapter 2

Modern Needs for Different Genetic Types

J.D. TURTON

1. INTRODUCTION

The aim of the livestock farmer should be to obtain or breed, and then to raise, the breed or type of stock that will produce most efficiently the products required for his needs, whether these needs are represented by income from a purely commercial operation, or whether, as in the case of the subsistence farmer in Third World countries, they are the means of survival, or better, of improvement of his standard of living.

The task of the animal breeder is to produce types of stock that maximize productivity in specific environments. In this context, productivity must be considered in economic terms, taking into account inputs of fixed and variable costs, the time scale of operations, production per unit of land (if applicable), and all the biological components of productivity, including reproductive rate, viability and longevity. Thus, in harsh environments, the ability to survive and produce modest amounts of draught power or milk may represent a near-optimum economic situation, whereas in developed countries with adequate sources of animal feeds and/or grassland, intensive methods of production are often the best option from the economic standpoint.

At the start of a breeding programme, one matter the breeder must consider is the possibility of environmental circumstances changing. Sometimes, a change can render a breeding aim obsolescent. The use of trypanotolerant cattle is a case in point. In large areas of Africa, cattle trypanosomiasis, transmitted by several species of the tsetse fly, *Glossina,* is enzootic, and either precludes the keeping of zebu cattle or cattle of European breeds, or makes it very risky. Two West African breeds, the N'Dama and West African Shorthorn, have a marked resistance, more correctly called tolerance, to trypanosomiasis, and can thrive in areas where zebu cattle would suffer high morbidity and mortality from the disease. But unimproved cattle of these two breeds are small, and have a relatively low growth rate. Indeed, it has been the custom for farmers to cross them with zebus in areas of low or no trypanosomiasis risk, in order to increase size. At present, a programme to increase beef production in tsetse infested areas of West Africa would have little option other than to work with one or both of these tolerant breeds, if measures against the tsetse fly or the disease itself could not be adopted. But such a breeding programme would not necessarily be the best approach if an effective method of trypanoprophylaxis (such as active immunization) were available. Thus, the choice of a breed for a particular situation can be a difficult one if there is the possibility of environmental change occurring. Sometimes, a programme can be modified to meet the new situation, as would be the case where crossbreeding was being carried out, but with single-breed selection programmes, flexibility is low or non-existent.

Chapter 2 references, p. 46

Changes in demand for a product, or a change in the type of product required, can also play havoc with inflexible programmes, but in some situations an inflexible programme is unavoidable.

Thus, the task of matching genotypes to environments often involves a complex of biological, economic and social variables. Also, as the above remarks indicate, genetic requirements are not necessarily static, so that the gene pool of a particular domestic species should ideally contain genes useful for a wider set of environmental circumstances or products than is required at a given time. It is partly for this reason that so much attention has been focused in recent years on the conservation of rare and endangered breeds and species. There are a number of instances of advantageous traits found in relatively unimproved breeds being incorporated by crossing into other breeds, although the best examples are not in cattle or buffaloes. Certain highly prolific breeds of sheep, such as the Finnish Landrace or Romanov, especially the former, have been used in this way, and there is currently much interest in highly prolific Chinese breeds of pigs. Also, the Booroola gene, a major gene for high ovulation rate in Australian Merino sheep, has attracted much recent interest. It is possible that this gene originated on the Indian subcontinent, and that sheep carrying it were imported to Australia in the 19th century.

In cattle, the genetically determined trait of double-muscling is of commercial interest, particularly in Italy, and the incidence of the trait is high in certain breeds.

This chapter will first summarize the effects of environmental stress on productivity, as a background to consideration of genetic differences in adaptation to such stress. This leads to discussion of genotype–environment interaction, which, when present, may indicate the necessity for having a range of genetic types, each optimal for a particular environment.

Buffaloes and cattle both produce milk and meat, and are used for work, and thus are in competition in some parts of the world. The role of the buffalo requires special consideration, and cattle and buffaloes will be discussed from the comparative standpoint. Some aspects of genetic resistance to diseases and parasites will be covered, and the importance of breed differences assessed. Finally, the effects of some major genes are outlined, and genetic differences in the composition of animal products are briefly put into perspective.

2. THE EFFECT OF ENVIRONMENTAL STRESS ON PRODUCTIVITY

The main stress factors for cattle and buffaloes are those of climate, and the most important factor is high temperature, either alone, or combined with high humidity. Cold is a factor which scarcely applies in the case of buffaloes, the great majority of which are in tropical or subtropical areas, but cold is a factor of some importance in cattle, particularly in parts of North America and the U.S.S.R. The importance of these stress factors, in the context of this chapter, is that some genotypes are better adapted than others to environmental extremes.

2.1. Heat

The effect of heat on performance has been extensively reviewed, a notable recent reference being Johnson (1982), from which much of the following is drawn. For a given level of heat stress, the depressant effect on performance increases as the genetic potential of the animals increases. For milk yield, Johnson states that, for Holstein-Friesians, good performance can be obtained if the average temperature–humidity index (THI) does not exceed 72 throughout the year. This index is: (average dry bulb temperature) +0.36 (dew-point temperature) +41.2, temperatures being in degrees Centigrade. Tropically adapted cattle and buffaloes can fully express their genetic potential at higher index values than Holstein-Friesians.

The weight gains of bovines are decreased at temperatures above the thermoneutral zone for the particular breed, because appetite, and hence feed intake, are depressed, and there is a similar effect on milk yield. Within the thermoneutral zone, an animal's heat production is constant and independent of the thermal environment. A lack of adaptation to high environmental temperatures is expressed also in poor reproductive performance. In many experiments, reproductive performance was shown to be negatively correlated with THI values. In particular, high temperature tends to lower conception rate, probably through its effect on hormone levels in blood. Environmental temperature also interacts with nutrition in its effect on performance. Fuquay (1981) has drawn attention to the fact that animals on a high plane of nutrition tend to be adversely affected by heat to a greater degree than those on a low plane, a finding that is not unexpected when one bears in mind that the animal's attempt to maintain thermoneutrality represents a balancing act with an equation which has heat production and absorption on one side, and heat dissipation on the other. In heat stress, there appears to be an increased protein demand, one which cannot be met under grazing conditions in the tropics.

2.2. Cold

The effects of cold stress on performance have been reviewed by Young (1981). Throughout the world, very large numbers of cattle are given little or no protection from sub-zero temperatures. In North America, there are 65 million beef cattle and 13 million dairy cattle in areas where the average January temperature is below 0 °C. Few large-scale beef operations provide substantial winter shelter for their animals, even in the Prairie Provinces of Canada, where mean daily temperatures range from –10° to –20 °C. Most humans would probably regard such conditions as being as far below their 'comfort zone' as extreme tropical heat, and yet cold is much less of an adaptation problem to cattle than heat. The reason for this is the levels at which the lower critical temperatures (CT) of cattle are found. Young defines the lower CT (the lower border of the zone of thermoneutrality) as the temperature below which an animal must increase its rate of heat production to maintain homeothermy, and gives values in a diagram. For store cattle and dry, pregnant cows, the lower CT is –10° to –20 °C, for growing and lactating dairy cows –20° to –30 °C, and for feedlot cattle –30° to –40 °C. Another reason why the effects of cold in cattle attract less attention than those of heat is that there is no good reason to bring heat-adapted cattle into cold areas, because their performance for milk and meat is generally much inferior to that of temperate breeds, whereas there is an incentive to use temperate cattle in the tropics, either as purebreds or crossbreds, because their additive genetic merit for milk and meat production exceeds, often to a very large extent, that of indigenous tropical cattle.

Nevertheless, as Young indicates in his review, low temperatures do adversely affect performance in cattle, because as temperatures decrease, proportionately more feed energy is diverted to maintenance. Although satisfactory weight gains in feedlot can be achieved over a wide range of temperatures, gains in winter can be up to 20% lower than those at other times of the year in spite of the fact that cold stimulates appetite, and investigations have shown that milk yield in dairy cows fed ad libitum begins to decline at –4 °C, and is markedly depressed at –23 °C. Other studies have indicated that

Chapter 2 references, p. 46

40–60% of seasonal variation in feedlot performance can be attributed to climatic factors, although only part of this is attributable to cold. Young concludes that cold stress poses important challenges and problems for the livestock industry, and that further long-term studies into cold adaptation are needed. Certainly, the effects of cold in cattle have been far less fully researched than those of heat.

3. *BOS INDICUS* VERSUS *BOS TAURUS* CATTLE

Most cattle in the tropics are *B. indicus*, and all cattle used in commercial farming in temperate regions are *B. taurus*. In subtropical areas, the use of zebu cattle in crossbreeding with *B. taurus* is common. Certain attributes of zebu cattle are responsible for their good adaptation to tropical environments. Robertshaw and Finch (1976) list the following as being responsible for zebus having better adaptation to heat than *B. taurus:*

(1) lower fasting metabolism, so that under heat stress, zebus have less metabolic heat to dissipate;
(2) more and larger sweat glands;
(3) a larger skin surface area, due to the presence of large, dependent skin flaps on the neck, dewlap and prepuce;
(4) very little subcutaneous fat; in zebus, fat tends to be deposited intramuscularly, and not subcutaneously; and
(5) a short, smooth coat.

In addition, zebus are less susceptible to insect worry than *B. taurus* cattle, have better resistance to the non-specific effects of ticks, and utilize low-quality forages more efficiently than *B. taurus* cattle (Turner, 1980). To these can be added the greater resistance of zebus to many specific diseases, particularly those caused by protozoa (e.g., anaplasmosis, babesiosis and East Coast fever).

4. GENOTYPE–ENVIRONMENT INTERACTION

This is an important factor in any argument as to maintaining a diversity of genetic types to cover the spectrum of environments in which livestock are kept. It is most simply explained by an example. If two breeds or types of cattle, A and B, are kept in two dissimilar environments, X and Y, then genotype–environment interaction occurs if the magnitude of the difference in performance of the two breeds in X differs significantly, in the statistical sense, from the magnitude of the difference in Y. The interaction may be manifested by a reversal of ranking of the breeds, A being better than B in one of the environments, and B being better than A in the other. Alternatively, no reversal in ranking may take place, only a change in the performance of one breed relative to the other.

In the analysis of experimental data, interaction can be detected by the inclusion of an interaction term in the statistical model, by estimating the genetic correlation between performance in two or more environments (a correlation substantially less than one indicating interaction), or by regression of trait values on environmental levels. Statistically, in the analysis of variance, interaction represents a breakdown in the additivity of the main effects in the model.

Interaction is not restricted to two factors in models with three or more factors, but such higher-order interactions, even though they may involve genotype and environment, plus one or more other factors, will not be considered here. When considering genotype–environment interaction in terms of the genetic correlation, it is helpful to remember that, as Robertson (1959) showed, the interaction consists of two parts, one attributable to the genetic correlation in performance between environments, and the other to unequal genetic standard deviations of the performance trait in the environments. Thus, part of the difference between an obtained (low) correlation and a high correlation, which would imply little or no interaction, may be due to differences in additive genetic variance in the two environments.

In considering genotype–environment interaction, it is important to remember that it is interactions which are both biologically and statistically significant that are of practical importance. Some interactions are of statistical significance, but, because their effect is small, are of little practical relevance. Robertson (1959) suggested that a genetic correlation of about 0.8 would signal a biologically significant interaction, and furthermore, that a useful experiment on genotype–environment interaction must be able to detect, as a significant deviation from unity, a genetic correlation of 0.6.

Genotype–environment interaction has implications for the efficiency with which selection can be carried out. If substantial interaction is present, then the relative or absolute ranking of animals for performance in one environment will not be an accurate predictor of their ranking in another environment, and this applies to individual selection (a performance test) and to family selection (a progeny or sib test). Genetic change in performance in one environment from response to selection based on performance in another environment is directly proportional to the genetic correlation between performance in the two environments (Dickerson, 1962). When interaction is substantial, selection should be carried out in the environments in which the animals will be kept, provided the environments are fairly predictable. If environmental variation is likely to be unpredictable in time or degree, then the breeder has little choice but to aim at general adaptability over a range of conditions. Unpredictability might take the form of major, uncontrolled variation in nutrient supply to an animal, or variable exposure to diseases or parasites. Dickerson (1962) makes the point that selecting for adaptability to several environments is similar to selecting for several traits simultaneously in the same environment, and that the genetic change (ΔG_t) in average performance in all environments from selecting in all environments simultaneously is dependent on the number, k, of environments and the correlation r_{ij} between phenotypic expression of the same genotype in different environments. The relationship is given by the following expression:

$$\frac{\Delta G_t \text{ when } k > 1}{\Delta G_t \text{ when } k = 1} = \sqrt{\left(\frac{k}{1 + (k-1)r_{ij}}\right)}$$

This indicates the degree to which the simultaneous selection procedure is superior to selecting in only one environment and then using the animals over k environments. The reader can check this by substituting figures in the formula. There are some limiting restrictions to proper use of the formula, but nevertheless it illustrates the general principle.

The evidence for the presence of interactions will now be considered. Genotype–environment interaction in animals was reviewed in depth by Pani and Lasley (1972). They summarized their conclusions for beef and dairy cattle as follows.

4.1. Beef cattle

Preweaning average daily gain (ADG): 'one expects differences in the relative magnitude of the genotypes in the sexes without altering their rank order for ADG.'

Chapter 2 references, p. 46

Weaning weight: 'the importance of interaction for weaning weight varies a great deal from one instance to another.'

Postweaning gain: 'In view of the varying results of work on genotype × nutrition interaction, it would be desirable to determine the importance of genotype × nutritional level interactions, using the genotypes likely to be used in a particular farm or area.'

Feed efficiency: 'genotype × environment interaction appears to be important for feed efficiency.'

Carcases: 'It appears that interaction effects are probably not important for carcase traits.'

4.2. Dairy cattle

Milk yield:

(a) 'Many reports show that sire × herd interactions are not important for milk yield.'

(b) 'The trend for higher heritability at higher levels of production is evident.'

(c) 'Interactions involving levels of production, type of housing and other differences in herd environments are unimportant.'

Warwick (1972) also reviewed the evidence that existed at that time. His opening words are worth quoting. 'There is relatively little scientific evidence on the existence of genotype–environment interactions in cattle and particularly on the ranges of environments and management systems through which they may be important to breeders. Looking at the situation broadly, we are sure they exist — even though perhaps the evidence is not tied up neatly in scientific papers.' The review showed that interactions for both growth and dairy performance occurred when the comparisons made were between *B. taurus* and *B. indicus*. In the case of studies involving only *B. taurus* cattle, significant interactions for growth traits were found in some studies, but not in others, and the general picture was that indicated by Warwick's opening remarks.

These reviews indicate that the existence of interactions, where environmental or genotypic differences are not marked, depends very much on individual circumstances, but Warwick's remarks concerning *B. indicus* and *B. taurus* cattle are an indication that the importance of interactions is likely to increase as divergence between environments or genotypes increases. It is unfortunate that, although the theoretical basis and implications of interaction have been determined, many of the studies in which genotype–environment interaction is considered do not give the reader information on the biological importance of the interactions, or their implications. We are not given data on the proportion of variance accounted for by interaction compared with other main effects, on genetic standard deviations in the environments, and the genetic correlations. Sometimes, this is because the studies were not designed specifically to detect and quantify interaction. Too often we are given only a statement that statistically significant interactions occurred. Some more recent studies will now be considered.

Several studies failed to find genotype–environment interaction for dairy performance traits (Kräusslich, 1974; Taneja and Garg, 1976; Danell, 1982; Powell and Dickinson, 1977; Mohammad et al., 1982) over a variety of situations in which differences in environment were not extreme. The most interesting instance was the work of Powell and Dickinson, who analysed data on 142 Holstein-Friesian bulls which had each sired at least 10 daughters in Mexico, and also had sire summaries (estimated breeding values) in the U.S.A. There was no interaction between sire and country, and the genetic correlation between the independent sire proofs in the two countries was 1.006. Laster et al. (1974) found that the effect of several climatic variables had similar effects in different types of crossbreds from Hereford and Aberdeen Angus cows mated to Hereford, Angus, Jersey, South Devon, Limousin, Simmental and Charolais bulls. Baker (1977) reported on data obtained by the U.K. Meat and Livestock Commission, which indicated that the ranking of sire breeds (Charolais, South Devon, Lincoln Red, Sussex, Hereford and Aberdeen Angus for growth rate was the same whether their progeny out of Friesian cows were kept on an intensive cereal–beef system or on an 18-month grass/cereal–beef system.

The existence of genotype–environment interaction was reported for dairy performance (Kretzschmar and Ross, 1976; Buvanendran and Petersen, 1980; Parekh and Pande, 1982), growth or feed efficiency (Ribeiro, 1977; Béranger, 1978; Keller and Brinks, 1978; Langholz, 1978; Burns et al., 1979; Geay and Robelin, 1979) and reproductive traits (Koger et al., 1979; Hansen et al., 1982). The results of some of these studies are of particular importance, and merit consideration in more detail.

Two of the studies showed quite remarkable interaction in the case of artificial insemination (AI) sires of European breeds, for which records of daughters' performance were available in their countries of origin and also in tropical countries. Buvanendran and Petersen (1980) analysed data on 230 Danish Jerseys exported from Denmark to Sri Lanka and on their half-sisters in Denmark. The genetic correlation between milk yields in the two environments was not significantly different from zero (0.08 ± 0.35), indicating the presence of substantial interaction. The heritability of milk yield in the daughters in Denmark was 0.11 ± 0.02, but that in Sri Lanka did not differ significantly from zero (0.22 ± 0.23).

Parekh and Pande (1982) analysed data on 14 Holstein-Friesian and 11 Jersey bulls in the U.S.A., whose semen had been used in India to produce crossbred progeny from Gir cows. The predicted differences (breeding values) of the bulls in the U.S.A. were known, and the authors estimated breeding values from the Indian data using several methods, including best linear unbiased prediction (BLUP). For the Holstein-Friesians, the rank correlations of the U.S. predicted differences (PD) with PD's based on Indian results (corrected for the effects of year and season) and Indian BLUP results were -0.69 ($P < 0.05$) and -0.77 ($P < 0.01$), indicating considerable interaction. For the Jerseys, the corresponding correlations were not significant. The results of these two studies require independent verification using data from other sources, but nevertheless they do cast doubt on the wisdom of using bulls with high breeding values, based on yields in temperate climates, to sire crossbred progeny in the tropics, and suggest that substantial sire–environment interactions can occur when environmental differences are extreme. Furthermore, it may well be that special 'tropical strains' of *B. taurus* sires, i.e., those ranking highest when evaluated on crossbred daughters in the tropics, may be needed.

After reviewing work on the meat production of bulls of European beef breeds (Charolais, Limousin and Maine Anjou) and Friesian bulls, Geay and Robelin (1979) concluded that there exists for each type of animal, and for each physiological age, a level of energy supply which maximizes food conversion efficiency. A restriction in energy supply generally results in a decrease in live-weight gain, and the magnitude of the decrease differs between genotypes. Thus, some breeds or types are better able to cope than others with an adverse change in feed supply, and so a diversity of types to cope with differing situations is desirable.

Béranger (1978) summarized the basis for genotype–nutrition interaction for feed conversion efficiency. If energy intake is reduced below the ad libitum level, feed efficiency decreases in animals with a high potential for protein growth, because they reduce their growth rate without much modification of the composition of gain. Energy level reduction increases feed efficiency in animals with a low potential for protein growth, high appetite and high fatten-

Chapter 2 references, p. 46

ing capacity, due to a decrease in fat deposition and energy content of gain. Thus, differences between types are reduced by restricted feeding.

Genotype–environment interactions for reproductive performance of Hereford cattle reared in the contrasting environments of Florida and Montana were reported by Koger et al. (1979) and Burns et al. (1979). Their results led these authors to conclude that genetic adaptation to environment can be important in commercial beef cattle production in the U.S.A., and should be considered in performance testing, inter-regional exchange of breeding stock and artificial insemination programmes.

Finally, as an example of the magnitude of interactions, the results of Hansen et al. (1982) are interesting. These authors studied postpartum traits in a 2 × 2 factorial experiment involving two breeds (Hereford and Holstein-Friesian) and two dietary treatments (high and low plane). After the first calving, the difference between the two breeds (Holstein minus Hereford) on the high level was 543 kg of fat corrected milk (FCM) and −13.9 days for service period, and on the low level 362 kg FCM and +64 days. The interactions were significant, and involved a reversal of ranking for service period. The interactions for FCM persisted after the second and third calvings.

The results of studies reported since the reviews of Pani and Lasley (1972) and Warwick (1972) have reinforced their conclusions, and, although more information is required, it seems reasonable to summarize in the following terms.

(1) When environmental or genotype differences are small, statistically significant interactions are usually absent, but if they occur are generally of minor biological importance. However, in some situations (European beef breeds) interactions may assume economic importance.

(2) Interactions occurring when there are moderate environmental or genotype differences may need to be taken into account when choosing genetic types.

(3) Where large environmental (tropics vs. temperate) or genotype (*B. taurus* vs. *B. indicus*) differences are involved, major interactions can occur. Such interactions could have major implications in crossbreeding programmes involving the use of frozen semen from *B. taurus* bulls.

When an interaction is important in biological and economic terms, it supports the maintenance of a diversity of genetic types, each well-suited to a particular set of environmental and economic circumstances.

5. THE ROLE OF THE BUFFALO IN ANIMAL PRODUCTION

The water buffalo (*Bos bubalis*) is an animal of great importance in the agriculture of Asia and Egypt, and in several countries outside these areas plays an important though minor role. The two types, the swamp and river buffaloes, differ in appearance and in chromosome number, the former having a diploid complement of 48 chromosomes and the latter 50. The two types hybridize, and hybrids of both sexes are fertile. Descriptions of the two types can be found in several publications, for example Ross Cockrill (1974) and NRC (1981). Swamp buffaloes are found from the Philippines westward up to India. They are primarily work animals, but are also used for meat, though rarely for milk production. They are compulsive wallowers in pools, rivers and muddy puddles, and their wallowing is a behavioural response to a physiological need — protection against heat. Buffaloes of both types are conspicuously different in outward appearance from zebu cattle, whose anatomical and physiological characters reflect their adaptation to tropical environments. The buffalo, with its rounded conformation, non-pendulous skin, sparse hair, and low density of sweat glands compared with cattle, is not particularly well-adapted to prolonged exposure to sunlight, and has adopted wallowing to make up for this deficiency.

River buffaloes are found farther west than swamp buffaloes, from India to the Middle East, and even into Europe (e.g., Italy, Bulgaria, Turkey, Greece, Yugoslavia and the U.S.S.R.). They have also been exported to Brazil, where there are some 400 000 animals, and to countries such as Trinidad, Venezuela, Colombia, Guyana, Costa Rica and Ecuador. The river buffalo is primarily a dairy type, although it is also used for work and for meat. In India, buffaloes have been kept mainly for milk, but are an important source of meat because of the ban on slaughter of cattle in all States except Kerala and West Bengal (Acharya, 1983). They are used for draught in rice-growing areas, but elsewhere cattle are the main draught animals. Like the swamp type it is a wallower, but tends to prefer clean water to mud. The traditional role of the buffalo is that of the universal provider in peasant agriculture, one that it fulfils admirably. The world population of buffaloes exceeds 130 million, of which about 48% are in India, 23% in China and 7.5% in Pakistan, these countries ranking first to third respectively in the size of their buffalo populations (Mahadevan, 1978). In India, buffalo numbers are increasing more rapidly than those of cattle. Of milk produced in India by animals other than goats, buffaloes produce 70%, although they comprise only 35% of the population of such animals (NRC, 1981).

In spite of the enormous number of buffaloes in existence, and the fact that they appear to satisfy a particular need, research and development work on buffaloes has been less in volume than that on cattle, although if one confines the comparison to tropical cattle it becomes less invidious. Since about 1978, interest in the buffalo, and consequently the resources allocated to its promotion, have increased. The interest of the Food and Agriculture Organization of the United Nations (FAO), which jointly sponsored a seminar on buffalo reproduction and AI in 1978, and the publication of the U.S. National Research Council referred to earlier, are evidence of this.

It is appropriate, therefore, to look more closely at the attributes of the buffalo in order to assess critically how well it fits its current role in agriculture. Bhattacharya (1978) has discussed several advantages of the species, which are listed here, and amplified.

(1) Adaptability. Buffaloes can maintain good bodily condition under environments, such as stubble fields and marshy areas, in which cattle cannot maintain condition.

(2) The milk yields of buffaloes are higher than those of unimproved, indigenous tropical cattle. Also, the milk of the buffalo has higher contents of fat and protein, and hence of total solids, than that of cattle. Values vary, but those in Table 2.1 will cover most situations. In underdeveloped tropical countries, the majority of people do not have ready access to refrigerated storage, nor are bulk sterilizing facilities readily available in rural communities. Raw milk is a product with a short shelf-life even under hygienic collection, and collection in rural conditions in the tropics is frequently not accompanied by a high standard of hygiene. As a result of these circumstances, much milk is processed locally into more durable products such as clarified butterfat, known in

TABLE 2.1

Milk composition of buffaloes and cattle

	Total solids(%)	Fat(%)	Protein(%)	Lactose(%)
Buffalo	17.5–18.5	7.6–9.0	4.0–4.5	4.6–4.8
Cattle	12.0–13.0	3.0–6.0	3.0–3.3	4.5–4.6

Chapter 2 references, p. 46

the Indian subcontinent as ghee. The very high fat content of buffalo milk makes it ideal for this. According to Srinivasan (1982), 43% of liquid milk in India is processed into ghee. Much of the liquid milk sold in the urban market in India as 'cow milk' is a mixture of milk from cattle and buffaloes, with added water, for example in the ratio 25 : 35 : 40 (Dairy India, 1983). A chart produced by the Indian National Dairy Development Board summarizes data on dairy production and products in India. It states that 97% of milk is produced by the rural sector, the remainder coming from urban dairy enterprises. The rural sector retains 54% of its milk for its own requirements. The great preponderance of the rural sector in milk production, the importance of products such as ghee, and the traditional preference of rural communities for the buffalo explain the dominance of the species for milk production in India.

(3) Buffaloes tend to thrive better than cattle on coarse, fibrous fodder. They have been reported as digesting and utilizing crude fibre and cellulose more efficiently than cattle, although not all research results are in agreement on this. Buffaloes are less discriminating grazers than cattle in some environments, and therefore have a greater food intake in these circumstances. There is some evidence that buffaloes retain food in the digestive tract for a longer time than cattle, and also that they have a higher rate of nitrogen retention. It has been suggested that their rumen physiology is more favourable to utilization of ammonia nitrogen than that of cattle, and that their cellulose digestion is less depressed by soluble carbohydrate than is the case in cattle. These differences go some way to accounting for the better adaptability of the buffalo to certain types of poor nutritional environment.

(4) Work. The buffalo is an excellent source of power for ploughing, harrowing and draught. It is unrivalled for use in paddy cultivation. Although slower than cattle for traction, it is more powerful. A study by Ross Cockrill (1968) showed the buffalo to be the most efficient and cheapest source of power in many Asian countries. In developing countries in which peasant farmers have little or no capital, and little chance of acquiring any, buffalo power would seem to have little to fear from the internal combustion engine for some time to come. The persistence of the buffalo in Balkan countries, the U.S.S.R. and Turkey suggests that it remains an efficient animal in the economic, ecological and social environments that persist in some countries not classed as developing.

(5) Buffaloes are tolerant of the non-specific effects of ectoparasites, although in this respect there is no evidence that they are superior to indigenous tropical cattle.

The principal debit item in the buffalo's account is its reproductive performance. As Mahadevan (1978) puts it, 'Low reproductive efficiency is accepted as a universal problem in buffaloes'. These problems comprise mainly of a late age at first calving, and a high incidence of anoestrus and silent oestrus. The buffalo also has the handicap of having a gestation period about one month longer than cattle, which increases the calving interval by this amount. Bhattacharya (1974) cites studies in which calving intervals varied from 409 days in Italy to 441 and 506 days in India, and to 488 and 585 days in Egypt. The buffalo also tends to be a seasonal breeder, with the main breeding season in the tropics coinciding with the cool and rainy seasons. However, it has been found possible to extend the breeding season by adopting intensive management practices (Nagarcenkar, 1979).

The development of satisfactory procedures for producing frozen buffalo semen is fairly recent (1976). In India, the processing technique uses a Tris–egg yolk–glycerol diluent, and freezing takes place, using liquid nitrogen, in 0.5-ml straws (Vasanth, 1979). The conception rates achieved appear low (40–50%) in comparison with those of cattle in Europe or the U.S.A., but are broadly in line with those achieved for cattle in India. In Pakistan, an egg yolk–lactose–glycerol diluent is used, and freezing of 0.6-ml straws in liquid nitrogen takes place (Chaudhry and Wierzbowski, 1979). Pregnancy rates are similar to those achieved in India. Thus, satisfactory techniques are now available for artificial breeding using frozen semen, and this is a matter of great importance for the success of any programme for the genetic improvement of buffaloes.

5.1. Buffaloes versus cattle

A number of studies have been reported in recent years comparing aspects of performance in buffaloes and cattle. These have been carried out in several countries, including India, Pakistan, Sri Lanka, Egypt, Italy, Australia, Papua-New Guinea, Yugoslavia and Iraq. The studies have not generally been designed comparisons in the statistical sense, and in some cases the breeds of cattle involved do not make a useful comparison for evaluating the relative merits of buffaloes and cattle in environments to which buffaloes are traditionally regarded as being well-suited. The question of interest is whether, in environments to which buffaloes are well-adapted, efforts should be directed exclusively toward the improvement of buffaloes, or whether cattle have a part to play in these areas, from which it follows that some resources should be devoted to the development and improvement of cattle along with buffaloes or instead of them.

In Egypt, dairy performance of buffaloes has been compared with that of Holstein-Friesian, Dutch Black Pied and Jersey cows and their crossbreds with Baladis or other breeds indigenous to Egypt (Fahmy et al., 1975; Kassab et al., 1977; El-Ghandour et al., 1979a,b,c; Hassan et al., 1979). In the studies involving purebred European cattle, it should come as no surprise that the milk yields of the cattle exceeded those of the buffaloes, because this is what one would expect under conditions in which it was considered feasible to keep cattle of breeds such as the Friesian and Jersey. For milk fat yield, the results were marginally in favour of buffaloes. In comparisons involving crossbreds with a high proportion of European inheritance, the results were similar to those obtained with purebred European cattle.

Comparisons of greater relevance would be those made under tropical conditions in which use of purebred European cattle, or their high-grade crosses with local breeds, would be unsuitable. A small number of such comparisons have been made in India and Pakistan, although they are comparisons between animals co-existing in these conditions by chance or design, rather than studies specifically set up to test hypotheses concerning the relative suitability of the two species.

Ishaq and Shah (1973, 1975) compared the performance of Nili-Ravi buffaloes and Sahiwal cows, based on data recorded over a period of about 9 years. These two breeds are leading dairy breeds in their respective species. The average daily milk yields were very similar (4.6 and 4.4 kg for the buffaloes and cattle respectively), but, as one would expect, the buffaloes had the advantage in milk fat content (6.7 vs. 4.31%), and hence in fat production. The reproductive comparison was in line with what the reader might expect from what has been said earlier, with buffaloes having the later age at first calving (1867 vs. 1156 days), and the lower calving rate (64.9 vs. 82.0%).

Data on 135 village herds in India were reported by Reddy et al. (1980), and their results are given in Table 2.2. Unfortunately, the type of crossbred was not specified, but, from inspection of the relative yields and fat content of the crossbreds and nondescripts, and a knowledge of current crossbreeding programmes in India, one would suspect that they contained a proportion of Jersey or Brown Swiss inheritance. The net cost of producing 1 kg of milk was lowest for the crossbreds (80.7 paise) and highest for the buffaloes

Chapter 2 references, p. 46

TABLE 2.2

Comparative performance of buffaloes and cattle

Type of animal	Lactation duration (days)	Calving interval (days)	Milk yield (kg)	Milk fat(%)
Crossbred cattle	292	370	2971	4.5
Local, adapted cattle (nondescripts)	242	420	874	4.0
Buffaloes	273	421	1617	6.5

(109.4 paise). In another study, Karan Swiss cattle (Brown Swiss × zebu), purebred zebus (Tharparkars, Sahiwals and Red Sindhis) and Murrah buffaloes at the National Dairy Research Institute, Karnal, India were compared in respect of economic efficiency for production of milk fat and total solids by Ram et al. (1976). They showed that the net costs of production were in the ratio 1 : 1.38 : 1.75 for Karan Swiss, zebus and Murrahs respectively for liquid milk, and 1 : 1.65 : 1.53 for fat. The authors comment that buffalo milk is preferred to milk from cattle by the dairy industry and the consumers, but point out that the Karan Swiss in their experiment was a more efficient producer. The conditions of the experiment were those of a research institute, which could be matched by good commercial practice, and under such conditions efficiency is important. But consumer preference is a powerful factor, and might well offset the greater efficiency of the *B. taurus* × *B. indicus* cross. However, such results do not threaten the position of the buffalo as the multipurpose animal most suitable for the peasant farmer.

Figures on the relative performance of buffaloes and cattle at the Indian National Dairy Research Institute have been summarized by Acharya (1983). These showed that for lactation milk yield the three leading dairy breeds of buffalo outperformed all but Rathi cattle, and somewhat surprisingly, the unweighted mean calving interval for the buffaloes was 36 days less than in the cattle.

The official viewpoint, as expressed by Acharya, is that crossbred types of cattle, such as the Karan Swiss, when kept under intensive management and on irrigated, cultivated fodder, are more efficient than the buffalo, both in dry matter requirement per kilogram of milk and in the costs of milk production. It is possible that under such conditions the optimum genetic type is the crossbred cow with some *B. taurus* inheritance, but more comprehensive information is needed before this statement can be made more strongly. For rural communities, the evidence is strong that the buffalo is the optimum type.

6. RESISTANCE TO DISEASES OR PARASITES

Breed differences occur in resistance/susceptibility to diseases. Susceptibility is the complement to resistance, and in this discussion of the subject, the term ‘resistance’ will be used. In connection with the desirability of maintaining a diversity of genetic types, disease resistance can only be considered a major factor if it is responsible for the preference of one breed or type over another. Although there is evidence of breed differences in resistance to a number of diseases in temperate climates, there is no clear-cut example of one breed displacing another because of its greater resistance to a specific disease. Major problems exist in evaluating disease resistance. In some cases, there is difficulty in establishing a highly repeatable method of infection or in initiating metabolic disease. Properly designed experiments are very expensive, and in the case of diseases with a low mortality, there is difficulty in delineating a satisfactory criterion of resistance. The binomial or multinomial nature of data on disease, animals being infected or not, or exhibiting disease subjectively classified into several discrete categories of severity, introduces problems of statistical analysis, for example in progeny testing, where large numbers of progeny are needed to attain a satisfactory level of accuracy. Hence, most disease resistance studies on cattle or buffaloes are in the nature of surveys of natural rates of incidence. Such surveys have a number of drawbacks. One does not know whether the disease challenge was of similar severity over all breeds surveyed, and environmental factors may have modified the incidence differently across breeds.

Cattle diseases for which breed differences have been reported in surveys are actinobacillosis and actinomycosis (Becker et al., 1964), mastitis (Grootenhuis, 1978; Grootenhuis et al., 1979; Philipson et al., 1980), milk fever (Poulton et al., 1962; Leech, 1976; Philipson et al., 1980), Johne's disease, grass tetany, brucellosis and foul in the foot (Leech, 1976), and acetonaemia (Leech, 1976; Philipson et al., 1980).

Ocular squamous carcinoma (cancer eye) is a condition which exhibits marked breed differences in incidence, the Hereford being the breed exhibiting the highest incidence. The condition is associated with a low degree of corneoscleral and circumocular pigmentation, which is characteristic of Herefords. Incidences of 12.1–36.9% in the U.S.A. were reported by Anderson (1963), and of 2.83% in Hereford × Shorthorn (HS) crossbreds in Australia vs. 0–0.22% in Brahman × HS, Africander × HS, Africander and Brahman cattle (Nishimura and Frisch, 1977). Nevertheless, the evident predisposition to the condition has not prevented the Hereford from becoming in many countries the dominant breed for beef production.

It is when one turns to the tropics that resistance can assume major importance, and as so often, the issue is one of *B. indicus* vs. *B. taurus*. The problems referred to above concerning quantitative evaluation are equally applicable to the tropics, and many known breed differences in resistance are the result of observations by veterinarians, rather than analyses of surveys or experiments. *B. taurus* cattle (other than N'Dama and West African Dwarf cattle, which are also *B. taurus*) are more susceptible than indigenous African and Indian cattle to a wide variety of protozoal diseases such as trypanosomiasis, babesiosis, anaplasmosis and East Coast fever, to rickettsial diseases such as heartwater, and to viral diseases such as rinderpest. The high susceptibility of European cattle to tropical diseases has, along with their poor heat tolerance, precluded their use in many tropical areas. In the days before development of a tissue culture vaccine for rinderpest, effective vaccines for cattle were prepared using strains of virus passaged in rabbits (lapinized virus vaccine) or in goats (goat virus vaccine). Marked breed differences in the incidence of adverse reactions to vaccination occurred. Such reactions took the form of high temperature and diarrhoea, sometimes resulting in death. European cattle reacted too severely to the goat virus vaccine, which was less attenuated than lapinized virus, to permit its use on them, and were vaccinated with lapinized virus. Similarly, in West Africa, West African Dwarf and N'Dama cattle reacted severely to goat virus, whereas zebus tolerated it well.

Another disease for which marked breed differences in resistance occur is infection with *Dermatophilus congolensis* (formerly known as streptothricosis). This is basically a skin disease, but in severe cases, marked loss of condition occurs, and death may ensue. In West Africa, the West African Dwarf cattle are much more resistant than White Fulanis. A marked difference in resistance in Cameroon and Madagascar was reported by Dumas et al. (1971). In indigenous cattle, the incidence was 5 and 6% at two stations, whereas in imported purebred Brahmans on the same stations it was 71 and 52%. The incidence was also high in halfbred and three-quarter bred Brahmans (34 and 51% respectively).

But the most notable, and most extensively reported, resistance to a specific disease is that exhibited by N'Dama and West African Dwarf cattle toward trypanosomiasis, as was mentioned briefly in the Introduction. This phenomenon is more correctly called trypanotolerance, as the cattle may carry trypanosomes in the blood without exhibiting obvious outward signs of disease. These breeds can survive without treatment in areas where other breeds rapidly succumb (Murray and Trail, 1982). In tsetse fly infested areas of the forest and guinea-savanna zones of West Africa, these two breeds reign supreme. In areas of low tsetse challenge, they are traditionally crossed with zebus to increase size. The trypanotolerance of the crossbreds is in direct relationship to the amount of West African Shorthorn or N'Dama inheritance in the cross.

In spite of the fact that the phenomenon of trypanotolerance has been documented for 50 years, no adequate quantitative genetic studies on its inheritance have been carried out. The problem lies in the fact that no simple quantitative test of tolerance exists. The only real attempt to develop such a test was made by Desowitz in 1959. He measured the oxygen consumption of trypanosomes of a rat-adapted strain of *Trypanosoma vivax* in a Warburg apparatus. The trypanosomes were suspended in serum from cattle free from trypanosomiasis or in serum from infected animals. The oxygen consumption of the trypanosomes was depressed by antibody to trypanosomes, and an antibody index was calculated which had a zero value if oxygen consumption in the presence of a test serum was the same as that of the control, and 100 when no oxygen was consumed, due to a high antibody titre in test serum. The results showed that there is a difference in immune response between the N'Dama (trypanotolerant) and the zebu (susceptible). When animals of these breeds have been born and raised in a tsetse infested area, they receive antibody from the dam's colostrum and natural exposure to the disease. Reinfection as adults (as in Desowitz's experiment) elicits a secondary immune response. In the N'Dama, the amount of such antibody produced (a hyperimmune response) is much greater than in the zebu. We know, therefore, that there is a marked between-breed difference in immune response. What we do not know, is how much genetic variation in immune response there is within the N'Dama breed. If substantial genetic variation exists, this could be exploited by selection provided a suitable quantitative test of immune response could be developed. The numerical dominance of the N'Dama and West African Shorthorn breeds in parts of West Africa is due to their trypanotolerance, and they constitute the best example in cattle of a breed 'selecting' itself for a specific environmental niche.

Some interest has been shown in the possibility of finding a biochemical genetic marker associated with trypanotolerance. For example, haemoglobin type (Queval and Petit, 1982) and the activity of erythrocyte glucose-6-phosphate dehydrogenase (Queval, 1982) have been studied in this way. There is also current interest in examining whether there is any association between trypanotolerance and antigens at the BoLA (bovine lymphocyte antigen) locus. The attraction of finding such relationships lies in the simplicity of identification of tolerant animals, and hence a selection programme based on the marker. However, studies on biochemical polymorphism and its relationship to performance or disease have been carried out for more than 20 years, and there is no example to cite of its being of any practical value in cattle or buffaloes.

In Australia, a difference between *B. taurus* cattle and purebred or crossbred *B. indicus* in the incidence of natural infection with infectious keratoconjunctivitis (pinkeye) has been reported by Frisch (1975). Four aetiological agents have been associated with the condition in Australia — the rickettsia *Moraxella bovis,* IBR virus, adenovirus and helminths of the *Thelazia* genus. In some beef herds, the incidence can be very high. In cattle at the Tropical Cattle Research Centre, Rockhampton, the incidence in Hereford × Shorthorn (HS), Africander × HS, Brahman × HS, Africander and Brahman cattle of different age groups was 43.3–72.5, 3.49–3.95, 5.7–8.4, 0–6.0 and 0% respectively, the differences of the HS from the other groups being highly significant. The disease significantly depressed body weight by up to 7.3%.

6.1. Tick resistance

Differences in resistance to the non-specific, debilitating effects of ticks occur between *B. indicus* and *B. taurus* cattle, and, within breeds, resistance to ticks is probably highly heritable. Heritability of resistance to infestation with the tick *Boophilus microplus* was estimated by Seifert (1971) and Wharton et al. (1970). In Shorthorn × Hereford (HS), Brahman × HS and Africander × HS cattle, Seifert estimated the pooled heritability in the Brahman and Africander crossbreds to be 0.82, based on dam–calf correlations for log tick counts, although values for the HS cattle and for earlier generations of crossbreds were not significantly different from zero. The heritability in the other study was 0.39 from dam–calf correlation. Resistance is generally tested by placing a standard number of larval ticks on animals, and counting how many of them reach maturity (one-host ticks such as *Boophilus microplus*), or finding the proportion of ticks that failed to engorge after a standard period. Most such work has been carried out in Australia with *B. microplus.* The resistance of Brahman cattle to this tick, measured by the percentage of larvae failing to survive to maturity on the host, was 99%, compared with 85% in cattle of British beef breeds, 98% in Jerseys, 93% in Guernseys, 89% in Australian Illawara Shorthorns, 85% in Friesians and 96% in Australian Milking Zebus (Utech et al., 1978).

Similar results for the lone star tick (*Amblyomma americanum*) were found by Strother et al. (1974) in that Herefords were less resistant than Brahmans and Brahman × Hereford crossbreds, and for the bush tick (*Haemaphysalis longicornis*) by Dicker and Barlow (1977), Brahman × Hereford cattle carrying significantly fewer adult ticks than Friesian × Hereford, Simmental × Hereford and Hereford cattle.

The extent to which ticks and intestinal helminths affect gains in body weight was studied by Turner and Short (1972) in an experiment with Hereford × Shorthorn (HS), Africander × HS and Brahman × HS cattle. Tick resistance accounted for 40% of the superiority in growth of Brahman × HS and Africander × HS cattle over the HS crossbreds. Resistance to the effects of helminths (mainly species involved in parasitic gastroenteritis, *Cooperia* spp. and *Haemonchus placei* being numerically dominant) accounted for none of the growth difference between the Africander × HS and HS, and for 25–40% of the difference between Brahman × HS and HS. The comparison of Brahman × HS with Africander × HS suggested that the latter type was more susceptible than the former to the effects of helminthiasis. There was a reversal of ranking of the two crosses for growth between animals given no anthelmintic treatment and treated animals. With no treatment, the Brahman crossbreds were superior, but in treated animals the Africander crossbreds were best. Results such as this support the conclusions drawn in the section on genotype–environment interaction.

Chapter 2 references, p. 46

7. CROSSBREEDING AND HETEROSIS

Maintenance of a diversity of genetic types permits the exploitation of heterosis for performance traits by means of crossing breeds or lines. Although several genetic models for heterosis have been proposed (for a review see Cunningham, 1982), experimental evidence and general opinion support the view that the dominance model is applicable in most circumstances in animals. With this model applied to a single locus, the degree of heterosis in a population depends on the proportion of heterozygotes in that population and the degree of dominance, the latter being the deviation of the heterozygote value for a trait from the point midway between the two homozygotes, as indicated below for a locus with two alleles, A_1 and A_2. The numbers indicate arbitrary values for the two homozygotes.

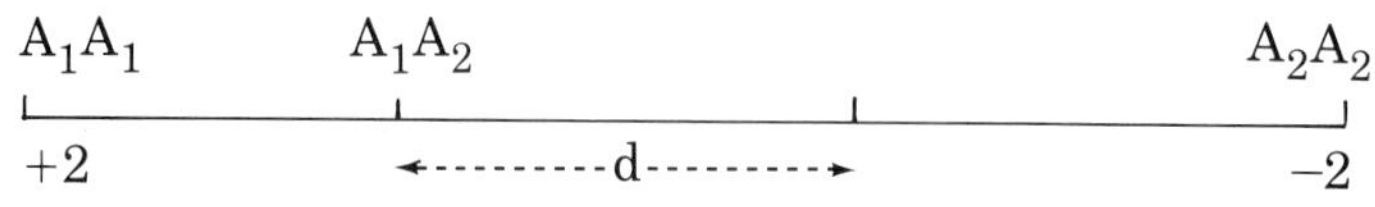

A_1A_1	A_1A_2		A_2A_2
+2	←---------d---------→		−2

d= the dominance deviation, i.e. the amount of dominance.

The model may be extended to *n* independent loci at which heterozygosity exists. So, for a particular trait for which heterosis can be exhibited, the amount of heterosis in a population tends to increase as the proportion of heterozygotes at the relevant loci increases, and that of heterozygous animals in the population increases. To state that the amount of heterosis increases as the genetic distance between parent breeds or lines increases is to resort to circularity of argument. Nevertheless, in endeavouring to exploit heterosis, the breeder seeks, albeit empirically, to find parent populations carrying alternative alleles at the loci controlling the particular trait in which he is interested.

Breeding programmes which aim to exploit heterosis by specific or rotational crossbreeding are constrained by the practical necessity of using breeds of similar genetic merit. If two breeds differ in additive genetic merit, as for example for the milk yield of a *B. taurus* dairy breed and a *B. indicus* breed, then the need to maintain substantial numbers of the lower producing breed in the case of a specific cross, and two crossbred populations differing widely in performance in the case of a rotational cross, means that the heterosis achieved overall is 'diluted', when the whole population is considered, by the lower additive genetic merit of the *B. indicus* herd in the case of specific crossing, and of the predominantly *B. indicus* cross in the rotation. A simple example is given below.

(1) Specific F_1 cross of breed A (higher additive genetic merit) with breed B (lower merit). The cross desired is A × B. Assume that frozen semen of breed A is used. The necessity of maintaining a herd of B animals means that only a part of the whole population can be F_1 (at best 50% if population size is to be maintained). Thus, on a population basis, any heterosis obtained is at least halved. No breeder is likely to import semen of a breed of low additive merit to produce crossbreds with his high-merit breed.

(2) Rotational crossing: assume the same two breeds.

Generations	Sire	Dam	Progeny
1	A	B	AB
2	B	AB	B(AB)
3	A	B(AB)	A(B(AB))
etc.			

After seven generations, the proportions of the two breeds reach equilibrium, and there are two herds, one with two-thirds of its inheritance from breed A, and the other with two-thirds from breed B. With A and B differing markedly in additive genetic merit, these two herds would also diverge markedly in performance, which would obviously be unacceptable. Not only would heterosis again be 'diluted' by the herd with low additive merit, but the farmer would naturally go over to mating continually to the breed of higher merit if adaptation was not a limiting factor, so breaking the rotation. (For those not familiar with the concept of additive genetic merit, this can be regarded as that part of an animal's genetic merit which is transmitted to its offspring; alternatively, it can be defined as the average (genetic) merit of a large number of progeny from mating a sire to a set of cows that is a random sample from the breed.)

In addition to the benefit of heterosis, crossbreeding exploits complementarity. By this is meant the combination in a cross of advantageous traits present in one constituent breed of a cross but not another, and also embraces the reduction of an undesirable effect found in a breed by a counterbalancing desirable effect in another.

The utilization of crossbreeding to increase net herd efficiency of meat production was reviewed by Cartwright and Hammack (1982), specifically with reference to beef production in Texas, but the conclusions they draw have general relevance, and are based on the results of a large body of experimental material. The fact that crossbreeding has become the dominant breeding system for beef in Texas testifies to its success. The point is stressed that, although heterosis for any production trait may be small, the cumulative effect of it on herd production can be substantial.

An important measure of herd productivity is the weight of calf produced per cow exposed to the bull (hereafter called calf production). In breeding systems which involve British or Continental European beef breeds, Cartwright and Hammack give approximate values for relative productivity in terms of calf production, with a purebreeding system rated as 100. For F_1, rotational, terminal crossing, and rotational + terminal systems, the values given were 105, 115, 115 and 120 respectively. For systems involving British and Continental European breeds and Brahmans or other zebu types, the corresponding values for the four crossing systems were 110, 125, 125 and 135.

In the same review, these authors summarize the basic conclusions to be drawn so far from the work carried out over the past 12 years at the U.S. Meat Animal Research Center, at Clay Center, Nebraska. This work had by 1982 involved 20 breeds and some 10 000 animals.

The conclusions were:

(1) Crossing of Hereford with Aberdeen Angus to produce F_1 calves resulted in a 5% increase in calf production.
(2) The use of sires of large breeds (i.e., some Continental European breeds) on Angus and Hereford cows increases the incidence of dystocia, and this offsets the advantage of the crossbred progeny for weaning weight.
(3) In the feedlot, large, rapidly growing types had feed efficiency similar to that of British breeds, but had a slightly higher yield of retail meat per carcass when fed to the same degree of finish.
(4) Eating quality of meat was remarkably similar in all breed types studied.
(5) Certain types of dam were more productive than the Angus × Hereford cross, most notably crossbred Brahmans, which had a 25% superiority for calf production to weaning, even in areas as far north as central Nebraska.

Cartwright (1982) gave approximate average heterosis in F_1 for a large number of traits, the values being condensed from numerous reviews which have appeared since 1962. Traits classed as exhibiting various degrees of

Chapter 2 references, p. 46

heterosis are as follows: medium (4–5%) — postweaning average daily gain and yearling weight; medium–high (8–9%) — ease of calving, weaning weight and milk yield; high (10–11%) — calving rate; very high (20–25%) — weight of calf weaned per cow.

Frisch and Vercoe (1982) have reviewed the work carried out in Australia at the Tropical Cattle Research Centre, Rockhampton, with the Brahman and Africander, the Hereford × Shorthorn (HS) cross, and the Africander × HS and Brahman × HS. They draw attention to the fact that the productivity of beef cattle in tropical Australia depends on two groups of factors, the first being related to production potential, and the second to resistance to environmental stress. Tropically adapted breeds, such as the Brahman and Africander, have a lower genetic potential for production than less adapted breeds such as the Hereford, i.e., they would have poorer performance, such as for growth, in a low stress environment as this would allow the Hereford to express much of its genetic potential. However, the tropically adapted breeds have superior resistance to environmental stress. Across breeds and probably within breeds, these two groups of factors are negatively correlated. Performance in any particular environment will depend on the resultant of these two groups. In developing crosses for a tropical environment, one seeks to combine the two groups of factors in such a way that performance is optimized for that environment.

Although a great deal of crossbreeding for milk production has been carried out, much of this has been between *B. taurus* and *B. indicus* breeds in the tropics, the motivation being the large increase in performance that occurs over that of the indigenous zebus due to the superiority of the imported *B. taurus* breeds for additive genetic merit. Possible heterosis from crossing diverse genetic types has not been uppermost in the minds of those planning crossbreeding in these circumstances.

Within temperate areas, crossbreeding has not been a marked feature of the dairy sector, except in so far as crossing breeds similar in appearance has been carried out to introduce superior additive genetic merit. The reason for this lies in the superior milk yield of the Friesian group of breeds, which dominate numerically the dairy population in much of the developed world. The introduction of genes from U.S. and Canadian Holstein-Friesians into Friesian 'strains' in other countries for this purpose has been an increasingly prominent feature of dairy cattle breeding in recent years. The differences in productivity of Friesian strains — Holstein-Friesians, Israeli Friesians, British Friesians, Polish Black and White Lowlands etc. — are being characterized in the study started in Poland in 1974, under the auspices of the FAO. In this study, Polish Black and White Lowland (PBWL) cows are being bred to bulls of Friesian strains from nine other countries. Under intensive management, the highest average milk yield in 305-day 1st lactations was achieved by cows sired by U.S. Holstein-Friesian bulls (5492 kg), and the lowest (4397 kg) by purebred PBWL bulls (Jasiorowski et al., 1983). Milk fat yield was highest for cows sired by Canadian Holstein-Friesians (204.8 kg), and lowest for PBWLs (177.1 kg). For percentages of constituents, the highest and lowest values were respectively as follows: milk fat — 4.14 (New Zealand and Dutch sires) and 3.69 (U.S.); protein — 3.62 (Dutch) and 3.40 (U.S.); total solids — 12.78 (Dutch) and 21.11 (U.S.); SNF — 8.68 (Dutch) and 8.42 (U.S.). The ranking of the types under less intensive, 'field' conditions was very similar (Stolzman et al., 1981).

Other reports on Friesian strains (see review by Turton, 1981) have indicated that crossing Dutch Black Pied (Dutch Friesian) cattle with Holstein-Friesians increases many body measurements, notably withers height, udder ground clearance and the distance between the teats. Scores for dairy type were improved, but scores for fleshiness and fat cover were lower in crossbreds than in Dutch Black Pied cattle.

The differences between Friesian strains are a reflection of the amount of selection carried out in the different countries and of the respective selection aims. The U.S. Holstein-Friesian is a dairy animal first and foremost, but Friesians in Europe, whilst being primarily milk producers, also participate in the beef sector, as crossbreds or purebreds. In western Europe, beef from the dairy herd accounts for 70% of home-produced beef. In Israel, where there is essentially only one breed, the Israeli Friesian, this must provide all the home-produced beef.

In the countries of the European Economic Community, animal and plant production is dominated by the system of subsidy payments which forms part of the Common Agricultural Policy. The desire on the part of dairy farmers to obtain high yields of milk and greater overall efficiency of production has encouraged the introduction of genes from U.S. and Canadian Holstein-Friesians. There is, however, a body of opinion that considers this to be to the detriment of meat production qualities. In 1980, the percentage of Holstein-Friesian genes in young bulls entering progeny testing in western Europe was very high in Italy, Switzerland, France, Belgium and the Schleswig-Holstein region of the F.R.G. (90, 91, 80, 75, and 72% respectively), followed by Denmark (53%), U.K. (26%), the Netherlands (24%), Sweden (16%) and the Irish Republic (8%). From small beginnings with imported semen or bulls, the percentage of Holstein-Friesian genes in the countries which now have high percentages increased at a rapid rate as half- and three-quarter-bred bulls came into service (Cunningham, 1983). The system of payment for milk has a marked effect on the situation. Payment purely on volume of liquid milk obviously favours the U.S. strain. If a system of payment based purely or wholly on milk fat yield were to be introduced, the results from Poland suggest that crossing with sires of the New Zealand strain would come into vogue. The present genetic diversity among the best Friesian strains is a strength, and would enable a fairly rapid response to occur (by crossing) to changes in market demand, and as demand can be manipulated, for example by the Common Agricultural Policy system of payments, it seems wise to encourage maintenance of the best of this diversity.

As regards heterosis in general between breeds of similar additive genetic merit, the conclusions of the review by Turton (1981) were that positive heterosis occurs for milk yield, but not for milk composition traits. Although crossing between non-Friesian breeds does take place, as for example occurred in the F.R.G. with American Brown Swiss and German Brown cattle, crossing in the dairy sector seems destined to be dominated by the desire to improve additive genetic merit, both in *B. taurus* × *B. indicus* crossing in the tropics, and by introducing Holstein-Friesian genes into European Friesians.

8. MAJOR GENES

One of the supporting arguments for maintaining a diversity of breeds, particularly breeds declining in popularity on the grounds of their lack of commercial competitiveness under prevailing conditions, is that some of them may possess genes likely to be of value in crossbreeding. In this connection, major genes would be of particular interest. The term 'major genes' implies genes, at one or a few loci, which control a substantial proportion of the variance of a trait. Such genes are easily detected because, when they segregate in a population, the distribution of values for the trait they control deviates from the Normal distribution, and, in the case of a single locus may be bi- or trimodal. However, in the case of the two species under discussion, there are only two instances, both in cattle, of such genes making a commercial impact: (1) double-muscling and (2) the compress and compact types. The compact type ap-

Chapter 2 references, p. 46

peared in the Shorthorn breed, and the comprest in Herefords.

Compact and comprest cattle excited considerable interest in the U.S.A. at one time. The story of these conditions has been described by Warwick (1958). In the late 1930's and early and mid-1940's, the two types came into prominence. Such animals had short legs, with a short, thick body, and the ability to fatten at small sizes. Thus, they represented a beef type much desired at the time. As Warwick wrote: 'Probably no hereditary characters — quantitative or qualitative — have ever caused so much concern and discussion, unfortunately at times bordering on hysteria.' Although possibly due to different genes in the two breeds, each condition proved to be inherited as a simple dominant.

However, research showed that compacts and comprests had few, if any, points of superiority over normal types in respect of carcass quality, and they had some serious shortcomings. Comprest homozygotes, for instance, exhibited an extreme form of dwarfism, often with bowed front legs, and few such calves lived more than a short time. Homozygous compacts were similar to the 'bulldog' calves found in the Dexter breed. Thus, the two types rapidly lost popularity, and faded from the North American scene.

8.1. Double-muscling

Double-muscled (DM) animals occur in several breeds, and specific names for the condition are known in several languages, e.g. the German *Doppelender*, the French *culard* and the Italian *doppia groppa.* It is, however, in two breeds, the Belgian Blue and White (also known as the Central and Upper Belgian) and the Piedmont that commercial conditions have encouraged breeders to select for increasing the incidence. The characteristics of the condition have been described by Ménissier (1974). As the name suggests, DM animals are characterized by hypertrophy of certain muscles, particularly of the shoulder and hindquarter, as a result of which their carcases have a higher than normal ratio of muscle to bone and fat. This muscular hypertrophy is accompanied by a reduction in superficial fat. The growth curve of DM animals differs from that of normal (i.e., non-double-muscled) animals, the growth rate being superior at young ages, but inferior after weaning. DM animals have a lower mature body weight than normals. The appetite of DM animals tends to be less than that of normals, hence they perform best on intensive diets. Genetic background has a modifying effect on the DM gene(s), and in breeds with a low growth potential, DM animals keep their early growth advantage for a longer time. The extra muscularity of DM cattle adds 20–30% to the monetary value of their carcases in certain European markets, most notably in Belgium. There is, however, a price to pay for this carcase advantage.

Calving difficulties are common with DM calves, and some calves have cardiac anomalies, macroglossia, and reduced development of respiratory muscles, which brings about respiratory distress. In females, fertility may be low, and puberty is late in both sexes. Testis size is often small.

In Belgium, the price paid for a 2-week-old DM calf is four times that paid for a normal calf (Hanset and Jandrain, 1979), and that for heifers and bulls (per kilogram live weight) is greater by factors of about 1.9 and 1.8. These authors give figures indicating that, in 1975, caesarian section was carried out in 48% of calvings of heifers and 25% of calvings of cows in the Belgian Blue and White breed. Such figures indicate both the difficulty the DM calf causes at birth and the premium the butcher is prepared to pay for DM carcases.

The mode of inheritance of the condition is not known with absolute certainty, but most probably it involves a single major autosomal gene with modifiers that affect its expression. The DM trait tends to be recessive and rare in dairy breeds and British beef breeds, but incompletely dominant with variable expression in continental European beef breeds.

TABLE 2.3

Percentages of double-muscled calves from different types of mating

	Sires		
Dams	Double-muscled	Semi-double-muscled	Normal
Double-muscled	87.5	50.0	11.1
Semi-double-muscled	47.3	28.6	0
Normal	15.8	0	1.0

Ménissier (1974) summarized the results of several studies on inheritance of the trait, and these are given in Table 2.3. He also delineated two situations in which the DM trait can be used to economic advantage. The first is the situation where, with purebreeding, the monetary advantage of DM cattle in meat production outweighs the disadvantages to female reproductive performance, as is the case with the Belgian Blue and White.

The other situation involves the breeding of strains to produce DM bulls for crossing with normal cows of other breeds. Here, apart from the production of some DM calves, the other calves produced tend to be heavier and have a better beef conformation than calves sired by normal bulls. This type of crossing takes place in southwest France, particularly with Charolais, Maine Anjou and Blonde d'Aquitaine sires.

9. COMPOSITION OF ANIMAL PRODUCTS

Genetic variation in product composition, particularly breed or strain differences, is a matter of relevance to meeting market demands in compositional traits, especially if the need should arise to respond fairly rapidly to changes in demand. The composition of some animal products is susceptible to change through manipulation of the diet, but genetic variation in product composition also exists. This topic was reviewed by Warwick (1980), and the ensuing discussion draws upon the findings of his review.

9.1. Milk

The composition of the milk of buffaloes and cattle was discussed briefly in Section 5, and consideration will now be given to differences at the breed level in cattle. Such differences are relatively large in respect of fat percentage, with the extreme in major breeds of European origin being represented by the Holstein-Friesian (about 3.6%) and the Jersey (about 5.2%). Milk yield and the percentages of constituents are inversely related phenotypically, and genetic correlations between them are small and mostly negative. Ratios between percentage components, e.g., protein/fat, show less between-breed variation than do gross percentages. The most conspicuous ratio variation is shown by Channel Island breeds, which have proportionately more fat and less lactose relative to other solids than is the case in other breeds. The difference between the Holstein-Friesian and the Jersey slightly exceeds 2 percentage units for total solids and is about 1.5 units for fat, but is only about 0.5 of a unit for protein and even less for lactose. Many *B. indicus* breeds have low milk yields, and their fat percentages are as high or higher than in Jerseys.

In the past, there has been little interest shown in changing milk composition in the U.S.A. and western Europe. This is partly because pricing struc-

Chapter 2 references, p. 46

tures have ignored composition, but also because *yields* of milk and its components have both increased with time, although *concentrations* of components have decreased. Selection for changing ratios of constituents would be an exceedingly slow process, and the incentive to attempt it has not been present.

Crossing with Jerseys enjoyed a vogue in the U.S.S.R. some years ago as a means of raising the low fat content of Russian Black Pied cattle (Turton, 1969), but lost its popularity because it was part and parcel of Lysenko's discredited ideas on breeding. Lysenko had an idiosyncratic and wholly erroneous view of inheritance, from which was derived the idea that when Jersey bulls are crossed with cows of breeds with a low milk fat content, a high fat content is maintained in the milk of the progeny whatever proportion of Jersey blood they contain, so that back-crossing of the crossbreds to bulls of low-fat breeds would not reduce fat content. Lysenko received enthusiastic support from the political establishment of the U.S.S.R. at the time, because his views were in accord with Marxist theory, and much crossing with Jerseys was carried out. From 1956 to 1964, several hundred crossbred Jersey bulls were distributed throughout the U.S.S.R. In 1965, after the political fall of Lysenko, a committee of the Academy of Sciences of the U.S.S.R. examined data which had been collected by Lysenko at the Gorki Leninskie experimental farm, and found that these data did not fit in with his hypothesis.

Variation among breeds in the relative proportions of different fatty acids is found, but genetic variance is probably small, and Warwick found no reports of attempts to change the proportions by selection. In this connection, it is worth mentioning that fatty acids are normally metabolized in the rumen, whereas in monogastric animals, fatty acids may go through the digestive process unchanged, and be stored in the tissues. However, the use of 'protected' fats in ruminants enables them to pass through the rumen unchanged.

9.2. Meat

There are large between-breed differences in the proportions of fat and lean in carcases of cattle that are slaughtered at similarly defined end-points. Differences in fatness of breeds are much less when slaughter is carried out at the same stage of maturity than at the same age or weight. This is, of course, a vast subject area when considered in detail. It is sufficient here to make the point that such variability is exploited, often in crossbreeding, in an attempt to optimize production efficiency for particular situations, and/or to produce carcases of a desired type. It is a good example of the commercial exploitation of genetic diversity.

Breed differences exist in the relative proportions of different fatty acids in carcase fat, but so far as cattle are concerned, the amount of research has been small. Johnson, Kinsman and Breidenstein (cited byWarwick, 1980) found several significant differences between Shorthorn, Aberdeen Angus, Charolais and Holstein-Friesian cattle in respect of the proportions of fatty acids with different numbers of carbon atoms. However, there seems no prospect of such differences being exploited commercially.

10. SMALL POPULATIONS — THEIR VULNERABILITY TO EXTINCTION

Alderson (1981) lists six breeds of cattle which have become extinct in the United Kingdom this century, and seven breeds considered to be endangered because of their small population size. For instance, the numbers of males and females used in purebreeding in 1979 were 79 and 7 respectively for the Gloucester breed, 61 and 9 for the Shetland, and 102 and 10 for the White

Park, all endangered breeds. In their procedure for registering a breed as 'rare', the United Kingdom Rare Breeds Survival Trust specifies as one of the conditions a population size of less than 750 breeding cattle, although breeding populations of less than 750 animals can be maintained without serious gene loss by applying special breeding programmes that minimize inbreeding. Examples of breed extinction and vulnerability have been reported in many countries (see FAO, 1981).

The loss of breeds represents loss of genes, some of which may not be present in any other breeds, and may have had potential value for exploitation in animal production. In many countries of the Third World, the problem is exacerbated by the fact that the organizational structures and funds for deliberate conservation do not always exist, and a small population has a much better chance of survival if it is bred using mating schemes designed to avoid or mitigate genetic dangers that beset small populations breeding in an unregulated manner. So consideration of these dangers and of the numerical definition of 'small' is appropriate here.

In small populations, two factors operate to reduce genetic variability — inbreeding and genetic drift. If the degree of inbreeding increases unduly, reproductive performance is likely to decrease, and this exacerbates the problem of survival for the population. Genetic drift is the random change in gene frequency in a population from generation to generation. A gene can be lost from a population because its possessors do not produce offspring, or gametes containing the gene are not involved in fertilization when the animals mate. Drift is greater in small than in large populations. Thus, a gene has a greater chance of being 'lost' from a small than from a large population.

10.1 Effective population size

The size of a population in breeding terms is usually smaller than its size determined at a census. The measure which the geneticist uses is 'effective population size', sometimes referred to as 'effective population number'. It is defined in two ways: (1) as the number of individuals in an idealized population (i.e., one mating in an idealized manner) that would give the same drift in one generation as the non-idealized population under consideration; (2) as the size of an idealized population that would give the same rate of inbreeding as the non-idealized population being considered.

An idealized population is one which is comprised of several lines which are never interbred and which are of the same population size. Furthermore, mating is random within lines, there is no mutation and selection, and generations do not overlap, i.e., there is no mating between individuals in different generations. Formulae have been developed for estimation of effective population size (N_e) for different situations, and many of these were reviewed by Hill (1972).

The value of N_e is affected by the numbers of breeding males and females in the population, and by the variance and covariance in family size (i.e., by variation in the number of progeny left by each sire and dam). If family sizes are kept equal, as is done deliberately in genetic control populations, N_e is larger than when it is not.

Pirchner (1983) gives an example relevant to the present discussion, based on use of the formula

$$N_e = \frac{4N_m N_f}{N_m + N_f} \tag{1}$$

where N_m and N_f are the numbers of breeding males and females respectively

Chapter 2 references, p. 46

in the population. This formula is appropriate for situations in which N_m and N_f differ markedly. For a breed with 1000 cows and 20 bulls, maintained as a closed herd, N_e is 78. If the number of bulls is reduced to 4, as would be feasible with AI, N_e becomes only 16.

It is possible to estimate N_e indirectly from the change in the frequency of selectively neutral alleles between two points in time ($t_1$and t_2). A neutral allele is one which does not confer on its possessor any advantage or disadvantage. It is difficult to prove selective neutrality, but many blood group alleles are assumed to be essentially neutral. The formula to use for estimating N_e is

$$\sigma^2_{\Delta_q} = 1 - (1 - \frac{1}{2N_e})^t \qquad (2)$$

where $\sigma^2_{\Delta_q}$ is the variance of gene frequency change, t is the number of generations elapsing between t_1 and t_2, and p and q are, in the simplest case, the frequencies of the alternative alleles at a two-allele locus (actually, for q (or p), the average of the frequencies at t_1 and t_2 is used, and $p = 1 - q$). Also, $\sigma^2_{\Delta q} = \Delta^2 - \Sigma s^2$, where Δ^2 is the squared difference in the frequencies of q between t_1 and t_2, and Σs^2 is the sum of the sampling error variances for q at t_1 and t_2. Thus, the left hand side of equation (2) can be quantified, and the equation can be solved by the use of logarithms.

In many small breed populations, information on such matters as family size and gene frequency changes is lacking, so that estimates of N_e have to be made using equation (1). The important statistic is the value of N_e below which a population is at risk of eventual extinction. This matter was discussed by Yamada (1981). Most dairy cattle populations in the developed world use AI extensively, so the ratio of the number of breeding females to the number of AI sires is very large, and N_e is quite small (10–50). For $N_e = 50$ and $N_e = 10$, the loss of genetic variation per generation is 1 and 5% respectively. Alderson (1981) gives data on the population sizes of several endangered breeds. The Kerry is listed as having 241 females and 13 males, which gives $N_e = 49$. This breed appears reasonably safe genetically, though any lack of interest in the breed could result in a reduction in the population size, and an increase in the risk of extinction. The distinction has to be made between the effects of genetic factors, which are predictable and tend to operate on a long time-scale, and factors which can cause a sudden drop in population size.

The Gloucester has $N_e = 25.7$ on the 1979 figures, and a drop in the number of sires from the 7 recorded in 1979 to say 4, due to disease, accident, etc., would reduce N_e to only 11.6. Such figures illustrate the problem. Populations deliberately bred with a relatively small number of sires, such as dairy cattle, can have quite small N_e values, but are in no danger of extinction because they have large numbers of females, the number of sires is kept small by design, and plenty of replacement sires are available. With endangered breeds, the number of breeding males may represent all available males, so that a sudden reduction in the number can have serious consequences; the number of breeding females may also be small. If the breeding of an endangered population is controlled, to equalize family size, reduce the rate of inbreeding increase, and narrow the ratio of females to males, then N_e can often be increased to a safe level.

11. FINALE

Genetic variation is the substrate of genetic improvement, whether such improvement is brought about by selection or by crossing to combine desirable genetically determined traits in the same animal. In a genetical utopia, nothing would be done to compromise the world's genetic resources. But in real life, it is neither practical nor economically feasible to guarantee the existence of all breeds and strains. Individual countries, the FAO, private organizations and individuals have done a great deal over the past decade or so to preserve rare and endangered breeds. Time alone will show whether such breeds have a role to play in providing superior germplasm for particular situations.

This chapter has tried to set out the reasons why it is desirable to maintain diversity, and to indicate how it is exploited. It has looked at a number of specific types of production and certain attributes of cattle and buffaloes with the intention of highlighting areas of current interest and importance.

We live in a time when man is clever enough to develop animal productivity to such an extent that he produces surpluses of certain commodities in, for example, the EEC, but not clever enough to find a way of transferring this surplus to those parts of the world where undernutrition is rife. The solution to low levels of animal production in Third World countries must lie, at least in part, in developing better production systems for animal feed, and types of animals that utilize such feed more efficiently.

In some parts of the world, the buffalo stands out as a well-adapted animal which must surely have considerable potential for improvement. In those tropical countries where crossing *B. taurus* with *B. indicus* has a role to play, genotype–environment interaction shows signs of being of importance, necessitating the evaluation of exotic sires in the environment where the crossbreds will be raised.

Resistance to diseases and parasites has always been a topic of interest to animal scientists, but, as has been indicated, there is only one good instance of resistance to a specific disease alone determining the choice of a breed, and information on within-breed genetic variation in resistance to disease is generally lacking, because of the difficulty of devising accurate quantitative indicators of disease resistance that do not involve reproducing the disease itself. From the practical standpoint, knowledge of such variation is important, as it is the key to whether efforts should be made to breed for resistance.The advantage that a hardy breed may have over a less hardy type for disease resistance may be small in respect of a single disease, but the advantage for several diseases is cumulative, rather in the way that the considerable heterosis for calf production builds up from modest advantages for each of its constituent traits.

The techniques of genetic engineering are now being used for investigative purposes in farm livestock, and, in laboratory mammals, genes have been transferred from one species to another, and have functioned in the recipient species. It is possible to 'cut' the DNA of chromosomes into segments, to determine the base sequences (the genetic code) of the DNA, and by DNA hybridization techniques to find where such segments are located in a chromosome. Thus, the basic technology exists to identify segments of DNA which can be followed through from parent to offspring, and to examine whether any such segments are associated with good performance for a trait. In this way, high-performance 'genes' could be empirically identified. The possibility exists for screening breeds for advantageous DNA segments. Such procedures would perhaps offer a way of searching minor or rare breeds for DNA segments of economic merit. In the meantime, and even when gene manipulation is possible, genetic diversity can be maintained from generation to generation by applying sound breeding programmes to livestock populations adapted to production systems around the world.

Chapter 2 references, p. 46

12. REFERENCES

Acharya, R.M., 1983. Breeding strategy for increased milk production. In: Dairy India 1983. P.R. Gupta, New Delhi, pp. 43–48

Alderson, G.L.H., 1981. The conservation of animal genetic resources in the United Kingdom. In: Animal Genetic Resources Conservation and Management. Proc. FAO/UNEP Technical Consultation Food and Agriculture Organization, Rome, pp. 53–76.

Anderson, D.E., 1963. Genetic aspects of cancer with special reference to cancer of the eye in the bovine. Ann. N. Y. Acad. Sci., 108: 948–962.

Baker, J.K., 1977. Notes on genotype–nutrition interaction. In: Crossbreeding Experiments and Strategy of Breed Utilization to Increase Beef Production. A seminar in the EEC Programme of Coordination of Research on Beef Production, Verden, F.R.G. 9–11 February 1976. Kirchberg, Commission of the European Communities Directorate General, Scientific and Technical Information and Information Management, pp. 414–423.

Becker, R.B., Wilcox, C.J., Simpson, C.F., Gilmore, L.O. and Fechheimer, N.S., 1964. Genetic aspects of actinomycosis and actinobacillosis in cattle. Technical Bulletin 670, Florida Agricultural Experiment Stations, 24 pp.

Béranger, C., 1978. Feed efficiency and genotype–nutrition interactions in growing animals, particularly in cattle for beef production. In: H. De Boer and J. Martin (Editors), Patterns of growth and Development in Cattle. A seminar in the EEC Programme of Coordination of Research on Beef Production, Ghent, 11–13 October 1974. Martinus Nijhoff, The Hague, pp. 383–391.

Bhattacharya, P., 1974. Reproduction. In: W. Ross Cockrill (Editor), The Husbandry and Health of the Domestic Buffalo. Food and Agriculture Organization, Rome, pp. 104–158.

Bhattacharya, P., 1978. Buffalo. In: G. Williamson and W.J.A. Payne, An Introduction to Animal Husbandry in the Tropics. Longman, London, pp. 398–435.

Burns, W.C., Koger, M., Butts, W.T., Pahnish, O.F. and Blackwell, R.L., 1979. Genotype by environment interaction in Hereford cattle. II. Birth and weaning traits. J. Anim. Sci., 49(2): 403–409.

Buvanendran, V. and Petersen, P.H., 1980. Genotype–environment interaction in milk production under Sri Lanka and Danish conditions. Acta Agric Scand., 30(4): 369–372.

Cartwright, T.C., 1982. Expression of heterosis in beef cattle. In: Proc. Third Conference, Australian Society of Animal Breeding and Genetics, pp. 62–66.

Cartwright, T.C. and Hammack, S.P., 1982. Utilizing crossbreeding to increase net herd efficiency. In: Proc. Third Conference, Australian Society of Animal Breeding and Genetics, pp. 44–49.

Chaudhry, M.S. and Wierzbowski, S., 1979. Semen freezing and artificial insemination in buffalo in Pakistan. In: Buffalo Reproduction and Artificial Insemination. Proc. Seminar sponsored by FAO/SIDA/Govt of India, held at National Dairy Research Institute, Karnal 132001, India, 4–15 December 1978. Food and Agriculture Organization, Rome, pp. 315–316.

Cunningham, E.P., 1982. The genetic basis of heterosis. 2nd World Congress on Genetics Applied to Livestock Production, 4–8 October 1982. 6. Round tables. Editorial Garsi, Madrid, pp. 109–205.

Cunningham, E.P., 1983. European Friesians — the Canadian and American invasion. Animal Genetic Resources Information, 1/83: 21–23.

Dairy India, 1983. P.R. Gupta, New Delhi, xvi + 501 pp.

Danell, B., 1982. Interaction between genotype and environment in sire evaluation for milk production. Acta Agric. Scand., 32(1): 33–46.

Desowitz, R.S., 1959. Studies on immunity and host–parasite relationships. 1. The immunological response of resistant and susceptible breeds of cattle to trypanosomal challenge. Ann. Trop. Med. Parasitol., 53: 293–313.

Dicker, R.W. and Barlow, R., 1977. The relative infestation levels of the bush tick in Zebu × European heifers. Third International Congress of the Society for the Advancement of Breeding Researches in Asia and Oceania, pp. 7–1 to 7–4.

Dickerson, G.E., 1962. Implications of genetic–environmental interaction in animal breeding. Anim. Prod., 4: 47–63.

Dumas, R., Lhoste, P., Chabeuf, N. and Blancou, J., 1971. Note sur la sensibilité héréditaire des bovins à la streptothricose. (Note on the hereditary susceptibility of cattle to streptothricosis.) Rev. Elev. Méd. Vét. Pays Trop., 24: 349–353.

El-Ghandour, M.A., El-Gazzar, H. and Youniss, N.A., 1979a. Studies on the buffaloe's and cow's milk in the upper part of Egypt. I. Effect of stage of lactation on milk yield and its composition. Research Bulletin 976, Faculty of Agriculture, Ain Shams University, 13 pp.

El-Ghandour, M.A., El-Gazzar, H. and Youniss, N.A., 1979b. Studies on the buffaloe's and cow's milk in the upper part of Egypt. II. Effect of season of the year on milk yield and its composition. Research Bulletin 977, Faculty of Agriculture, Ain Shams University, 12 pp.

El-Ghandour, M.A., El-Gazzar, H. and Youniss, N.A., 1979c. Studies on the buffaloe's and cow's milk in the upper part of Egypt. III. Effect of age on milk yield and its composition. Research Bulletin 978, Faculty of Agriculture, Ain Shams University, 19 pp.

Fahmy, S.K., Shaheen, M.A., Youssef, F.M. and Soliman, A., 1975. A comparative study of herd

milk production in Friesian and buffaloes. Agric. Res. Rev., 53(6): 19–32.
FAO, 1981. Animal Genetic Resources Conservation and Management. Proc. FAO/UNEP Technical Consultation, Food and Agriculture Organization, Rome, 388 pp.
Frisch, J.E., 1975. The relative incidence and effect of bovine keratoconjunctivitis in *Bos indicus*, and *Bos taurus* cattle. Anim. Prod., 21(3): 265–274.
Frisch, J.E. and Vercoe, J.E., 1982. Consideration of adaptive and productive components of productivity in breeding beef cattle for tropical Australia. 2nd World Congress on Genetics Applied to Livestock Production, 4–8 October 1982. 6. Round tables. Editorial Garsi, Madrid, pp. 307–321.
Fuquay, J.W., 1981. Heat stress as it affects animal production. J. Anim. Sci., 52: 164–174.
Geay, Y. and Robelin, J., 1979. Variation of meat production capacity in cattle due to genotype and level of feeding: genotype–nutrition interaction. Livestock Prod. Sci., 6: 263–276.
Grootenhuis, G., 1978. Verschil in Vatbaarheid voor mastitis tussen het FH- en het MYR-veeras. (Differences in susceptibility to mastitis between Dutch Black Pied and Meuse-Rhine-Yssel cattle breeds.) Tijdschrijft voor Diergeneeskunde, 103(23): 1270–1276.
Grootenhuis, G., Oldenbroek, J.K. and Van den Berg, J., 1979. Differences in mastitis susceptibility between Holstein-Friesian, Dutch Friesian and Dutch Red and White cows. Correlation between parameters for mastitis and for production. Vet. Q., 1(1): 37–46.
Hansen, P.J., Baik, D.H., Rutledge, J.J. and Hauser, E.R., 1982. Genotype × environmental interactions on reproductive traits of females. II. Postpartum reproduction as influenced by genotype, dietary regimen, level of milk production and parity. J. Anim. Sci., 55: 1458–1472.
Hanset, R. and Jandrain, M., 1979. Selection for double-muscling and calving problems. in: B. Hoffman, I.L. Mason and J. Schmidt (Editors), Calving Problems and Early Viability of the Calf. Martinus Nijhoff, The Hague, pp. 91–104.
Hassan, A., El-Komy, A. and Badawy, A., 1979. Seasonal variations in body reactions, daily milk yield and milk composition of crossbred cows and buffaloes. Ind. J. Dairy Sci., 32(3): 264–269.
Hill, W.G., 1972. Estimation of genetic change. 1. General theory and design of control populations. Anim. Breeding Abstr., 40(1): 1–15.
Ishaq, S.M. and Shah, S.K., 1973. Comparative performance of Nili-Ravi buffaloes and Sahiwal cows as dairy animals. In: Proc. Seminar on Dairy Research, Pakistan, Agricultural Research Council, pp. 144–146.
Ishaq, S.M. and Shah, S.K., 1975. Comparative performance of buffaloes and Sahiwal cows as dairy animals. Agric. Pakistan, 26(1): 75–88.
Jasiorowski, H., Reklewski, Z. and Stolzman, M., 1983. Testing of different strains of Friesian cattle in Poland. 1. Milk performance of F_1 paternal Friesian strain crosses under intensive feeding conditions. Livestock Prod. Sci., 10(2): 109–122.
Johnson, H.D., 1982. Role of physiology in cattle production in the tropics. In: M.K. Yousef (Editor), Animal Production in the Tropics. Praeger Publishers, New York, pp. 3–28.
Kassab, S.A., Afifi, Y., El-Santiel, G. and Mahmoud, S., 1977. Some environmental factors affecting milk yield from buffalo and cross-Jersey cows. J. Agric. Res., Tanta University, 3(1): 29–35.
Keller, D.G. and Brinks, J.S., 1978. Inbreeding by environment interactions for weaning weight in Hereford cattle. J. Anim. Sci., 46(1): 48–53.
Koger, M., Burns, W.C., Pahnish, O.F. and Butts, W.T., 1979. Genotype by environment interactions in Hereford cattle. I. Reproductive traits. J. Anim. Sci., 49(2): 396–402.
Kraüsslich, H., 1974. Comparison of daughters of Holstein-Friesian and German Black and White bulls under different environmental conditions. In: Proc. Working Symposium on Breed Evaluation and Crossing Experiments with Farm Animals, Zeist, 1974. Research Institute for Animal Husbandry 'Schoonoord', pp. 199–205.
Kretzschmar, B. and Ross, K., 1976. Genotyp–Umwelt-Interaktionen und deren Auswirkungen auf die Genauigkeit der Zuchwertschätzung von Besamungsbullen. (Genotype–environment interactions and their effects on the accuracy of breeding value estimation of AI bulls.) Tierzucht, 30: 542–546.
Langholz, J.-J., 1978. Effect of breed and interaction with nutrition. In: Patterns of Growth and Development in Cattle. A Seminar in the EEC Programme of Coordination of Research on Beef Production, Ghent, 11–13 October 1977. Martinus Nijhoff, The Hague, pp. 461–480.
Laster, D.B., Bond, T.E. and Cundiff, L.V., 1974. Climatic–breed interactions in beef cattle. Proc. International Livestock Environment Symposium, 17–19 April 1974, University of Nebraska, Lincoln. American Society of Agricultural Engineers, pp. 301–304.
Leech, F.B., 1976. Some biological factors affecting survival, with particular relation to farm animals. Br. Vet. J., 132(4): 335–345.
Mahadevan, P., 1978. Water buffalo research—possible future trends. World Anim. Rev., 25: 2–7.
Ménissier, F., 1974. Hypertrophie musculaire d'origine génétique chez les bovins: description, transmission, emploi pour l'amélioration de la production de viande. (Muscular hypertrophy of genetic origin in cattle: description, transmission and use for improvement of meat production.) 1st World Congress on Genetics Applied to Livestock Production, Vol. 1. Editorial Garsi, Madrid, pp. 85–107.
Mohammad, W.A., Lee, A.J. and Grossman, M., 1982. Genotype–environment interaction in sire

evaluation. J. Dairy Sci., 65(5): 857–860.

Murray, M. and Trail, J.C.M., 1982. Trypanotolerance: genetics, environmental influences and mechanisms. 2nd World Congress on Genetics Applied to Livestock Production, 4–8 October 1982. 6. Round tables. Editorial Garsi, Madrid, pp. 293–306.

Nagarcenkar, R., 1979. Riverine buffaloes of India and possibilities of genetic improvement vis-a-vis cattle . In: Buffalo Reproduction and Artificial Insemination. Proc. Seminar sponsored by FAO/SIDA/Govt of India, held at National Dairy Research Institute, Karnal 132001 India, 4–15 December 1978. Food and Agriculture Organization of the United Nations, Rome, pp. 97–128.

Nishimura, H. and Frisch, J.E., 1977. Eye cancer and circumocular pigmentation in *Bos taurus, Bos indicus* and crossbred cattle. Aust. J. Exp. Agric. Anim. Husbandry, 17(88): 709–711.

NRC, 1981. The Water Buffalo: New Prospects for an Underutilized Animal. National Research Council, National Academy Press, Washington, DC., 116 pp.

Pani, S.N. and Lasley, J.F., 1972. Genotype × environment interactions in animals. Research Bulletin 992, Agricultural Experiment Station, University of Missouri-Columbia, 103 pp.

Parekh, H.K.B. and Pande, A.B., 1982. Genetic evaluation of exotic sires under different environment and their accuracy. 2nd World Congress on Genetics Applied to Livestock Production, 4–8 October 1982. 7. Symposia (1). Editorial Garsi, Madrid, pp. 170–177.

Philipson, J., Thafvelin, B. and Hedebro-Velander, I., 1980. Genetisk analys av sjukdomsdata. (Genetic analysis of disease data.) Svensk Veterinartidning, 32(8): 233–235.

Pirchner, F., 1983. Population Genetics in Animal Breeding (2nd Edition). Plenum Press, New York, 414 pp.

Poulton, B.R., Anderson, M.J. and Dell, J.C., 1962. The relationship of various hereditary and environmental factors to the incidence of milk fever (parturient paresis) in dairy cows. Bulletin 604 Maine Agricultural Experiment Station, 22 pp.

Powell, R.L. and Dickinson, F.N., 1977. Progeny tests of sires in the United States and Mexico. J. Dairy Sci., 60(11): 1768–1772.

Queval, R., 1982. La glucose-6-phosphate déshydrogénase érythrocytaire chez les races bovines trypanosensibles et trypanotolérantes de l'Ouest Africain. (Erythrocyte glucose-6-phosphate dehydrogenase in West African cattle breeds susceptible to and tolerant of trypanosomes.) Rev. Elev. Med. Vét. Pays Trop., 35(2): 131–136.

Queval, R. and Petit, J.-P., 1982. Polymorphisme biochimique de l'hémoglobine de populations bovines trypanosensibles, trypanotolérantes et de leur croisement dans l'Ouest-Africain. (Biochemical polymorphism of haemoglobin in trypanosusceptible and trypanotolerant cattle and their crossbreds in West Africa.) Rev. Elev. Méd. Vét. Pays Trop., 35(2): 137–146.

Ram, K., Kulwant Singh and Tomer O.S., 1976. Economic efficiency of Brown Swiss crosses, zebu cattle and Murrah buffaloes for production of milk fat and milk solids. Ind. J. Anim. Sci., 46(6): 269–273.

Reddy, Y.V.R., Venkataraman, T.G. and Sampath, S.R., 1980. Efficiency of cross-bred cows in the cost of milk production. Livestock Adviser, 5(1): 5–8.

Ribeiro, J.A.R., 1977. The effects of genotype × location interaction on various production traits in two selections of Hereford cattle. Dissertation Abstr. Int. B, 38(2): 428.

Robertshaw, D. and Finch, V., 1976. The effects of climate on the productivity of beef cattle. In: A.J. Smith (Editor), Beef Cattle Production in Developing Countries. Centre for Tropical Veterinary Medicine, Edinburgh, pp. 280–293.

Robertson, A., 1959. The sampling variance of the genetic correlation coefficient. Biometrics, 15: 469–485.

Ross Cockrill, W., 1968. The draught buffalo (*Bubalus bubalis*). The Veterinarian, 5: 265–272.

Ross Cockrill, W. (Editor), 1974. The Husbandry and Health of the Domestic Buffalo. Food and Agriculture Organization, Rome, 993 pp.

Seifert, G.W., 1971. Variations between and within breeds of cattle in resistance to field infestations of the cattle tick (*Boophilus microplus*). Aust. J. Agric. Res., 22: 159–168.

Srinivasan, M.R., 1982. Developments in dairy products manufacture. In: Research in Animal Production. Indian Council of Agricultural Research, New Delhi, pp. 392–403.

Stolzman, M., Jasiorowski, H., Reklewski, Z., Zarnecki, A. and Kalinowska, G., 1981. Friesian cattle in Poland — preliminary results of testing different strains. *World Anim. Rev.*, 38: 9–15.

Strother, G.R., Burns, E.C. and Smart, L.I., 1974. Resistance of purebred Brahman, Hereford and Brahman × Hereford crossbred cattle to the lone star tick, *Amblyomma americanum* (Acarina: Ixodidae). J. Med. Entomol., 11(5): 559–563.

Taneja, V.K. and Garg, R.C., 1976. Genotype–environment interaction for milk yield in dairy cattle. Ind. J. Dairy Sci., 29(2): 145–146.

Turner, H.G. and Short, A.J., 1972. Effects of field infestation of gastrointestinal helminths and of the cattle tick (*Boophilus microplus*) on growth of three breeds of cattle. Aust. J. Agric. Res., 23; 177–193.

Turner, J.W., 1980. Genetic and biological aspects of zebu adaptability. J. Anim. Sci., 50: 1201–1214.

Turton, J.D., 1969. Recent research in cattle breeding and production in the USSR - a review. Anim. Breeding Abstr., 37: 347–391.

Turton, J.D., 1981. Crossbreeding of dairy cattle — a selective review. Anim. Breeding Abstr.

49(5): 293–300.
Utech, K.B.W., Wharton, R.H. and Kerr, J.D., 1978. Resistance to *Boophilus microplus* (Canestrini) in different breeds of cattle. Aust. J. Agric. Res., 29(4): 885–895.
Vasanth, J.K., 1979. Note on freezing of buffalo semen and fertility. In: Buffalo reproduction and artificial insemination. Proc. Seminar sponsored by FAO/SIDA/Govt of India, held at National Dairy Research Institute, Karnal 132001. India, 4–15 December 1978. Food and Agriculture Organization, Rome, pp. 304–314.
Warwick, E.J., 1958. Fifty years of progress in breeding beef cattle. J. Anim. Sci., 17: 922–943.
Warwick, E.J., 1972. Genotype–environment interactions in cattle. World Rev. Anim. Prod., 8: 33–38.
Warwick, E.J., 1980. Effect of genetic factors on the nutrient composition of animal products. Anim. Breeding Abstr., 48(12): 843–858.
Wharton, R.H., Utech, K.B.W. and Turner, H.G., 1970. Resistance to the cattle tick *Boophilus microplus* in a herd of Australian Illawarra Shorthorn cattle: its assessment and heritability. Aust. J. Agric. Res., 21: 163–181.
Yamada, Y., 1981. The importance of mating systems in the conservation of animal genetic resources. In: Animal Genetic Resources Conservation and Management. Proc. FAO/UNEP Technical Consultation, Food and Agriculture Organization, Rome, pp. 268–278.
Young, B.A., 1981. Cold stress as it affects animal production. J. Anim. Sci., 52: 154–163.

Chapter 3

Domestication: A Forward Step in civilization

W.J.A. PAYNE

1. INTRODUCTION

We do not know how man first domesticated livestock. We can only theorize. Possibly the most interesting known facts are that domestication is a recent phenomenon in man's sojourn on Earth and that it is not a simple or short-term procedure; as contemporary efforts to domesticate additional species, such as the eland, demonstrate. The earliest evidence to date suggests that dogs were the first animals to be domesticated, some 12 000–14 000 years ago (Turnbull and Reed, 1974). However, it has not been predators that have become the major group of domesticated animals, but ruminant species of the family Bovidae — cattle, sheep, goats, yaks and buffaloes (World Animal Science, Vol. A1). The most likely reason for this situation is that ruminants possess a major biological advantage from man's point of view: they can utilize roughage feeds that humans find inedible, to produce foods such as milk and meat considered desirable and nutritious by man.

2. THE ORIGIN OF CATTLE AND BUFFALOES

The Bovidae belong to the order Artiodactyla, or even-toed ungulates. They are the dominant family of hoofed mammals and one of the most recent to evolve. There is, however, some disagreement between authorities as to how the genera within the subfamily Bovinae, that includes cattle and buffaloes, should be classified. One accepted method (Fig. 3.1) suggests that all types of cattle, yaks and bison evolved from one group of common ancestors and all buffaloes from another. Because there is no continuous fossil record by which the evolution of these groups can be traced, the classification in Fig. 3.1 could change if and when additional evidence becomes available. It is likely, given the geographical distribution of present wild species, that the centre of origin of the Bovidae was in the Asian tropics or subtropics.

2.1. The wild ancestors

2.1.1. Cattle

If it is accepted that *Bos taurus* and *Bos indicus* cattle are variants of the same species, and this is likely as they possess the same number of chromosomes ($2n = 60$) and interbreed freely, then there are three distinct species of domesticated cattle in the world. The most numerous and important are the large number of breeds of *B. taurus* and *B. indicus* — the common domestic cattle bred in most countries. The other two species — the Bali and the mithan — are at present only of local importance. The Bali (*Bibos banteng*:

Chapter 3 references, p. 71

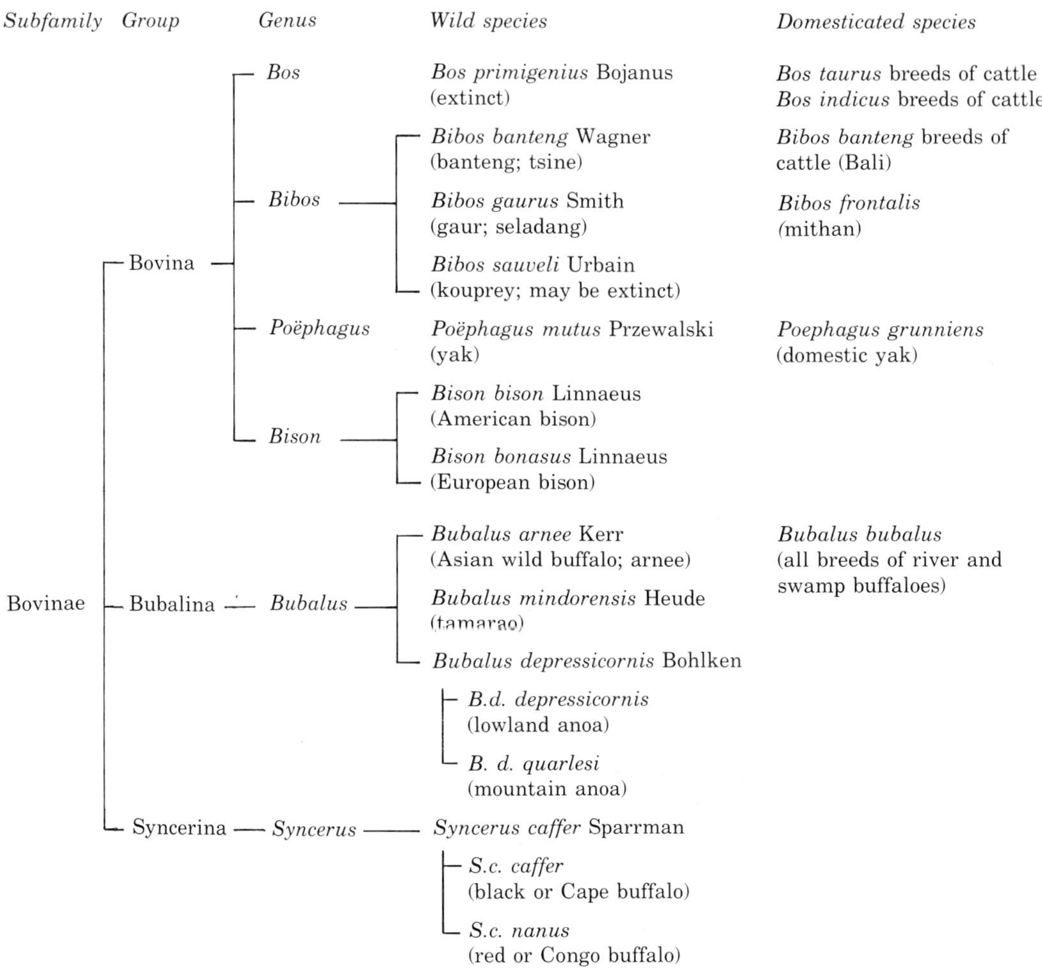

Figure 3.1. Wild and domesticated species within the subfamily Bovinae.

synonyms *Bos (Bibos) banteng, Bos banteng, Bos javanicus, Bos javanicus domesticus* and *Bos sondaicus*) is found primarily in Indonesia, though limited numbers have been imported into Australia, the Philippines and Malaysia; some having become feral in northern Australia. The mithan (*Bibos frontalis*: synonyms *Bos (Bibos) frontalis, Bos frontalis* and *Bos gaurus frontalis*) has an even more limited distribution in the hill country that separates India and Bangladesh from Burma and in the highland area between India and Tibet and China.

***Bos taurus* and *Bos indicus*.** There are no surviving wild ancestors of *B. taurus* and *B. indicus*. . It is believed that they are descended from wild cattle, designated zoologically as *Bos primigenius* and variously named urus, ur, thur and auroch, that once ranged over Eurasia from the Asian Pacific shore to the Atlantic coast of Europe and were also found in the Nile delta region now known as Egypt and on the North African littoral (Fig. 3.2). As might be expected when a species has such an extensive range, there were at least three, geographically based, different races of *B. primigenius*. The North African race, designated as *Bos primigenius opisthonomus*, and known from both fossil and archaeological records, apparently became extinct in Egypt some 3400

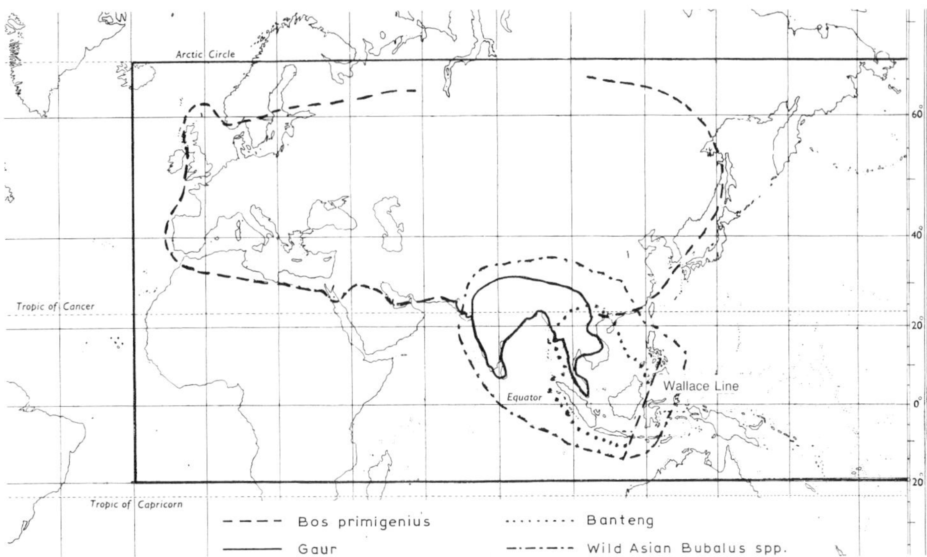

Fig. 3.2. Approximate limits of the distribution of *Bos primigenius* (– – –), the gaur (—), the banteng (. . .) and wild Asian *Bubalus* spp. (– · –).

years ago, but probably survived in some areas of the North African littoral for several more centuries. *Bos primigenius namadicus,* the Asiatic race whose fossil remains have been found at sites as far apart as the Lebanon and China, was, according to archaeological and historical evidence, still hunted in western Asia some 2800 years ago and possibly survived in isolated areas until more recent times. The European race, *Bos primigenius primigenius,* depicted in French and Spanish cave paintings and of which there are many fossil records, survived in the forests of northern Europe until the 17th century, the last known survivor being killed in Poland in 1627.

Bali cattle (*Bibos banteng*). Authorities generally agree that Bali cattle are a domesticated form of the wild banteng (*Bibos banteng*) that in historical times was widely distributed throughout Southeast Asia from Burma, through Thailand and central and southern Indo-China to Malaysia and some, but not necessarily all, of the Indonesian islands located west of the Wallace line (Fig. 3.2). Today, however, the banteng though still extant has a much more restricted distribution and can be considered to be an endangered species.

Mithan (*Bibos frontalis*). There are three theories as to the origin of the mithan. First, that it is a domestic survival of an extinct wild species, secondly that it is a crossbred between *Bos taurus* and/or *Bos indicus* cattle and the wild gaur, and thirdly that it is a domesticated gaur. To date there is no evidence of a wild ancestor, other than the gaur. As the result of evidence available at the time, this author (Payne, 1970) suggested that the mithan was a crossbred, but at around the same time Fischer (1969) showed that the mithan was identical with the gaur in karotype ($2n = 58$) and Gray (1972) noted that domestic cattle and the gaur are not completely interfertile. It is now generally considered that the mithan is a domesticated gaur. The gaur, though now very restricted in habitat and numbers, once ranged over much of India and across mainland Southeast Asia from the Indian border to Indo-China and Malaysia (Fig. 3.2), sharing some part of the southeastern habitat with the banteng.

2.1.2. Buffaloes

As far as is known the African buffalo (*Syncerus caffer*) has never been effec-

Chapter 3 references, p. 71

tively domesticated, although attempts at domestication have been made in the past and in recent times. All domestic buffaloes in Africa have been introduced from Asia, either in historical times or very recently and it can be categorically stated that all domesticated buffalo breeds throughout the world have originated from wild Asian species.

There are three wild species extant today (Fig. 3.1): the arnee (*Bubalus arnee*), the tamarao (*Bubalus mindorensis*) and two races of the anoa (*Bubalus depressicornis*). All three species are endangered; the tamarao and anoa more than the arnee.

The arnee is only found in national parks and reserves in India, Nepal and Burma, but fossil and archaeological records show that it was once widely distributed from southern China and Southeast Asia to western Asia and even as recently as the 19th century this buffalo was hunted in districts of India, Sri Lanka and several Southeast Asian countries (Fig. 3.2).

The tamarao is a small species found only in the island of Mindoro in the Philippines, whilst the anoa is also a small species found only in the island of Sulawesi in Indonesia, where one race (*B. depressicornis depressicornis*) inhabits lowland areas and another (*B. depressicornis quarlesi*) lives in mountainous districts.

Ross Cockrill (1984) suggested that all domestic buffalo breeds have been derived from the arnee and that historical reports of wild buffalo in Southeast Asian offshore islands refer only to feral buffaloes, descendants of domestic buffalo that were probably introduced into the islands by man, possibly the Malays or their predecessors on the Southeast Asian mainland. The presence of distinct species of buffaloes in the widely separated islands of Mindoro and Sulawesi does suggest, however, that not all swamp breeds of domestic buffalo in Southeast Asian offshore islands are necessarily descended from introduced arnee and that some may be the descendants of buffalo species that are now extinct or of crossbreds between introduced arnee-type buffaloes from mainland Southeast Asia and indigenous but now extinct species. If there are still separate species of buffalo on two offshore islands it is quite possible, or even probable, that wild species existed in islands other than Mindoro and Sulawesi and were exterminated at some time in the past by man. Nevertheless, it can be accepted that the arnee has probably made the major contribution to the genotype of all swamp buffalo breeds and is the sole progenitor of river buffalo breeds.

2.2. Centres of domestication

2.2.1. Cattle

Domestic cattle may be classified into two major groups: humpless (*Bos taurus*) and humped (*Bos indicus*), and presently available evidence suggests that the earliest domestic cattle were of the longhorn humpless type.

Humpless cattle. In studies of the early domestication of cattle two distinct humpless types are recognized: the longhorn and the shorthorn. Most authorities consider that the centre of domestication of longhorn humpless cattle was in western Asia (probably in a region formed by parts of modern Turkey, Iraq and Iran (Fig. 3.3)), and that domestication occurred some 8000–9000 years ago. If this was the case then longhorn humpless cattle are derived from the Asiatic form of the auroch (*Bos primigenius namadicus*). There are, however, authorities who suggest that there were several centres of domestication (Kolesnik, 1936), and in particular there are those who consider that longhorn humpless cattle were domesticated quite independently in southeastern Europe (Reed, 1977), their ancestors being the European type of auroch.

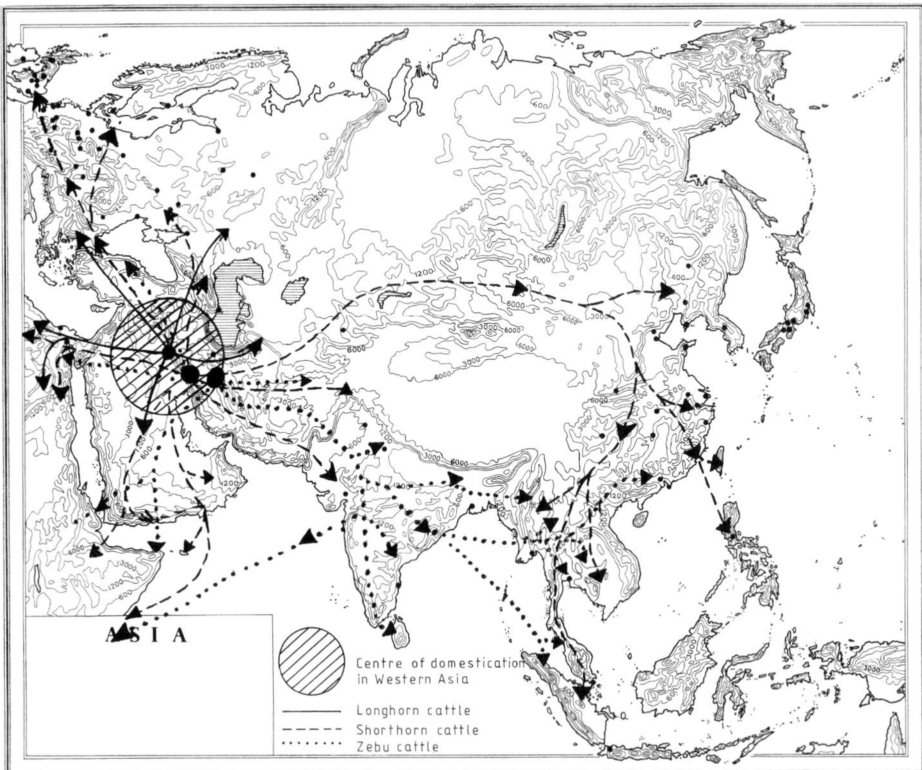

Fig. 3.3. Possible migratory routes of domestic cattle in Asia. After: Payne (1970).

About 5000 years ago the first records appeared in Mesopotamia of a generally smaller, shorthorned type of humpless domestic cattle. Epstein and Mason (1984) consider that the development of the characteristics that differentiate the shorthorn from the longhorn humpless domestic cattle can be explained as the natural outcome of the domestication process and of selection by man. In particular, the general superior milk production of the shorthorn humpless type probably resulted from selection for milk production in an environment where the new and growing urban centres in Mesopotamia provided a ready market for the sale of milk.

Humped cattle. There are two types of humped cattle: cervico-thoracic, in which the hump is located on the posterior part of the neck, above the 6th/7th cervical to 4th/5th thoracic vertebrae, and thoracic, in which the hump is situated on the shoulder above the 1st–9th thoracic vertebrae. The humps consist of muscle and connective tissue in which variable quantities of fat are embedded; the overall composition depending upon breed, individuality and the condition of the animal. Both types of humped cattle are usually designated as 'zebu', but in Africa cervico-thoracic, humped cattle are generally called 'sanga'. Zebu cattle are in general better acclimatized to tropical and subtropical environments than European-type humpless cattle, though no more so than tropical humpless type breeds such as the West African N'Dama.

Zebu cattle appear to have originated in the southeastern districts of the western Asia region in which longhorn cattle were first domesticated. The earliest evidence of their existence as domestic animals being found in northern Baluchistan and adjacent areas and dated about 5000–6000 years ago (Payne, 1970; Epstein and Mason, 1984). There are authorities (Marshall, 1931; Johnson, 1951), who have argued that the diversity of zebu cattle types

Chapter 3 references, p. 71

and their geographical distribution support a theory that the Indian subcontinent was the centre of origin of zebu cattle, but present evidence suggests that zebu cattle were taken into the subcontinent by migrating peoples from western Asia.

To summarize, present available evidence suggests that the centre of origin of the first domesticated longhorn humpless, shorthorn humpless and zebu cattle was western Asia, though there are as yet unproven claims that there were additional centres of domestication of longhorn humpless cattle. The shorthorn humpless and zebu cattle were probably derived, possibly partly by selection by man, from longhorn humpless cattle some 2000–3000 years after the longhorns were first domesticated; the shorthorn humpless in the thickly populated areas of Mesopotamia and the zebu in the warmer and drier climates within the region of domestication.

Bali cattle (*Bibos banteng*). The exact centre of domestication of Bali cattle and the period of time during which it was undertaken are matters for conjecture, but domestication must have taken place in the region inhabited by the banteng and is likely to have occurred during the agricultural revolution in Southeast Asia when man started to engage in agriculture rather than in food gathering.

In historical times the banteng is known to have inhabited a region that extended from Burma, through Thailand, central and southern Indo-China, to western Malaysia and the Indonesian islands west of the Wallace line (Fig. 3.2.). Banteng from mainland Southeast Asia probably reached Borneo and the Indonesian islands west of the Wallace line when these islands were connected to western Malaysia during glacial periods; some 40 000–70 000 years ago.

As the largest concentration of Bali cattle is found in the island of Bali (Payne and Rollinson, 1973) it would be reasonable to assume that the centre of domestication was Bali or an adjacent island. Strong support for a centre of origin somewhere in this area is provided by blood haemoglobin studies. Namikawa and Widodo (1978) reported that the Hbb-X component of cattle haemoglobin was generally found in the blood of the indigenous cattle of Southeast Asia and they suggested that the high incidence of Hbb-X in Southeast Asian cattle was the result of a gene flow from Bali cattle. Namikawa (1981) has since reported on the geographical distribution of alleles of the Hbb locus in Southeast Asian and eastern Asian cattle and their phylogeny has been analysed quantitatively on the basis of polymorphism at that locus which involves three characteristic alleles originating from *B. taurus*, *B. indicus* and *Bibos banteng* cattle. Some of the results of these studies are shown in Table 3.1. These demonstrate that the proportion of genes originating in Bali cattle are highest within the island of Bali, whilst the further away other Southeast Asian breeds are from Bali the less genes they possess that are similar to those of the Bali.

This evidence does not prove that the centre of domestication of Bali cattle was in the island of Bali, but it does suggest that it was in the area that includes the islands of Java, Madura and Bali. It is of some interest that Payne and Rollinson (1976) suggested on the basis of morphological evidence, before the haemoglobin data was available, that Madurese cattle were possibly derived from crosses between Bali and other breeds. What is surprising is the relative high incidence of Hbb-X in indigenous cattle from Palawan and Mindoro islands in the Philippine archipelago, suggesting that there should be a reconsideration of the accepted origin of indigenous Philippine cattle.

Other explanations of the data provided in Table 3.1 are that Bali cattle were more widely distributed in the past and interbred with introduced cattle at different rates or that cattle of other origins were interbred with the wild banteng. One reason why there are few genes from *B. taurus* and *B. indicus*

TABLE 3.1

Estimated proportion of genes originating from *Bos taurus*, *Bos indicus* and *Bibos banteng* cattle

Breed	Location	Proportion of genes originating from:		
		Bos taurus (Northern or European cattle)	*Bos indicus* (Zebu cattle)	*Bibos banteng* (Bali cattle)
Holstein (for comparison)		1.000	0.000	0.000
Thai	Northern Thailand	0.123	0.823	0.054
Thai	Southern Thailand	0.539	0.346	0.115
Kedah-Kelantan	West Malaysia	0.604	0.285	0.111
Philippine native	Luzon	0.107	0.723	0.170
Philippine native	Palawan: Mindoro	0.109	0.641	0.250
Sumatran	Padang, Sumatra	0.236	0.569	0.194
Madurese	Madura	0.456	0.328	0.217
Javanese	East Java	0.374	0.395	0.231
Bali	Bali	0.084	0.292	0.791

Source: Namikawa (1981)

cattle in Bali cattle may be because in the past it was the colonial power's policy not to allow the introduction of other types of cattle into the island of Bali whilst they were freely introduced elsewhere in Indonesia. It is quite certain that crossbreeding between domestic cattle and wild cattle, including the banteng, was in the past an acceptable husbandry practice in several Southeast Asian countries. For instance, Raffles (1816) noted that domestic cows in Java were driven into the forest in anticipation that they would mate with banteng in order to improve the breed.

Wharton (1969), in a study of the banteng, concluded that the species prefers semi-open forest land and avoids dense evergreen forests. The islands of Java and Bali would have provided a very suitable habitat for the banteng after the end of the last glacial period as the length of the dry season increased and relatively open monsoon forests covered the lowlands (Rollinson, 1984), so that when human societies in these islands abandoned their nomadic or semi-nomadic life of gathering food in the forest for some form of agriculture there could have been large populations of banteng in the area, providing the kind of conditions required for domestication.

The earliest evidence to date in Southeast Asia of some form of agriculture (rice culture) is at a site in Non Nok Tha in northeastern Thailand where cattle bones have also been found (Higham and Leach, 1971). This site was possibly occupied by agriculturists 7000 years ago and no later than 5500 years ago, but the evidence available suggests that the bones were probably those of *Bos indicus*. Until archaeological or other evidence becomes available from Indonesian islands it is impossible to be certain as to when agriculture began in this area but the scanty evidence available from the region suggests that domestication of banteng may have occurred within the last 5000 years.

The mithan (*Bibos frontalis*). If the mithan is a domesticated gaur, then its centre of origin must have been within the area over which the gaur ranged in the past. This was, as mentioned previously, the forested areas of southern India, some parts of central, north and northeastern India, Nepal, Bhutan, eastern Bangladesh, Burma and as far into Southeast Asia as Malaya (Gee, 1964). As the mithan population, estimated to be of the order of 150 000, is now

Chapter 3 references, p. 71

concentrated in Bhutan, Arunachal Pradesh and the Naga, Manipur and Mizo hills in northeastern India, eastern Bangladesh and the Patkoi, Chin and Arakan hills in Burma (Simoons, 1984) in cool forest areas with an elevation of 600–2700 m, it is concluded, although there are no fossil, archaeological or historical records available, that the centre of domestication must have been somewhere in this region. The fact that the mithan is used by swidden farming peoples primarily for ceremonial sacrifice (Simoons and Simoons, 1968), whereas other types of cattle in surrounding regions are used primarily for work and milk production purposes, provides some support for the conclusion that the centre of domestication was somewhere in the region occupied by the swidden farming peoples.There is no evidence at the present time as to when domestication of the mithan took place.

2.2.2. Buffaloes

Evidence on the first domestication of the buffalo is very limited. According to Ross Cockrill (1984) it is generally agreed that buffalo were first domesticated about 4500 years ago and that the centre of domestication was either Mesopotamia during the Akkadian dynasty or the valley of the Indus during the Harappa/Mohenjo Daro civilizations. As the largest number and diversity of river buffalo breeds are to be found in the Indian subcontinent, it is probable that the valley of the Indus was the earliest centre of river buffalo domestication, particularly as Boehmer (1974) stated that there is evidence from Mesopotamia that suggests that buffalo were introduced on two occasions, separated by approximately a 2000-year interval in which there is no evidence of the presence of domestic buffalo.

There is also a possibility that there was a separate centre of buffalo domestication in China in the Yangtze and/or Yellow River valley as there is evidence of the use of domestic buffaloes during the Shang dynasty (c. 3500 years ago) and domestication could have occurred at a much earlier date.

As swamp buffaloes are considered to be more similar to the wild arnee than are river buffaloes it has been assumed that they were domesticated at a later date. If this was so, then there must have been more than one centre of domestication and it is possible that there were a number of different centres of domestication of swamp buffaloes in Southeast Asia. This possibility is supported by the fact that there were wild and/or feral buffaloes in widely separated Southeast Asian countries in the immediate past. The statement by Ross Cockrill (1984) that the swamp buffalo was introduced into island Southeast Asia by migrants fom mainland Asia and that all wild buffalo were in reality feral buffalo can be questioned in view of historical accounts of wild buffalo in Southeast Asia, the diversity in swamp buffalo types and the presence today of different species of wild buffalo in some offshore Southeast Asian islands.

To summarize, present evidence suggests that buffaloes were first domesticated in the Indus valley in the Indian subcontinent about 4000–5000 years ago, but that there may have been separate centres of domestication in Mesopotamia and China and of swamp buffaloes in several different Southeast Asian countries.

3. DISPERSAL OF CATTLE FROM CENTRES OF DOMESTICATION

Dispersal of domestic cattle from centres of domestication was confined to the Eurasian land mass, the continent of Africa and offshore islands until the end of the 16th century; however, with the advent of the era of European discovery, cattle were dispersed to the Americas, Australasia and the oceanic islands.

3.1. The Eurasian land mass, Africa and offshore islands

Evidence as to the dispersal of longhorn humpless, shorthorn humpless and zebu types of cattle throughout this vast area will be considered separately and their contribution to today's breeds assessed. There has been a very limited dispersal of Bali cattle and virtually no dispersal of the mithan.

3.1.1. Longhorn humpless cattle

Western Asia was a region, during the historical period in which longhorn humpless cattle appear to have been domesticated, where there was a constant flux of peoples. They lived in societies that were probably somewhat similar in organization and culture to the pastoral societies of Sub-Saharan Africa, prior to the 20th century. Included, were peoples of Semitic, Hamitic, Vedic Aryan, Ural Altaic and possibly other cultures.

Historical and anthropological evidence suggests that the Semitic and Hamitic peoples migrated with their livestock westward towards the eastern Mediterranean littoral, and from there southwestward into Africa and northwestward towards southeastern Europe. The Vedic Aryan peoples migrated southeastward into the Indian subcontinent and northwestward and northward into Europe and Eurasia, whilst the Ural Altaic peoples migrated north and eastward into Asia. The presence and continuous movements of these peoples, together with their livestock, provided a unique opportunity for the dispersal and spread of domestic longhorn cattle to most of the Old World and Africa.

Africa. The earliest records of the presence of domesticated longhorn humpless cattle in Africa are dated about 7000 years ago (Faulkner and Epstein, 1957) and it is possible that these cattle interbred with indigenous wild cattle. They arrived in northeast Africa during a minor wet, climatic phase (5000–2350 BC), when according to Butzer (1961) the desert retreated 100–250 km towards the centre of the Sahara and pastoral migrations were not so circumscribed by arid conditions as they would be today. From what is now Egypt, Hamitic peoples, together with their livestock, migrated westward along the North African littoral, south and southwestward across the Sahara via the Tibesti and Tassili highlands and southwards along the Nile to East Africa (Fig. 3.4). Although there are no Hamitic longhorn cattle in these regions today, their past presence is attested by numerous rock engravings and drawings, archaeological and historical evidence and Sanga cattle breeds; descendants of crosses between longhorn and zebu cattle. Although Mount Elgon on the Kenya/Uganda border is the furthest south that rock drawings of longhorn cattle have been found to date, Ford (personal communication) reported that in an area adjacent to the Zambesi river there were a small number of trypanotolerant cattle, locally known as Binga, that appeared to be a dwarf form of Hamitic longhorn. Thus it is possible that longhorn humpless cattle were taken as far south as the Zambesi river.

When the Hamitic peoples migrating along the North African littoral reached the area that is now known as Morocco, it is believed that some proceeded northward into Europe (Fig. 3.4). Curson and Thornton (1936) suggested that many Portuguese and Andalusian breeds have been derived from the Hamitic longhorn as have possibly some longhorn breeds in France and Britain. In West Africa, the N'Dama, a trypanotolerant breed, has definitely been derived from the Hamitic longhorn as has the Kouri breed found around the shores of Lake Chad. It is possible that Kouri cattle are descended from

Chapter 3 references, p. 71

Hamitic longhorn that accompanied peoples who migrated across the Sahara via the Tibesti and Tassili highlands (Fig. 3.4).

Europe. There is ample archaeological and historical evidence of the past presence of longhorn, humpless cattle throughout the northern Mediterranean littoral, the Balkans, central and western Europe. As Epstein and Mason (1984) point out, Highland cattle — a breed still extant in the U.K. — show few differences in conformation from Etruscan sculptures of longhorn cattle made 2000–3000 years ago. It is likely that the first longhorn humpless cattle were introduced into Europe by at least two routes; from North Africa into Portugal, Spain and beyond and from western Asia into the Balkans and/or central Europe and beyond (Figs 3.3 and 3.4). It is also probable that there were more recent migrations of peoples owning longhorn humpless cattle from Asia into

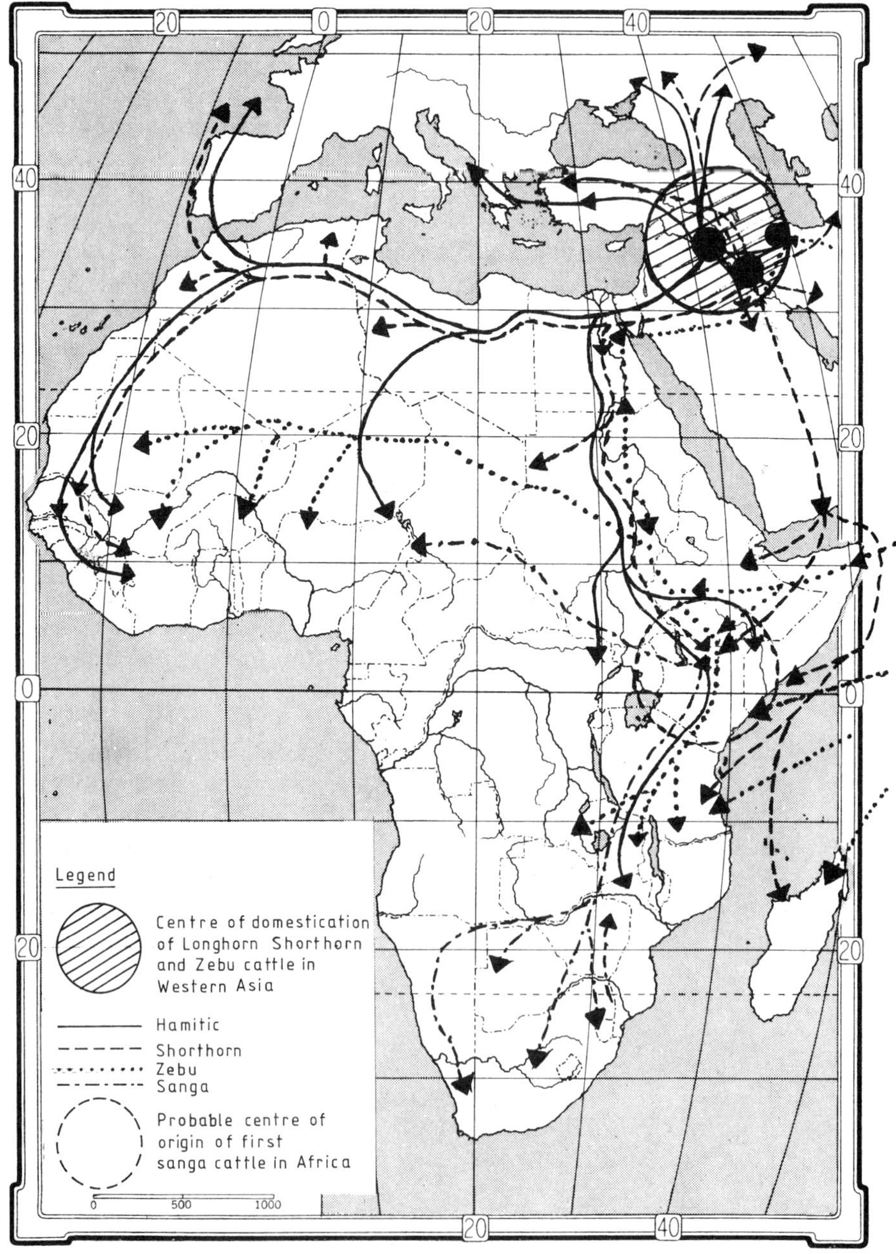

Fig. 3.4. Possibly migratory routes of domestic cattle in Africa. After: Payne (1964).

central and southern Europe. Although there are few longhorn breeds in Europe today there is no doubt that the longhorn, intermingled and crossbred with more recent shorthorn types, has contributed in a greater or lesser measure to the genetic make-up of many modern European breeds.

If there was a separate centre of domestication of longhorn cattle in southeastern Europe, then some modern breeds of European cattle may have been derived from both the Asiatic and the European races of *Bos primigenius* as well as from shorthorn humpless cattle.

Asia. The available evidence suggests that from a centre of domestication in western Asia, longhorn cattle were taken by migrating people, south and southeastward into Mesopotamia and Arabia, east and southeastward into the Indian subcontinent and north and northeastward into southern Russia, the Caucasus and central Asia (Fig. 3.3). Rock engravings of cattle with long lyre-shaped horns, dated at 4000–5000 years old, have been found in central Arabia, whilst numerous works of art of approximately the same age, depicting longhorn-type cattle, have been discovered in Mesopotamia. Fossils considered to be those of longhorn cattle have been uncovered in the Quetta valley in Pakistan, whilst numbers of seals and statuettes depicting longhorn cattle, dated at 4000–4500 years old, have been found in the ruins of the Mohenjo Daro and Harappa civilizations of Vedic speaking peoples in the Indus valley.

Although there is quite early evidence (c. 5000 years ago) of the presence of longhorn cattle in Anau, Turkestan, and Mongolian cattle appear to have been partially derived from longhorn types, the spread of longhorns north and eastward does not appear to have been as rapid as it was elsewhere. The earliest evidence of the presence of longhorn cattle in the steppes of southern Russia and in the northern Caucasus being dated about 2000 years ago.

3.1.2. Shorthorn humpless cattle

As stated previously the earliest evidence of the occurrence of domesticated shorthorn humpless cattle comes from Mesopotamia, dated some 5000 years ago. As these cattle were probably superior to longhorn cattle in some respects, such as milk production, and were smaller and thus needed less feed, they were apparently taken along more or less the same migratory routes as the longhorn cattle, permanently replacing the latter in many regions of Asia, Africa and Europe.

Africa. These cattle were brought into Egypt at least 4500 years ago and by 1700–1500 BC they were the predominant breed in Lower Egypt (Faulkner and Epstein, 1957). From Egypt they were taken by migrating pastoralists along the North African littoral and southwards into Upper Egypt, Ethiopia, the Sudan and beyond (Fig. 3.4). Modern Egyptian cattle are of the shorthorn humpless type, as are existing breeds in Libya, Tunisia, Algeria and Morocco. Some migrating pastoralists with their cattle reached West Africa (Fig. 3.4) and these cattle are considered to be progenitors of the West African Dwarf Shorthorn breed. The latter is a trypanotolerant breed, though tolerance is not so marked as in the N'Dama breed, possibly because less time has elapsed since these cattle arrived in the West African environment. In Ethiopia, the Sudan and further south, shorthorn humpless cattle have been replaced by zebu and sanga breeds, though remnant groups survived in the Nuba mountains, southern Sudan and Uganda until relatively recent times (Payne, 1970), and Alberro and Halle-Mariam (1982) stated that there are still shorthorn humpless cattle kept by the Sheko people in mountainous territory on the Ethiopian Sudanese border.

It is probable that shorthorn humpless cattle were also introduced from southern Arabia to the Horn of Africa, the offshore islands along the East

Chapter 3 references, p. 71

African coast and possibly the East African mainland (Fig. 3.4). An isolated breed of shorthorn type cattle are still owned by the Quarra in Oman and similar cattle are found on the island of Socotra. Tradition has it that such cattle were found on the island of Pemba in historical times and on the island of Mafia, off the coast of Tanzania up until the 1920's (Payne, 1970). A small shorthorn type of cattle also existed in Madagascar prior to the influx of zebu cattle (Dechambre, 1951).

Europe. These cattle were either brought very quickly into Europe or there were separate selections of shorthorns from domesticated longhorn humpless cattle within Europe, as the earliest evidence of their existence in Europe is dated at about the same time as evidence for their domestication in Mesopotamia. There is no doubt that they became widely dispersed and that in northern Europe the type became smaller.

They may have been brought into Europe by several routes; along the northern littoral of the Mediterranean, through the Balkans or the plains of central Europe or even from the North African littoral by land and/or sea to Spain, France and the British Islands (Figs 3.3 and 3.4). whatever the route and whatever their subsequent history there is no doubt that they are the progenitors of some of the most productive European cattle breeds, such as the Friesian, Jersey, Shorthorn and Brown Swiss.

Asia. Shorthorn humpless cattle replaced longhorns throughout western Asia and were in their turn partially replaced by zebu or zebu × shorthorn crossbred cattle. The majority of shorthorn-type cattle in western Asia today are remnant breeds such as the Jaulan in the Golan hills of Syria, but there are substantial numbers of a breed known as the Kurdi in the mountainous areas of northern Iraq, southeastern Turkey and northwestern Iran. Shorthorn cattle were also taken east and northeastward into Tibet and China, possibly by the Ural Altaic-speaking peoples who invaded China about 4500 years ago (Fig. 3.3). From China they were probably taken south, southwest and southeast by migrating peoples into Burma, Thailand, Malaysia, Vietnam and Laos where they interbred with zebu cattle that were introduced from the Indian subcontinent (Fig. 3.3). All breeds in these countries today are of a crossbred type similar to the sanga cattle of Africa (Payne, 1970), but also possessing some *Bos (Bibos)* spp. genes (Namikawa, 1981). They were also introduced from China to offshore islands such as Taiwan and the Philippines and it is possible that small numbers were introduced into Indonesia from mainland Southeast Asia. It is likely that shorthorn-type cattle were also introduced into India, though evidence for this is scanty. There is a breed known as the Siri, found today in Bhutan, Nepal, Sikkim and northern India that appears to be of mixed zebu × shorthorn humpless ancestry but the shorthorn ancestors may have been introduced southward from Tibet and not northward from the Indian subcontinent.

3.1.3. Zebu cattle

On present available evidence it is assumed by this author that zebu-type cattle evolved from previously domesticated cattle somewhere in western Asia, but wherever the origin there is no doubt that once the zebu was established in the Indian subcontinent it spread very rapidly. This may be because zebu cattle are more resistant to rinderpest and to some external parasites than other cattle and more able to acclimatize to arid and tropical climates. Zebu breeds have, in historical times, been spreading in tropical Africa in somewhat similar circumstances at the expense of other types of domestic cattle.

As previously stated, two types of humped cattle are designated as 'zebu': cervico-thoracic or neck-humped and thoracic or chest-humped. Neck-humped cattle appear to be an intermediate type between humpless and chest humped cattle as Slijper (1951) has shown that crossbreds of the latter types tend to possess neck humps. Payne (1970) suggested that all neck-humped zebu should be designated as 'sanga', as this is a term used in Africa for these cattle, whilst more recently Mason has proposed that they be termed 'zeboid' (Epstein and Mason, 1984).

Available evidence suggests that the earliest zebu-type cattle were neck-humped and that for reasons unknown the chest-humped characteristic was selected for by the pastoralists so that chest-humped cattle are of a more recent origin. Epstein and Mason (1984) theorized that pastoralists were selecting for a hump that contained additional fat. Whatever the reason, the evolution of the neck-humped zebu apparently occurred towards the east and/or south of the western Asia centre of domestication, as chest-humped zebu were introduced into the Indian subcontinent long before they were introduced into Africa.

The domestication scenario in western Asia appears to be that from longhorn humpless cattle have originated, probably partly due to selection by pastoralists, first shorthorn humpless cattle, then neck-humped cattle and finally chest-humped cattle and at certain periods in history two or more of these cattle types must have co-existed in the same region. This scenario does not, of course, preclude additional centres of selection of shorthorn humpless or chest-humped cattle outside western Asia. In addition, for century after century different peoples migrated from or through western Asia so that each cattle type in turn was introduced into the lands to the north, east, south and west of western Asia. Dispersal of the neck- and chest-humped zebu cattle was no exception as they were introduced into the remainder of Asia, Africa and Europe, but as their special characteristics were advantageous in hot and dry climates, introductions into southern and southeast Asia were more successful than introductions into northern Asia and Europe where somewhat better acclimatized longhorn and shorthorn humpless cattle were already established in number.

Africa. Neck- and chest-humped cattle were introduced into Africa in successive waves, and at different times from different regions of Asia (Fig. 3.4). Available evidence suggests that some neck-humped cattle were introduced into Egypt both along the land bridge from western Asia and across the sea from southern Arabia via Somalia and Ethiopia, but they could not have been introduced in large numbers as they did not significantly affect the composition of the shorthorn humpless cattle population of Egypt (Payne, 1970). Chest-humped zebu cattle were not introduced into Africa until about 1500 years ago according to Epstein and Mason (1984). It is likely, however, that there were small-scale introductions over a long period, but after the Arab invasion (c. AD 669) the numbers probably increased very rapidly. Cattle were apparently imported through ports all along the East African coast from the Red Sea to the Zambesi river by Indian and Arab traders. These importations were most numerous in the north and persisted almost until modern times.

The first introductions would have had little influence on the composition of the pastoralist's herds of longhorn and shorthorn humpless cattle in Ethiopia and Northeastern and East Africa, but gradually as more zebu cattle arrived and particularly after chest-humped zebu were introduced in number the composition of the herds must have changed, with a predominance of crossbred neck-humped or sanga cattle. As stated previously, these cattle must have been better acclimatized to the tropical environment of northeastern and East Africa than the longhorn and shorthorn cattle and they were probably less susceptible to rinderpest, a disease that they may have introduced from Asia. Thus Ethiopia and northeastern and East Africa was probably the major centre of origin of sanga cattle in Africa.

Chapter 3 references, p. 71

The establishment of herds of sanga cattle in this region must have taken place during a period when there were pressures on the local pastoralists, who were possibly a people somewhat similair to the Hottentots, to migrate; the migration routes being dictated to a very large extent by the availability of feed and water and the location of the tsetse fly (*Glossinia* spp.). These pastoralists, together with their sanga cattle, were followed by others in southward migrations, whilst at a later date other migrating pastoralists introduced chest-humped zebu into Central Africa (Fig. 3.4). These migrations have been described in detail by Payne (1964), and have determined the present distribution of sanga and zebu cattle breeds in Central and southern Africa.

As chest-humped zebu cattle continued to arrive in East Africa the composition of the herds changed yet again towards a preponderance of the zebu types. Posnansky (personal communication) stated that there is evidence that Small East African Zebu cattle were already quite numerous in the Rift valley of Kenya some 400–500 years ago. However, there is also evidence that quite large numbers of sanga cattle were still present in East Africa until comparatively modern times (Payne, 1964) but that they almost entirely disappeared during the rinderpest pandemic at the end of the last century.

The Ankole cattle of western Uganda and Tanzania, Rwanda and Burundi, a sanga breed, were probably introduced some 400–700 years ago from Ethiopia (Epstein, 1957).

There were also migrations of pastoralists together with their sanga and zebu cattle from East Africa to West Africa in comparatively recent times (c. AD 1500), across the savannas between the rain forest and the Sahel (Fig. 3.4). As a consequence sanga and zebu cattle were introduced into West Africa where they interbred with the local humpless to produce the mixture of humpless, sanga and zebu breeds found in West Africa today (Payne, 1970).

Asia. Until very recent times the major breeds in western Asia were either of the sanga or zebu type, but European breeds have now been introduced. Sanga breeds, such as the Damascus, Lebanese and Iranian are found in the northern and more fertile areas — Syria, Lebanon, southern Turkey and Iran — whilst zebu breeds such as the Iraqi and the Southern Arabia Zebu dominate in the less fertile and more tropical areas — southern Iraq and Arabia.

Zebu breeds are found throughout the Indian subcontinent and in Sri Lanka, whilst zebu breeds from the subcontinent were introduced in the past into Burma, Thailand, Malaysia, Laos, Kampuchea and Vietnam, presumably during the period when Hinduism was spreading throughout Southeast Asia (Fig. 3.3). Cattle breeds in the Philippines and Indonesia also demonstrate the presence of zebu genes, but it is not at present clear as to whether zebu cattle were first introduced to these countries in the distant past when Hinduism was spreading or in more recent times. In Southeast Asia the introduced zebu cattle interbred with shorthorn humpless cattle introduced from China by migrating peoples (Fig. 3.3) so that all cattle breeds in Southeast Asia today are of the sanga type, though those closer to the littoral appear to exhibit more zebu characteristics than those further north and inland. Indeed, some zebu cattle must have been taken north into China as Epstein (1969) stated that the cattle in southern China exhibit some influence of zebu genes, but that their presence in the cattle tends to disappear towards the north. In adddition, cattle breeds in Southeast Asia and the offshore islands of the Philippines and Indonesia also possess some *Bos (bibos)* spp. genes (Namikawa, 1981) and are thus in this way different from the sanga breeds of Africa or western Asia.

3.2. The Americas, Australasia and the oceanic islands

There were no cattle in the Americas until the era of European exploration and colonization. On his second voyage in 1493 Colombus introduced cattle into the island of San Domingo. These were the first cattle to arrive in the Western Hemisphere. In 1521, 28 years later, Don Gregoria de Villalobos transferred cattle from Santa Domingo to Vera Cruz, Mexico. These were the first cattle to be introduced to the North American continent and were of the longhorn humpless type.

3.2.1. The Americas

The majority of cattle originally introduced into the Americas, first by the Spanish and then by the Portuguese, were of the longhorn humpless type, but within 100 years cattle of the shorthorn humpless type were introduced by British (Jamestown, 1607), Dutch (New York, 1625) and Swedish (Delaware) settlers. An account of later introductions has been provided by Bowling (1942).

North European breeds spread rapidly throughout North America, but they were not able to acclimatize to conditions in the south and southwest as well as the longhorns introduced by the Spanish. The latter, however, produced beef of poor quality and ranchers eventually introduced other types of cattle. It is believed that zebu cattle were first introduced to North America in 1849, when a Dr Davis of Fairfield County, South Carolina imported two bulls from Mysore, India. Other importations of zebu cattle followed, and zebu were crossed with the northern European breeds, so that by the beginning of the 20th century there were a number of ranchers owning zebu and/or crossbred cattle. Importations were, directly or indirectly, first from the Indian subcontinent and later from Mexico and Brazil.

The introduction of zebu and crossbreeding with humpless cattle culminated in the 20th century in the development of the American Brahman breed — a composite of many Indian breeds — and a number of semi-stabilized crossbred breeds, of which the Santa Gertrudis is probably the best known. A detailed account of the importation of zebu cattle into North America and the varied crossbreeding programmes that were developed is provided by Payne (1970).

Today, although there are some zebu and crossbred zebu cattle in the northern regions of North America, these cattle are mainly confined to the south and the southwest of the continent and are entirely used for beef production. An experimental effort in the 1940's and 1950's to introduce zebu genes into dairy herds failed, and has not been repeated.

Until relatively recent times the majority of cattle in the tropical regions of the Caribbean and Latin America were of the humpless type, descendants of introduced Spanish and Portuguese cattle. They were known as criollos. In more temperate regions, however, the descendants of the first introduced cattle were rapidly replaced by northern European breeds.

Towards the end of the 19th century there were large-scale importations of zebu cattle from the Indian subcontinent into Brazil and later into other countries. As a consequence there are today, in Brazil and elsewhere in tropical Latin America, Gir, Nellore and Kankrej breeds together with a composite zebu breed known as the Indú-Brasil, and crossbreds between these breeds, the criollo and other imported breeds. There have also been large-scale importations of the American Brahman and North American crossbred zebu breeds.

The situation today is that northern European breeds are dominant in the temperate regions, whilst zebu and crossbred zebu breeds of various origin are dominant in tropical regions. Criollos have declined in number but in some regions criollo or crossbred criollo cattle are still of some importance.

Chapter 3 references, p. 71

3.2.2. Australasia and the oceanic islands

There were no cattle, or for that matter many mammals in Australia and the oceanic islands before European settlement. In general, northern European cattle, particularly British breeds, were first introduced, but small numbers of zebu-type cattle were also imported, particularly in countries where sugar cane was grown, and Bali cattle were introduced into northern Australia.

Somewhat later than in the Americas, an interest in the utilization of zebu-type cattle in the tropical regions developed and by the middle of the 20th century there were importations of zebu cattle by ranchers and by government organizations in Australia. These included Red Sindhi and Sahiwal cattle from Pakistan, American Brahman and crossbred zebu breeds such as the Santa Gertrudis from the U.S.A. and Africander cattle.

In a period of 30–50 years zebu and crossbred zebu breeds have become widely distributed in tropical Australia and it is likely that they will ultimately replace the British beef breeds. In addition, indigenous crossbred zebu breeds such as the Droughtmaster have been evolved. As in the Americas the North European breeds remain dominant in the more temperate areas of Australia and in New Zealand, though unlike the situation in North America a crossbred zebu milking breed — the Australian Milking Zebu (AMZ) — is being promoted in tropical regions.

In the oceanic islands zebu or crossbred zebu cattle are slowly replacing European breeds, where there is beef cattle ranching, but generally northern European breeds are still used for milk production purposes.

3.3. Bali cattle

As stated previously, as far as is known there has been a very limited dispersal of Bali cattle. There is evidence that they were imported into other Indonesian islands and particularly into Sulawesi, Java and Timor during the first decades of this century. In 1849 Bali cattle were imported into the Coburg peninsula in northern Australia and went feral. About 1000 head were present in the 1970's (Kirby, 1979). Importations were also made into Singapore for slaughter purposes and an importation of breeding stock was made into mainland Malaysia in 1951 (Devendra et al., 1973), from where small numbers were introduced into Sarawak, Brunei and Sabah. The author saw Bali cattle in Luzon in the Philippines in the 1960's, but it is not known exactly when these cattle were imported.

4. DISPERSAL OF BUFFALOES FROM CENTRES OF DOMESTICATION

There is relatively little information as to the dispersal of buffaloes from their centre(s) of domestication. What is certain is that past dispersal of buffaloes was much slower and more limited than that of cattle and that they were not widely dispersed until very recent times.

If buffaloes were first domesticated in the Indian subcontinent or even if there were separate centres of domestication in China, Southeast Asia and Mesopotamia, what little evidence is available suggests that dispersal was more widespread in eastern than in western Asia up until 1000 years ago (Ross Cockrill, 1984). According to Epstein (1971) buffaloes were first introduced into Egypt about 1000 years ago, but did not disperse to other African countries. There is evidence that they were present in Turkey at about the same period, were numerous in Italy by the 12th century and in southeastern Europe by the 14th century. Buffaloes were introduced into western Europe in mediaeval times but they never became established.

From the 16th to the 18th century the Portuguese made frequent importations of buffaloes into East Africa from Sri Lanka and India, but these all failed and it was not until the present century that successful importations were made into any African country other than Egypt. There are now small, thriving herds in Mozambique, Nigeria, Tanzania and Uganda.

The first buffaloes were introduced into the Americas around 1890 (Ross Cockrill, 1984) and since then many introductions have been made into the Caribbean and South America. Today there are possibly 500 000 buffaloes in Brazil and smaller numbers in Venezuela, Colombia, Peru, Bolivia, French Guiana, Guyana, Surinam, Trinidad, Costa Rica and Panama. Trinidad has been a major centre for the dispersal of buffaloes into neighbouring countries. In the 1970's buffaloes from Guam were introduced in Florida and Louisiana in North America.

In Asia the Spanish imported buffaloes into Guam from the Philippines soon after settlement. Buffaloes were first introduced into Australia in 1826, where there is now a large feral population, and into New Guinea at the beginning of the 20th century.

5. PRESENT DISTRIBUTION OF CATTLE AND BUFFALOES

5.1. Cattle

The present distribution of cattle in the world, by regions and within continents, is shown in Table 3.2. Approximately two-thirds of the world population of cattle are to be found in the Old World and one-third in the Americas, Australasia and the oceanic islands. Slightly more than half the world's cattle population are in the tropics. If the U.S.S.R. is excluded, as part is in Europe and part in Asia, America is the continent with the most cattle, followed by Asia, Africa, Europe and Australia. More than half of all Asian cattle are to be found within the Indian subcontinent (18.5% of the world population).

Cattle are still increasing in number (at the global rate of 6% between 1973 and 1983 (Table 3.2)), but the increase is not spread evenly throughout the world. It is quite rapid in some of the least developed countries and in the poorest continent — Africa — and least in countries with well-developed cattle industries such as those in North America, Europe and Australasia, where the emphasis is on production per animal. There have also been increases in cattle numbers in regions where the cattle industry was not previously well-developed, but where national income has recently increased very rapidly, such as some oil-rich countries in western Asia and newly industrialized countries in eastern Asia (Table 3.2).

In the world at present there is approximately 11 ha of land available per head of cattle (Table 3.2), but the variation from region to region is wide; from 1.8 ha per head in the Indian subcontinent to 216 ha per head in the humid region of Central Africa. Cattle populations remain low in the latter region as much of it is infested with tsetse fly, but in general cattle are not as numerous in the very humid regions of the tropical world as they are in the drier regions.

Thus not only have cattle been dispersed all over the world and the world population very substantially increased since the 16th century, but numbers are still increasing, particularly in tropical and subtropical regions.

5.2. Buffaloes

Unlike cattle, buffaloes are not widely dispersed across the world as 97% of the total world population are still to be found in Asia (Table 3.3.) and more

Chapter 3 references, p. 71

TABLE 3.2

World distribution of cattle in 1973 and 1983

Continent	Region	1973 ('000 head)	1983 ('000 head)	1983 as % 1973	As % total 1983	Area ('000 ha)	ha per head of cattle
Africa	North	7 517	6 986	93		575 289	
	Northeast	26 968	30 393	113		188 156	
	East	24 108	31 258	130		181 795	
	Sahelian	30 875	40 271	130		842 088	
	West	18 513	20 838	113		260 601	
	Central (humid)	1 132	1 379	122		298 313	216.3
	Central (drier)	11 480	13 370	116		330 996	
	Southern	16 300	19 336	119		269 341	
	Offshore islands	9 668	10 501	109		59 916	
	Total	146 561	174 332	119	14.2	3 006 495	17.2
Americas	North	161 192	160 691	100		2 131 186	
	Central	10 232	11 662	114		52 276	
	Caribbean	10 750	10 785	100		23 860	
	South (temperate)	67 640	67 851	100		371 223	
	South (tropical)	124 487	138 342	111		1 172 248	
	Andean	6 677	7 404	111		238 380	
	Total	380 978	396 735	104	32.4	3 989 173	10.1
Asia	Western	15 991	21 368	137		153 884	
	Southwestern	1 752	1 784	102		300 316	
	Indian subcontinent	226 579	243 149	107	18.5	448 894	1.8
	Southeast	26 637	26 812	101		449 349	
	Central	11 329	14 796	131		386 050	
	Eastern	5 702	7 348	129		59 237	
	China	63 348	57 450	91		959 696	
	Total	351 356	372 707	106	30.4	2 757 426	7.4
U.S.S.R.		104 006	117 186	113	9.6	2 240 220	19.1
Europe		133 848	133 317	100	10.9	487 084	3.7
Australasia	Australia	29 101	22 764	78		768 685	
	New Zealand	9 088	7 800	86		26 868	
	Oceanic islands	517	573	111		55 400	
		38 706	31 137	80	2.5	850 953	27.3
World		1 155 455	1 225 414	106		13 331 351	10.9

Source: FAO (1984)

than 80% within two Asian regions — the Indian subcontinent and Southeast Asia.

Although the FAO (1984) data provided in Table 3.3 underestimates the total number of buffaloes in Africa, the Americas, Australasia and the oceanic islands, the overall scenario is that small increases in buffalo populations in these continents and regions during the last decade have been overshadowed by substantial decreases in China, central Asia and western Asia and some decrease in Southeast Asia. The only substantial increase in buffalo population has been in Brazil but this has still been small compared with the decreases in Asia.

6. POSSIBLE FUTURE CHANGES IN CATTLE AND BUFFALO POPULATIONS

6.1. Cattle

As the area of land available per head of cattle decreases, and in some regions it is already very limited (Table 3.2), whilst at the same time the human population continues to increase, it will become essential to improve the productivity of cattle so that total numbers can be restricted. Thus it is likely that the rate of increase in cattle numbers in countries with a developing cattle industry will tend to decrease as is happening at the present time in countries with well-developed cattle industries. This means that it will become necessary to develop cattle types that are adapted to adverse en-

TABLE 3.3

World distribution of buffaloes in 1973 and 1983

Continent	Region	1973 ('000 head)	1983 ('000 head)	1983 as % 1973	As % total 1983
Africa	North (Egypt)	2 135	2 393	112	1.93
Americas	Caribbean (Trinidad)	7	8		
	South (Brazil)	145	570		
	Total	152	578	380	0.47
Asia	Western	1 323	1 050	79	
	Indian subcontinent	73 989	82 551	112	66.47
	Southeast	19 616	17 874	91	14.39
	Central	480	253	53	
	Eastern	1	1	100	
	China	29 929	18 750	63	
	Total	125 338	120 479	96	97.00
U.S.S.R.		429	320	75	0.25
Europe		417	433	104	0.35
Oceania		1	1	100	(insignificant)
World		128 472	124 204	97	

Note: Small numbers of buffalo recently introduced into African and American countries are not recorded in the FAO statistics.
Source: FAO (1984).

vironmental conditions; particularly in the tropics. Possible future scenarios in each continent are briefly discussed below.

Africa. A decline in pastoralism in the Sahel and North and northeastern Africa is inevitable due to a number of different causes, and it is probable that this husbandry system will ultimately be confined to the driest areas, in which the role of camels, sheep and goats may become more important than that of cattle. In those regions where the rainfall is somewhat higher and/or better distributed and there is no tsetse fly, various forms of agro-pastoralism are likely to expand, creating a demand for working-type cattle that can also produce reasonable quantities of milk. The cattle required are likely to be some type of crossbred, either indigenous zebu and/or sanga crossed with an introduced milking zebu breed such as the Sahiwal or indigenous zebu and/or sanga crossed with a European milking breed. In the drier and more stressful regions the percentage of European milking breed genes would be nil or very low, but in less stressful regions crossbreds with a higher percentage of European milking breed genes could probably be utilized. In highland areas crossbreds with a high percentage of European milking breed genes, or purebred European milking cattle, could be used.

In regions infested with tsetse fly, particularly in West and Central Africa, there is likely to be increased use of trypanotolerant breeds such as the N'Dama and the West African Shorthorn and increased research into the nature of trypanotolerance and its inheritance. The introduction of N'Dama into other regions such as East Africa has already begun and will probably accelerate.

Thus future changes in the cattle population of Africa are likely to include a slower overall rate of increase, a decline in numbers of pastoralist owned cattle, an increase in the numbers of working and milking cattle, increases in the number of crossbred types and a wider use of trypanotolerant cattle.

Chapter 3 references, p. 71

Americas. The numbers of cattle in the temperate areas of North and South America are likely to stabilize or slowly decline as productivity per animal and per unit area of land continue to improve. However, in some of the humid tropical regions cattle numbers will probably increase, due to the increasing use of improved and acclimatized zebu and crossbred zebu cattle, the development of more suitable pasture husbandry methods in the wet tropics and the likely development of agro-sylvo-pastoral and/or sylvo-pastoral systems in forest regions.

Asia. In western Asia the use of purebred European milking breeds and the upgrading of indigenous breeds for milk production using European milking breeds are likely to continue while the present rate of increase in cattle numbers will probably decline.

In the Indian subcontinent, present trends towards crossbreeding indigenous zebu with introduced European type milking breeds will continue, with the gradual development of new, partially stabilized crossbred breeds. Improvements in productivity and limited land availability will ultimately lead to the stabilization or even a reduction in total cattle numbers. In the hill areas of northern India, Nepal, Bhutan, Bangladesh and neighbouring Southeast Asian countries the utility of the mithan for crossbreeding and the production of lean meat should be explored.

Throughout Southeast Asia there is an increasing demand for milk and crossbred milking types of cattle are slowly increasing in number. These include crossbreds between the indigenous breeds and introduced European-type milking breeds and imported zebu milking breeds such as the Sahiwal and their crossbreds with European milking breeds. There may also be an increasing use of Bali type cattle as these exhibit high reproductive rates and produce very lean meat, highly prized in Southeast Asian culinary cultures.

Australasia. In the more temperate regions cattle numbers are likely to stabilize or slowly decline, whilst in the tropical regions zebu and/or zebu crossbreds will probably replace temperate-type beef cattle.

Europe. Improvements in the productivity of dairy cattle and consumer demand for leaner meat are likely to lead to a decline in the total number of cattle and less diversity in breeds.

6.2. Buffaloes

A decline in the buffalo population of Asia is likely to continue for the present, as mechanization of agriculture accelerates, but numbers may ultimately stabilize and even begin to increase as the advantages of river buffaloes for milk production in wet tropical regions are more appreciated and exploited. In addition buffaloes are beginning to be exploited for meat production purposes and not only for work and milk production.

The dispersal of buffaloes to suitable regions in Africa and the Americas, particularly those in which there are seasonally flooded grasslands, is likely to continue and will probably accelerate. Thus although, in the immediate future, the world buffalo population may continue to slowly decline, dispersal is likely to become worldwide.

7. SUMMARY

(1) Wild and domesticated species within the subfamily Bovinae, to which both cattle and buffaloes belong, are listed and one accepted method of

classification of the wild and domesticated species is depicted.

(2) There are three distinct species of domesticated cattle. The most numerous and important are the large number of different breed of *Bos taurus* and *B. indicus* cattle, accepted to be variants of the same species. The other two are the Bali (*Bibos banteng*) and the mithan (*Bibos frontalis*)

(3) There are no surviving ancestors of *B. taurus* and *B. indicus*. It is believed that they are descended from wild cattle, designated zoologically as *Bos primigenius,* that once ranged throughout Eurasia and the North African littoral. Bali cattle are a domesticated form of the wild banteng (*Bibos banteng*), whilst it is now considered that the mithan is a domesticated gaur (*Bibos gaurus*).

(4) All domesticated buffalo breeds have originated from wild Asian species. It is generally accepted that river buffalo have originated solely from the arnee (*Bubalus arnee*), but swamp buffaloes in Southeast Asia may also possess genes derived from other wild buffalo species.

(5) The probable centres of domestication are discussed. The first domesticated cattle were of the longhorn humpless (*B. taurus*) type and domestication probably first occurred in western Asia some 8000–9000 years ago. It is considered that shorthorn humpless (*B. taurus*) cattle and neck- and chest-humped zebu (*B. indicus*) cattle were derived, possibly partly by selection by man, from longhorn humpless cattle in different regions of western Asia, some 2000–3000 years after longhorns were first domesticated. There is strong support from blood haemoglobin studies that the centre of domestication of Bali cattle was somewhere in the vicinity of the island of Bali, and it is probable that the Mithan was domesticated in the region in which it is found today.

(6) Available evidence suggests that the valley of the Indus, in the Indian subcontinent was the centre of domestication of river buffalo, but there is some possibility that swamp buffalo were domesticated at more than one centre in Southeast Asia and/or China.

(7) The dispersal of the different types of cattle from centres of domestication and the effect that dispersals have had on the composition of existing breeds is discussed at length. Until the end of the 16th century dispersal was confined to the Eurasian land mass and Africa, but with the advent of the era of European discovery cattle were further dispersed to the Americas, Australasia and the oceanic islands.

(8) Dispersal of buffaloes has been much more limited than that of cattle and what is known as to the dispersal is discussed in detail.

(9) Details are provided of the present distribution of cattle and buffaloes in regions within continents and finally some possible future changes in cattle and buffalo distribution are briefly discussed.

8. REFERENCES

Alberro, M. and Halle-Mariam, S., 1982. The indigenous cattle of Ethiopia. Part I. World Anim. Rev., 42: 27–34.

Boehmer, R.M. von, 1974. The appearance of the water buffalo in Mesopotamian history and its Sumerian characteristics. (In German.) Z. Assyriol. 64: 1–19.

Bowling, G.A., 1942. The introduction of cattle into Colonial North America. J. Dairy Sci., 25: 129.

Butzer, K.W., 1961. A history of land use in arid regions, Dudley Stamp (Editor), Publication No. 17, UNESCO, Paris, p. 31.

Curson, H.H. and Thornton, R.W., 1936. A contribution to the study of African native cattle. Onderstepoort J. Vet. Sci. Anim. Husbandry, 7: 613.

Dechambre, E., 1951. Origines des animaux domestiques de Madagascar. Terre Vie, 98: 187–196.

Devendra, C.T., Choo, L.K. and Pathmasingam, M., 1973. The productivity of Bali cattle in Malaysia. Malaysian Agric. J., 49(2): 182.

Epstein, H., 1957. The sanga cattle of East Africa. E. Afr. Agric. J., 22(3): 149.

Epstein, H., 1969. Domestic Animals of China. Commonwealth Agricultural Bureaux, Farnham Royal, U.K.
Epstein, H., 1971. The Origin of Domestic Animals in Africa. Africana, New York.
Epstein, H. and Mason, I.L., 1984. Cattle. In: I.L. Mason (Editor) Evolution of domesticated animals. Longman, London.
FAO, 1984. Production yearbook, 37. Food and Agriculture Organization, Rome.
Faulkner, D.E. and Epstein, H., 1957 The indigenous cattle of the British dependent territories in Africa, with material on certain other countries. Pub. Col. Adv. Comm. Agric. Anim. Hlth., For., No. 5, HMSO, London.
Fischer, H., 1969. Die chromosomensätze des Bali-rindes (*Bibos banteng*) und des Gayal (*Bibos frontalis*). Z. Tierz. ZüchtBiol., 86: 52–57.
Gee, E.R., 1964. The wild life of India. Collins, London.
Gray, A.P., 1972. Mammalian Hybrids. A check-list with bibliography. Commonwealth Agricultural Bureaux, Farnham Royal, U.K.
Higham, C.F.W. and Leach, B.F., 1971. An early centre of bovine husbandry in Southeast Asia. Science, 172: 54–56.
Johnson, C.W., 1951. The origin and domestication of *Bos indicus*. The Cattleman, 38(2): 17–53.
Kirby, G.W.M., 1979. Bali cattle in Australia. World Anim. Rev., 31: 24–29.
Kolesnik, N.N., 1936. Origin and geographic distribution of cattle. Izv. Akad. Nauk, S.S.S.R., 375. Abstract: Anim. Breeding Abstr., 34: 90 (1966).
Marshall, J. 1931. Mohenjo-daro and the Indus civilisation. 3 vols. Arthur Probsthain, London.
Namikawa, T. 1981. Geographic distribution of bovine haemoglobin-beta (Hbb) alleles and the phylogenetic analysis of the cattle in Eastern Asia. Z. Tierz. ZüchtBiol., 98: 151–159
Namikawa, T. and Widodo, W., 1978. Electrophoretic variations of haemoglobin and serum albumin in the Indonesian cattle including Bali cattle (*Bos banteng*). Jap. J. Zootech. Sci., 49: 817–827.
Payne, W.J.A., 1964. The origin of domestic cattle in Africa. Empire J. Exp. Agric., 32(126): 97–113.
Payne, W.J.A., 1970. Cattle Production in the Tropics, Vol. 1, Breeds and breeding. Longman, London.
Payne, W.J.A. and Rollinson, D.H.L., 1973. Bali cattle. World Anim. Rev., (7): 13–21.
Payne, W.J.A. and Rollinson, D.H.L., 1976. Madura cattle. Z. Tierz. ZüchtBiol., 93: 89–100.
Raffles, T.S., 1816. The History of Java, 2 vols. Reprinted 1965, Historical Reprints OUP, Kuala Lumpur.
Reed, C.A. (Editor), 1977. Origins of Agriculture. Monton Publishers, The Hague and Paris.
Rollinson, D.H.L., 1984. Bali cattle. In: I.L. Mason (Editor), Evolution of domesticated animals. Longman, London.
Ross Cockrill, W., 1984. Water buffalo. In: I.L. Mason (Editor), Evolution of domesticated animals. Longman, London.
Simoons, F.J., 1984. Gayal or mithan. In: I.L. Mason (Editor), Evolution of domesticated animals. Longman, London.
Simoons, F.J. and Simoons, E.S., 1968. A Ceremonial Ox of India. University of Wisconsin Press, Madison, Milwaukee.
Slijper, E.J., 1951. On the hump of the zebu and zebu crosses. Hemara Zoa., 58:(1–2): 112.
Turnbull, P.F. and Reed, C.A., 1974. The fauna from the terminal Pleistocene of Palegawra cave, a Zarzian occupation site in northeastern Iraq. Fieldiana Anthropol. 63(3): 81–146.
Wharton, C.H., 1969. Man, fire and wild cattle in Southeast Asia. In: Proc. 8th Annual Tall Timbers Fire Ecology Conference 14–15 March 1968, Tallahassee, Florida, pp. 107–167.

Chapter 4

Cattle Genetic Resources of West Africa

PHILIPPE LHOSTE

1. INTRODUCTION

The cattle of West Africa are characterized by a large genetic and phenotypic diversity ranging from the zebu (*Bos indicus*) to the humpless or taurine (*Bos taurus*) with numerous intermediary types. If a classic distinction (Epstein, 1983) is made—a distinction between the areas where zebus are bred in a hot environment and humpless cattle in a temperate climate — this must be modified in the case of West Africa where zebu cattle are to be found in the driest areas, such as the Sahel, and the humpless in more humid, tsetse-infested areas. In the intermediary areas different crossbreed populations (zebu × humpless) have developed, and the incidents of crossbreeding are still very pronounced in certain areas according to ecological or socio-economic factors or to factors related to production methods.

The equally standard distinction (Doutressoulle, 1947; Leclercq, 1976) between the Sahelo-Sudanian area north of the 14th parallel N, devoted to the breeding of the zebu, and the Sudano-Guinean area south of the 14th parallel, devoted to the breeding of humpless cattle, is equally unsatisfactory because, as shown later, the reality is more complex and fluid. Recent phenomena, such as the drought of 1972–83 in West Africa, or the development of cultivated areas in certain regions have brought about herd movements and important modifications in the distribution of different genetic types.

Nevertheless, the distribution of cattle in Africa still shows a genetic stratification strikingly linked to ecological features:

(1) In the dry region, zebu cattle of a fairly large size, adapted to the heat, to long distances, and to sustaining themselves on poor fodder predominate. The zebu are restricted towards the south, in particular by trypanosomiasis, but equally by diseases related to the damp environment such as blood and gastrointestinal parasitism, skin diseases, diseases transmitted by ticks, etc.

(2) In the humid region, cattle are mainly of the humpless type, smaller in size, adapted to this particular range of diseases, and especially trypanotolerant. Certain populations have been able to survive in this environment, regarded as unfavourable to breeding, for centuries without any veterinary care at all. In total these humpless cattle are numerically far inferior to the zebu and their breeding area is not strictly continuous. Both in the forest region areas and in the humid savanna areas, one finds regions either devoid of cattle or very sparsely populated, for a variety of reasons: sanitary, historical, ecological, etc. Frequently these are also regions where the human population is sparse, or very unevenly spread.

(3) In the regions between those of the humpless and those of the zebu cattle, corresponding approximately to the Sudanian ecological zone, types, populations or breeds issuing from the crossbreeding of the zebu and the

Chapter 4 references, p. 88

humpless cattle are found. The process that occurs in the majority of cases is that the humpless breed is absorbed by the zebu: the zebu being the bigger animal. The new populations thus obtained reveal qualities favourable to breeding and to the needs of agriculture: build, an aptitude to work, acceptable meat value, etc. However, this trend, uncontrolled, would threaten the existence of certain humpless breeds whose genetic characteristics particularly favour adaptability to the environment.

2. CATTLE NUMBERS

The area of study covered by this chapter is intentionally limited to the 15 countries normally considered to constitute West Africa; i.e., those countries situated south of the Sahara and east of Cameroon and Chad, which form part of Central Africa. The 15 countries under consideration are, in alphabetical order (see Fig. 4.1): Benin, Gambia, Ghana, Guinea, Guinea Bissau, Ivory Coast, Liberia, Mali, Mauritania, Niger, Nigeria, Senegal, Sierra Leone, Togo and Upper Volta.

Table 4.1 shows the cattle populations (according to the FAO yearbook) for the years 1970 and 1981; the size of each country and their human populations are also listed.

Taking the area of West Africa as a whole, the first facts to note are that the bovine livestock numbers around 32 600 000 head of cattle: that is 19% of the total African cattle population or 2.7% on a worldwide basis. For the human population, these proportions become 30% of the African population, and 2.3% of the world population, whereas the surface area represents 20% of Africa and 4.6% of the world.

So it can be stated that in West Africa the average density of both the human and the cattle populations is lower than the world average, which is rather surprising as the majority of the countries in this area are regarded as cattle-breeding countries. In fact the cattle density (seen as the number of head per square kilometre) appears to vary greatly from one country to another, as

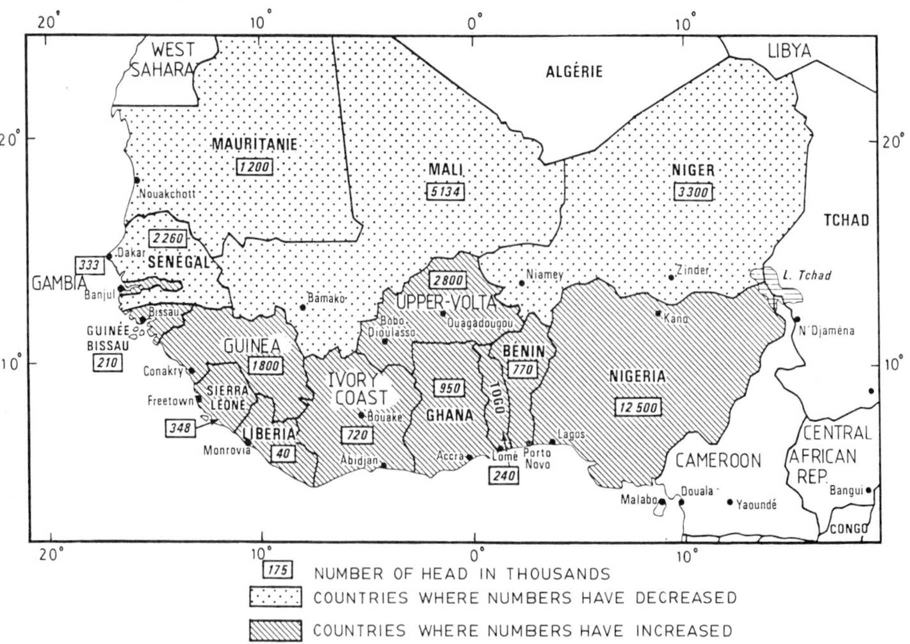

Fig. 4.1. Cattle numbers in West Africa (according to FAO Yearbook, 1981).

TABLE 4.1

Cattle population per country 1970–81.

Country		Area ('000 km^2)	Inhabitants ('000)	Cattle ('000 head)
Benin	1970	112.6	2 646	549
	1981	–	3 640	770
Ivory coast	1970	322.5	5 341	408
	1981	–	8 298	720
Gambia	1970	11.3	449	247
	1981	–	619	333
Ghana	1970	238.5	8 614	902
	1981	–	12 063	950
Guinea	1970	245.8	3 921	1 300
	1981	–	5 147	1 800
Guinea Bissau	1970	36.1	487	190
	1981	–	583	210
Upper Volta	1970	274.2	5 413	2 550
	1981	–	7 094	2 800
Liberia	1970	111.4	1 393	28
	1981	–	2 038	40
Mali	1970	1 240	5 362	5 400
	1981	–	7 136	5 134
Mauritania	1970	1 030.7	1 245	2 003
	1981	–	1 681	1 200
Niger	1970	1 267	4 008	4 077
	1981	–	5 479	3 300
Nigeria	1970	923.8	56 346	11 183
	1981	–	79 680	12 500
Senegal	1970	196.2	4 267	2 557
	1981	–	5 811	2 260
Sierra Leone	1970	71.7	2 692	296
	1981	–	3 571	348
Togo	1970	56.8	2 020	187
	1981	–	2 705	240
Totals				
West	1970	6 138.6	104 204	31 877
Africa	1981	–	145 545	32 605
Africa	1970	30 331	354 825	150 232
	1981	–	484 355	170 930
World	1970	133 920	3 696 640	1 088 613
	1981	–	4 513 440	1 209 833

Source: FAO.

shown in Table 4.2. With an average for the whole area of 5.3 head of cattle per km^2, one can note the following extremes: 29.5 head per km^2 in the Gambia, 0.3 head per km^2 in Liberia and 1 head per km^2 in Mauritania. Thus three groups of countries present themselves for consideration:

(1) Countries with a relatively high density (higher than the average for the whole area): these are mainly either the Sudano-Guinean countries (the Gambia, Guinea Bissau, Nigeria) or the Sahelo-Sudanian ones (Senegal, Upper Volta).

(2) Countries with a low density: Ghana, Mali, Togo and Sierra Leone.

(3) Countries with a very low density: Ivory Coast, Liberia, Mauritania and Niger.

It is evident that among the countries with a lower density of cattle farming two contrasting situations clearly exist:

(1) The Sahelian countries, such as Mauritania and Niger, that include regions of subdesert. Within these countries a big difference is found between

Chapter 4 references, p. 88

TABLE 4.2

Cattle densities

Country	Head of cattle per inhabitant		Head of cattle per km^2
	1970	1981	1981
Benin	0.21	0.21	6.8
Ivory Coast	0.08	0.09	2
Gambia	0.55	0.54	29.50
Ghana	0.10	0.08	4
Guinea	0.33	0.35	7.30
Guinea Bissau	0.39	0.36	5.8
Upper Volta	0.47	0.39	10.2
Liberia	0.02	0.02	0.3
Mali	1.01	0.72	4.1
Mauritania	1.61	0.71	1
Niger	1.02	0.60	2.6
Nigeria	0.2	0.16	13.5
Senegal	0.6	0.39	11.5
Sierra Leone	0.11	0.1	4.8
Togo	0.09	0.09	4.23
Averages			
West Africa	0.31	0.22	5.3
Africa	0.42	0.35	5.6

the south where both livestock and crop cultivation are concentrated and the extremely dry north where herds do exist but only in precarious conditions.

(2) The Guinean countries with their equatorial climate, like Liberia, where cattle farming is not common because of the forest that dominates the environment.

2.1. Recent evolution of cattle population (see Table 4.3)

The years of reference (1970 and 1981) considered in table 4.1 were chosen to encompass the decade of drought endured by West Africa in the 1970's. These observations show the character of the recent numerical evolution of cattle populations. In 11 of the countries the numbers increased (by an average of 16% over the 11 years); in 4 countries the numbers diminished (by an average of 15%). Figure 4.1, while showing the number of cattle in each coun-

TABLE 4.3

Cattle number variations 1970–81

Countries where numbers have increased		Countries where numbers have decreased	
Benin	+ 40%	Mali	− 5%
Ivory Coast	+ 76%	Mauritania	− 40%
Gambia	+ 35%	Niger	− 19%
Ghana	+ 5%	Senegal	− 12%
Guinea	+ 38%		
Guinea Bissau	+ 11%	Mean	− 15%
Upper Volta	+ 10%		
Liberia	+ 43%		
Nigeria	+ 12%		
Sierra Leone	+ 18%		
Togo	+ 28%		
Average	+ 16%		

try in 1981, also illustrates this trend; increase or decrease between 1970 and 1981.

It thus appears that the four Sahelian countries: Mali, Mauritania, Niger and Senegal, saw their cattle populations decrease, while an increase in bovine livestock was being realized in the countries to the south of the area, which were less affected by drought. Certain countries show high increases (for example, Ivory Coast up 76% in 11 years) which were only made possible by the influx of very high numbers of cattle brought in from the neighbouring Sahelian countries (from Mali and Upper Volta in the case of Ivory Coast).

The ratio of cattle numbers to human population presented in Table 4.2 is a relevant pointer: it can be seen that in the case of the Sahelian countries it falls sharply, by 30–40% in general, during the period under consideration; and even by 50% in the case of Mauritania. In the majority of countries throughout the Guinean area, a general equilibrium can be noted between the increase of the human and the cattle populations.

These figures illustrate an extreme variability in the cattle densities of West African countries. While this variability is indeed marked in relation to each country, it is yet more pronounced at a regional level in certain contrasting countries (Niger, Mali, Guinea, etc.).

Equally evident is a very clear tendency for the cattle herds to make their way south, in particular because of the drought in the 1970's. This evolution is an important factor in the economic equilibrium of these regions, in the sustaining of certain pastoral societies and in the genetic evolution of the cattle herds concerned.

3. PRINCIPAL CATTLE GENETIC TYPES

In the presentation of genetic types of West African cattle the now standard basis for classification of the African bovine breeds, clarified in a recent study (CIPEA/ILCA, 1979) and conforming to Mason's previous propositions (1951), has been used. Thus two cattle groups are distinguishable, according to the absence or the presence of the hump: the taurine (humpless), *Bos taurus* and the zebu (humped cattle), *Bos indicus*.

The crossbreeds of these two principal groups are numerous and definitely fertile, which would justify *B. indicus* and *B. taurus* being considered as two subspecies, and not two different species.

Mason (1951) suggests four principal groups: I — the kouri of lake Chad, II — the humpless, III — the crossbreeds, and IV — the zebus. Although indeed of a type different to the other humpless cattle of the region, the kouri is here classed with them and no study will be made of this particular type (large animals with giant horns) which lives in the region of Lake Chad, on the border of our area of study. (See Epstein, 1983, for further information on the kouri.)

Let us rapidly take stock of the actual state and evolution of the different genetic types, without going into a detailed description of the various African cattle breeds, which other works, to which reference can be made, have dealt with in more detail.

Figure 4.2 shows the localization of the different breeds and Figs 4.3–4.8 illustrate the principal genetic types.

3.1. Humpless cattle

The humpless cattle constitute the trypanotolerant cattle group: a group which can be divided into two principal types: (1) the humpless longhorns which make up a relatively homogeneous group considered as one breed — the

Chapter 4 references, p. 88

N'Dama; and (2) the shorthorns, distinguishable into two subgroups and several different breeds, or populations, often with names which differ from one country to another.

In a joint study of trypanotolerant livestock undertaken by the Food and Agriculture Organization of the United Nations (OAA/FAO), the International Livestock Center for Africa (CIPEA/ILCA) and the United Nations Environment Programme (PNUE/UNEP) the actual state of this livestock in 1978 was detailed (ILCA, 1979 and FAO, 1980).

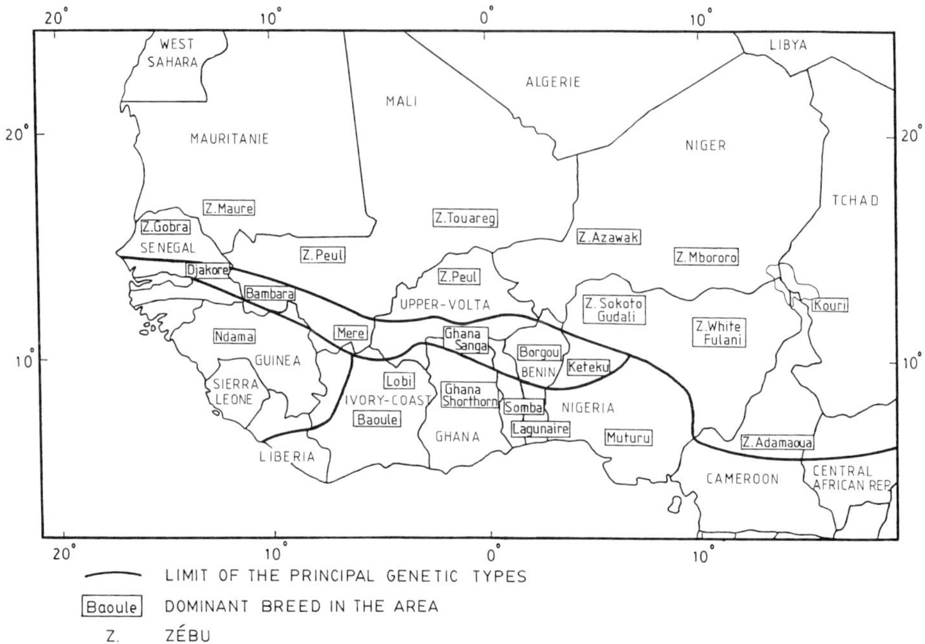

Fig. 4.2. The location of the principal West African cattle breeds.

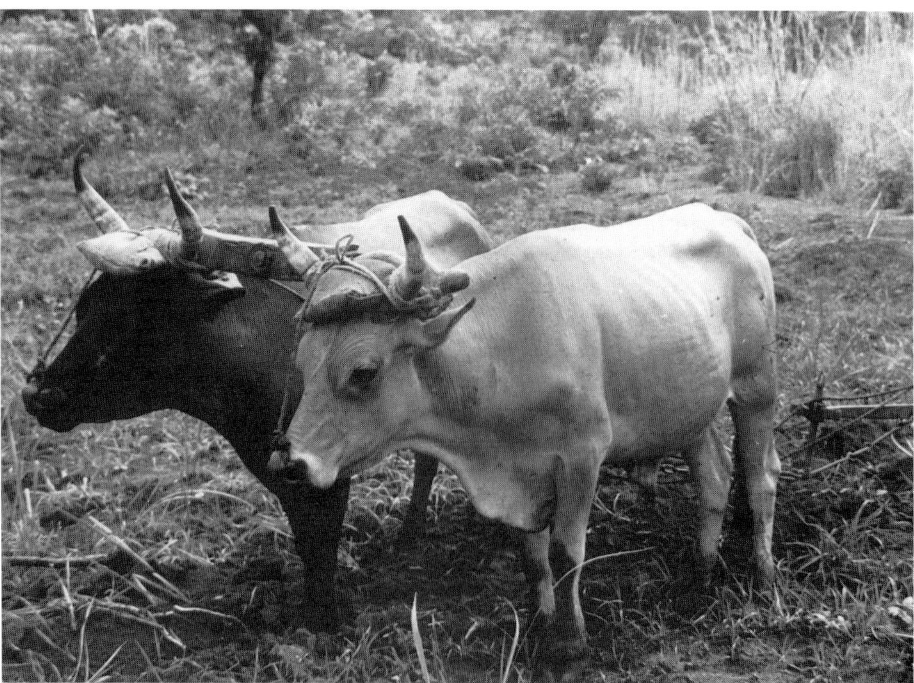

Fig. 4.3. Humpless N'Dama oxen used for draught in Upper Guinea.

3.1.1. The N'Dama breed. West African humpless longhorned cattle (Fig. 4.3)

The N'Dama type of humpless cattle form the largest group of trypanotolerant cattle with nearly 4 million head in West Africa (1983). The natural extent of this breed's region is found in the countries neighbouring Guinea, where it has spread out from its centre in the Guinean massif of Fouta Djallon. In addition the breed has diffused widely from its place of origin. The area of natural extension comprises eight countries (see Fig. 4.2): four countries where the N'Dama is very widely dominant: Guinea, Guinea Bissau, the Gambia and Sierra Leone; two countries where the N'Dama is in contact with the dominant zebu: Mali and Senegal (in these countries one naturally finds N'Dama × zebu crossbreeds); and two Guinean countries where the N'Dama is in contact with the humpless shorthorns; Liberia and Ivory Coast. As Ivory Coast took in a lot of zebu during the 1970's, the N'Dama and the humpless shorthorns traditionally found in this country are now in contact with the zebu in the north.

The N'Dama breed has been introduced into numerous other West African and Central African countries and is found in various natural environments. Towards the equatorial region, it has adapted to the Guinean forest in Sierra Leone, Upper Guinea, Liberia and Ivory Coast. Towards the Sudanian area it is naturally found up to the 1000 mm isohyet (approximately) in the Gambia, eastern Senegal and southern Mali. All of this demonstrates interesting qualities of adaptability which have been exploited with diverse introductions into several regions. The N'Dama breed, traditionally managed by the 'Fula' people* is a mixed race, bred for its meat and its milk. In traditional farming the cows are systematically milked. The breed has been used since the 1920's for farm cultivation in Upper Guinea and has proved valuable as a draught animal in spite of its relatively small size (see Fig. 4.3). It is equally well-adapted to different systems of farming, such as the ranching system (in Zaïre, Congo, Nigeria, Ivory Coast), the 'métayage' system (Central African Republic, Congo, etc.), and farming in the palm plantations (Ivory Coast, Benin, Liberia, etc,).

3.1.2. The humpless West African Shorthorn (Figs 4.4 and 4.5)

The situation of the humpless shorthorns presents a more complex picture than that of the N'Dama. Their original breeding areas comprise the coastal countries from Liberia to Cameroon, with in addition some areas in the south of Mali and Upper Volta. This means that there is practically no overlap between the natural breeding areas of the N'Dama and the humpless shorthorns, as Fig. 4.2 illustrates. The division line passes through Liberia, Ivory Coast and Mali; to the northwest of this line the N'Dama are to be found, to the east the humpless shorthorns. The fairly recent diffusion of N'Dama into practically every country in this area and the use of N'Dama bulls to improve other herds has meant the recent introduction of a certain amount of crossbreeding between the two subgroups.

Humpless shorthorn cattle can be divided into two types: the dwarf type and the larger savanna type. The following is the classification of humpless shorthorns (with principal locations):

(1) Dwarf West African Shorthorn (Fig. 4.4)
lagune (Ivory Coast)
or lagunaire (Togo, Benin)
or lagoon cattle (Ghana)
or 'Dahomey' (Zaïre)

---

* 'Fula': name given to the Fulani or Peul people in the Fouta Djallon in Guinea.

Chapter 4 references, p. 88

(2) Forest Muturu (Liberia) or Nigerian Dwarf Shorthorn

(3) Savanna West African Shorthorn (Fig. 4.5)
Baoulé or Lobi (Ivory Coast)
Ghana shorthorn (Ghana)
Somba (Togo, Benin)

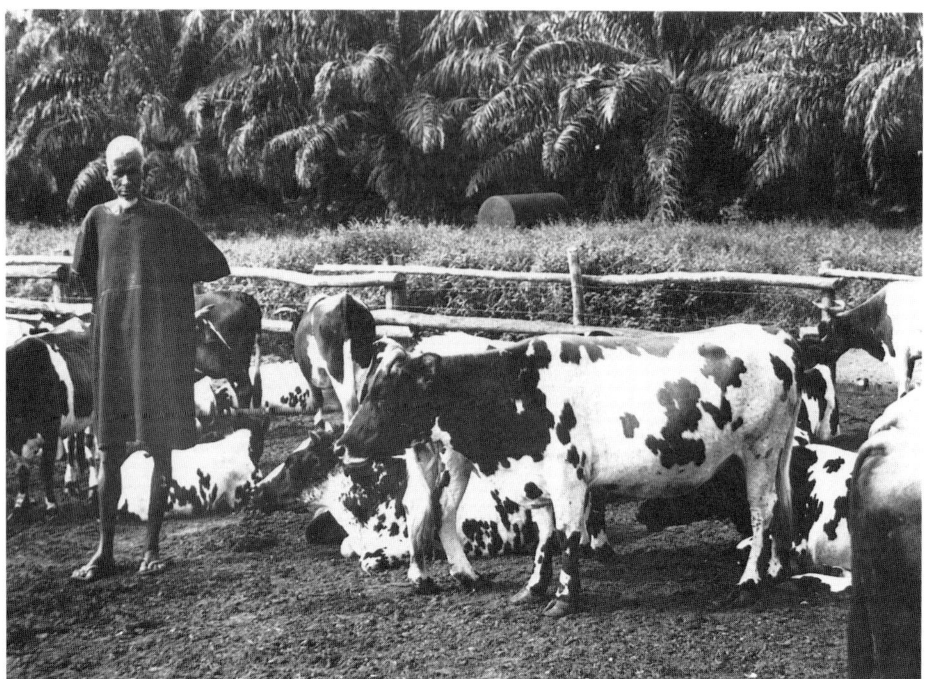

Fig. 4.4. Herd of a humpless dwarf shorthorn race, Ivory Coast.

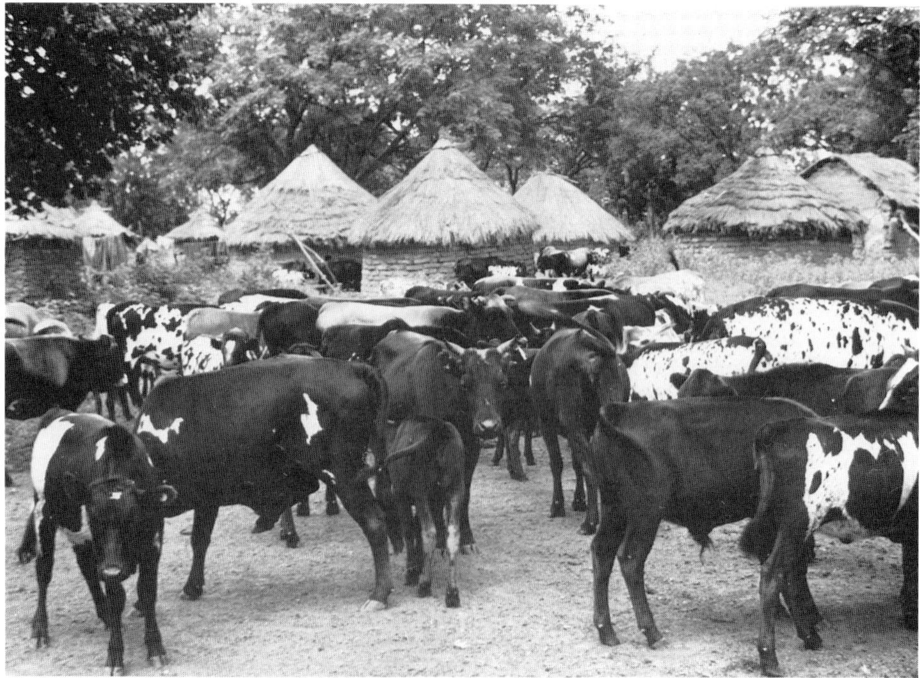

Fig. 4.5. Village herd of humpless shorthorns: Baoulé race, Ivory Coast.

Savana Muturu (Nigeria)
Daoyo, Namshi, Bakosi, Kirdi, Kapsiki (Cameroon)

These two populations total about 1 700 000 head and the numbers for the principal breeding countries, in order of importance (CIPEA/ILCA, 1979), are shown in Table 4.4.
These numbers are rough estimates because in the majority of these countries no count has been made which distinguishes between the genetic types (humpless, crossbreed or zebu).

The humpless Dwarf cattle situated in the coastal area have been little studied and seem to be more and more in danger of extinction. They are very small animals (90 cm at withers), and show a remarkable adaptability to the damp environment. The general tendency seems to be to crossbreed them with the larger breeds.

The savanna shorthorns are more numerous but equally under threat of absorption, because the process of crossbreeding with the zebu has been accelerating throughout the 1970's with the increased need for draught animals for farm cultivation, and with the descent of the zebus from the Sahel as a result of the drought. At the beginning of the 1980's the principal, relatively pure, centre of the breed seemed still to exist in an area towards the north of Ghana, the northeast of Ivory Coast, and the south of Upper Volta. The size of these animals is small (90–100 cm at withers). The farming methods are varied and the adaptability of these breeds is a positive factor although they have been less exported and transferred than the N'Damas. Mention can, however, be made of some successful introductions in Central Africa: Baoulé in the Central African Republic, the lagune breed (named 'Dahomey' in Zaïre) in Zaïre, Congo and Gabon.

3.2. The zebu × humpless crossbreeds (Figs 4.6 and 4.7)

Between the dry area, devoted to the breeding of zebus, and the humid area where the humpless cattle are to be found, in a belt of varying width, an area is developing of zebu × humpless crossbreeding. This phenomenon seems to have been increasing since 1972 on account of the exceptional migrations of zebu cattle, which, because of the years of drought, have been seeking new pastures. The form the crossbreeding takes most commonly is, in fact, zebu bull × humpless cow (or a cow already crossbred), as breeders seek matings that increase the size of the animal, either to provide animal traction or for meat.

The number of these West African crossbreeds was estimated at around 2 500 000 in 1978 (CIPEA/ILCA, 1979); they occupy a continuous band from Senegal to Nigeria, a band that goes through southern Mali, Upper Volta, northern Ivory Coast, Ghana, Togo and Benin. This band borders the 900 mm

TABLE 4.4

Numbers of shorthorn and dwarf cattle in principal West African breeding countries

Shorthorns		Dwarfs	
Ghana	616 000	Nigeria (Muturu)	38 000
Upper Volta	484 000	Benin (Lagunaire)	20 000
Ivory Coast	250 000	Liberia (Muturu)	15 000
Togo	144 000		
Nigeria	82 000		
Benin	75 000		

Chapter 4 references, p. 88

isohyet and corresponds to the Sudanian ecological area — an area of considerable cultivation.

Two distinct groups of zebu × humpless crossbreeds can be defined according to whether the humpless breed is represented by a N'Dama, or by a humpless shorthorn.

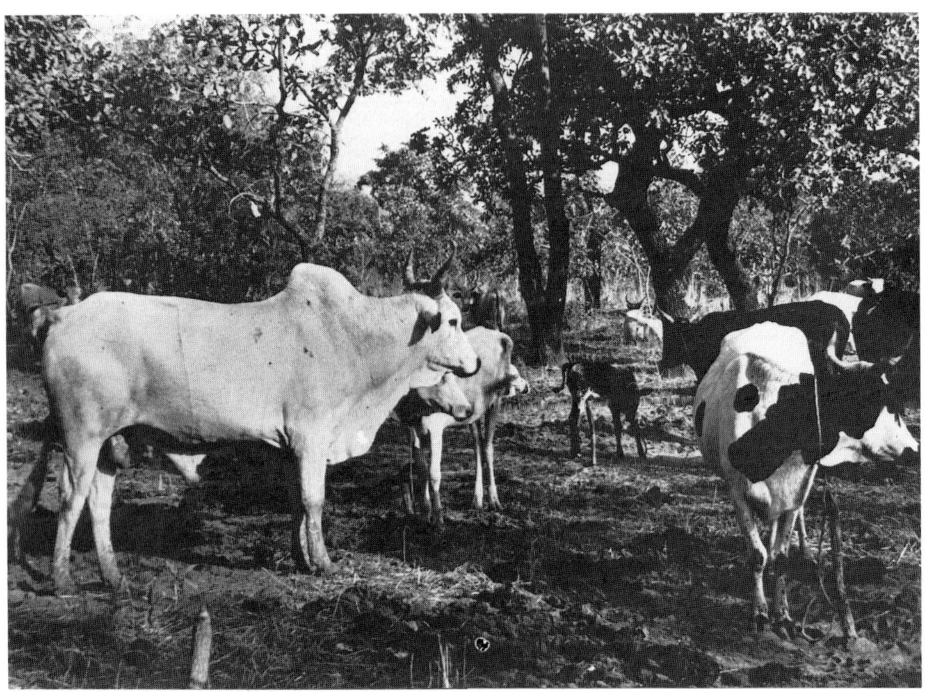

Fig. 4.6. Zebu (White Fulani race) × humpless (Somba race) for crossbreeding in Benin.

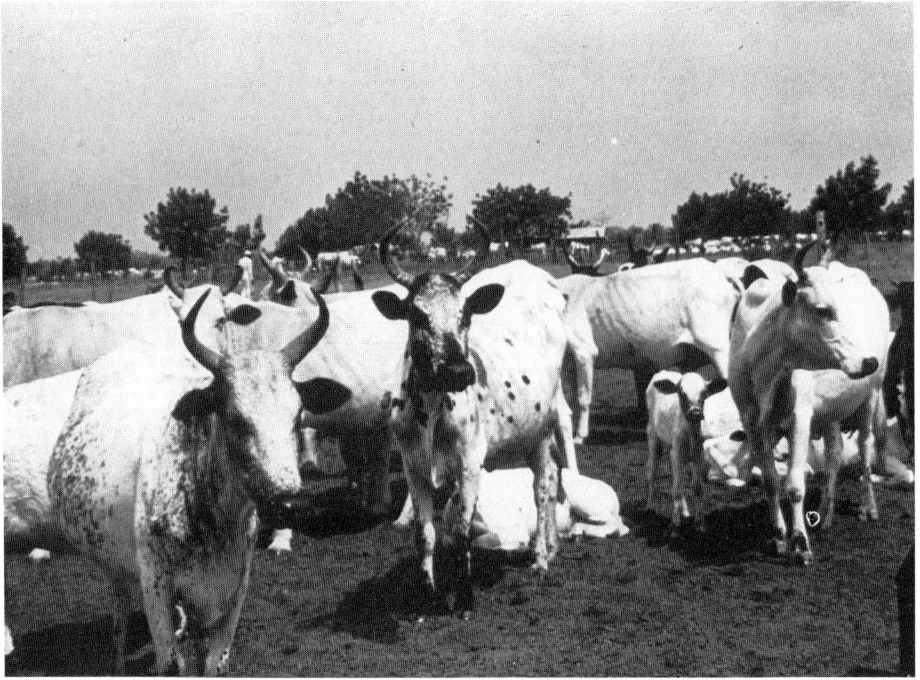

Fig. 4.7. Crossbred 'Ghana Sanga' herd in Ghana (Accra Plain).

3.2.1. The zebu × N'Dama crossbreed

This crossbreed is essentially found in the west of the study area: The Djakoré in Senegal (Gobra zebu × N'Dama cross) and the Bambara in Mali. These animals are very valuable for draught power and it is in this crossbreeding area that the most significant and the most evolving association between crop cultivation and animal farming is to be found.

3.2.2. The zebu × humpless shorthorn crossbreed

These constitute a group of cattle herds that are named: Mere in Burkina Faso and Ivory Coast, Sanga (or Ghana Sanga) in Ghana (Fig. 4.7), Borgou in Benin and Keteku in Nigeria. Those populations which are relatively stable (Borgou, Sanga) are considered simply as humpless cattle by certain authors.

While awaiting confirmation from genetic analysis or from other methods, it seems very probable, in particular in the case of the Borgou, that they result from former crossbreeding between the Somba breed of humpless shorthorn and the zebus to be found in the north of Benin. The genesis of the Keteku and of the Ghana Sanga would appear to be the same. Phenotypically, the Borgou, the Keteku and the Ghana Sanga are closely related. The dominant colour is white, spotted with black to a greater or smaller degree. These animals are more and more frequently to be found in the south of the coastal countries if the environment is suitable; this is the case in Ghana (on the Accra plain), in Togo and in Benin. These new cattle populations that are expanding in the coastal regions are tending to either absorb or eliminate the humpless Dwarf (the lagune breed) from their traditional breeding areas.

3.3. The zebu

Numerically the zebus constitute the majority of the African livestock. Their arrival in several waves on this continent came in all likelihood later than that of the humpless cattle which they displaced or replaced in certain cases.

The classification of West African zebus remains a matter of debate. Mason (1951) proposes four principal groups based on the length of the horns:

(1) short-horned zebu, e.g., Maure, Touareg, Azawak zebus
(2) medium-horned zebu, e.g., Zebus of Adamawa
(3) lyre-horned zebu, e.g., Peul zebu of Senegal, Sudan, etc, and
(4) long lyre-horned zebu, e.g., Red Mbororo zebu.

Leclercq (1976) divides the West African zebus into two principal subgroups: (1) the Sahelian short-horned zebu and (2) the Peul zebu. In the latter subgroup the zebus have varying horns and are of different sizes. In fact the genetic types in the African zebu population are often quite badly stabilized and there is a large variability within each race; in addition, as these animals are very mobile, there is a sizeable genetic flux and numerous intermediary types can be found, especially among the Fulani. In contrast certain breeds, such as the Red Mbororo zebu, display considerable homogeneity, but this is somewhat exceptional.

3.3.1. Classification and brief description

Reviewing rapidly the West African zebu breeds, let us not dwell on the now standard descriptions of their appearances (Joshi, 1957; Leclercq, 1976 and others); taking into account the diversity of the genetic types and the availability of more detailed material, only one photograph of a zebu (Fig. 4.8) is included here.

The zebu considered typically Sahelian are represented by the short-horned breeds: the Maure zebu in Mauritania, the Touareg zebu in Mali, the Azawak zebu in Niger, and the Arabe (or Choa) zebu in Chad. Naturally these cattle

Chapter 4 references, p. 88

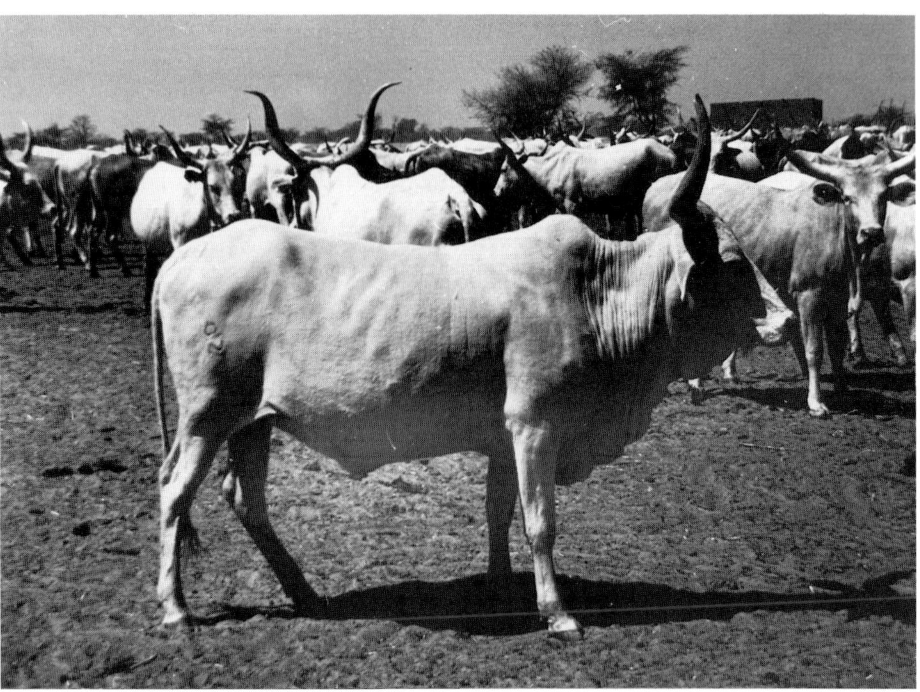

Fig. 4.8. Gobra zebu in Senegal (Ferlo).

populations have spread out from their regions of origin into neighbouring countries: the Maure zebus into Mali, the Touareg zebus into Niger and Upper Volta, etc. Therefore the actual dividing lines between these groups are not easy to specify.

Fulani zebus are basically to be found in the northern Sudanian and southern Sahelian regions, but they are moving more and more frequently into the Sudano-Guinean area. The breed is made up of varied ethnic groups.

The Gobra zebu of Senegal is a quite homogeneous type (Fig. 4.8) with high lyre-shaped horns, which lives in northern Senegal and constitutes the majority of this country's livestock. It is a good meat-producing animal.

Fulani zebus of Mali, and Nigeria form an important group of cattle herds of irregular appearance. They are medium-sized animals with moderate thin horns. The herds consist of animals which are multi-form rather than of several breeds.

The Gudali zebus of Sokoto in northwest Nigeria could be included in the preceding herds, but they do form a more identifiable group — short-horned, heavier and more powerful.

The White Fulani zebus of Nigeria are a type of Peul zebu, resembling in appearance the Gobra zebu, but the breeding areas of these two breeds are completely separate.

The Mbororo zebu is a particular breed (large animals with big horns and mahogany-coloured coats), originating from Niger. The population has partly moved into Nigeria, into Cameroon, and into the Central African Republic, in which countries they can now be found in large numbers. Thus therefore they exist in areas south of the 10th parallel N, and this justifies rectification of any simple notions (using as a dividing line the 14th parallel N, for example, or the too precise Sahelian area).

These herds, looked after by Mbororo breeders (a people related to the Fulani), demonstrate a remarkable adaptation to an environment which is quite different from that of their native region; they live in the Sudano-Guinean area, almost in contact with the tsetse fly, the breeders accepting certain losses due to pathological problems (parasitism, trypanosomiasis, etc.) in order to profit from a greater abundance of food in areas where the climate is more favourable to animal food production, and where there are fewer animals.

The most striking element concerning the distribution of West African cattle populations would seem to be the recent increase in genetic flux and in particular to enormous penetration made by the zebu into the most humid area in the south of West Africa.

4. GENETIC IMPROVEMENT IN TRADITIONAL CATTLE BREEDING

A certain number of programmes to improve local breeds have been developed for West African cattle. The FAO study (Joshi, 1957) on 'African cattle, types and breeds' mentions certain aid facilities — livestock services, animal breeding stations, etc. — which worked together, to a greater or lesser extent, for the improvement and management of cattle genetic resources. As a general rule, action taken in the sphere of traditional cattle farming has more often than not remained restricted to the following areas:

(1) systematic veterinary prophylaxis: programmes of vaccination against the principal epizootic diseases such as rinderpest, pleuropneumonia, anthrax;

(2) veterinary care in cases of illness, or when requested by the breeders;

(3) monitoring of population numbers (more or less reliable), and of animal movements permitting, to a certain extent, records to be kept of, if not regulation of, the concentration of cattle over more or less sizeable areas; and

(4) occasional food supplements (minerals, proteins, etc.).

In the area of genetic management the little effort that has been made has been essentially left in the hands of the breeders; the sort of endeavours undertaken in this area being:

(1) mass selection in the herds , by means of the castration of males that are judged substandard;

(2) the diffusion of 'selected' sires coming from the livestock improvement centres of the stations or the ranches; or

(3) more rarely, efforts to organize the breeders. The breeds which have mainly been the object of the genetic amelioration programmes are: the N'Dama breed and the Baoulé breed among the trypanotolerant cattle, and the Gobra zebu in Senegal, the Azawak zebu in Niger and the zebu of Adamawa among the zebu cattle.

These genetic amelioration programmes were usually conceived in the past with a view to selective farming based on improvement centres (stations, breeding centres, etc.) and to diffusion of improved male sires into the surrounding farming areas. This general idea was put into practice for example in Ferlo (Senegal) with the Gobra zebu, In Sierra Leone and in Ivory Coast with the humpless N'Dama, etc. The N'Dama breed has been the object of numerous selection or multiplication programmes in Guinea, in Senegal (the Kolda station in Casamance), in Ivory Coast (The Animal Production Research Center of Minankro-Bouake), in Mali (the Yanfolila ranch), and in Nigeria (various ranches) etc.

This sort of conventional programme for genetic amelioration poses various problems. The diffusion of sires which have been improved on the stations into the breeding areas is not trouble-free (sanitary problems arise in particular), and it is not certain that genetic progress obtained so slowly in a controlled environment (station or centre for improvement and multiplication) is propagated into the breeding areas. A certain number of examples in different countries seem to illustrate clearly the illusion, still too widespread, that genetic improvement results from the diffusion of a few improved sires into

Chapter 4 references, p. 88

large cattle populations. However, the introduction of an animal can produce an opportunity to make contact with the breeder and lead to sustained action in relation to performance control and mass selection; therefore the induced or complementary effects of certain actions of this sort must not be neglected.

When considering genetic improvement in the context of the existing farms, the very restrictive character of a naturally harsh environment must be taken into account. This environment strongly imposes natural selection, which tends to check efforts for genetic amelioration that are not accompanied by changes in farming conditions. There is, however, a large genetic variability which could be better exploited with a view to adapting the 'animal genetic material' to the natural conditions (food resources, sanitary conditions), and to the various systems of farming. Serious reflection ought perhaps to be given to this possibility with the aim of organizing and controlling the schemas of genetic stratification and maintaining a certain balance between the different genetic resources of the cattle.

It should be noted that on the whole extremely little has been done for the humpless shorthorns, in particular the lagunes, in spite of the repeated recommendations of the FAO and of the UNEP for a conservation programme. These humpless cattle are few in number and are threatened with absorption. The lagune type of humpless Dwarf is most in danger, being much fewer in number than the savanna shorthorn; however, the latter find themselves at the present time in areas where the development of crop cultivation, the progressive descent of the zebu and the demand for heavier cattle for draught, tends to put into doubt their continued breeding and their genetic purity.

In the case of the Baoulé breed, an example of a Savanna shorthorn, an exemplary programme can be mentioned that was carried out in the village communities in the north of Ivory Coast. In this programme, research working for development led to sustained work with around 10 000 head of cattle, with performance checks and notations of all herd events, adapted to the conditions of the rural environment. Methods of recording, of building up a databank and of computer processing information were perfected. This study led to a better understanding of farming systems and to original thought on the possibilities for genetic amelioration in village environments (Landais, 1983).

The crossbred types (Djakoré, Borgou, Mere, Sanga, etc.), which are becoming more and more important in terms of the association of crop cultivation with animal breeding, have been the object of virtually no genetic or zootechnic studies.

Crossbreeding the zebu with the humpless cattle seems to be an effective way of exploiting interracial variabilities; the humpless cattle are indeed good crossbreeding 'material', providing suitable mothers, of medium size and satisfactory fertility etc. So the classic problem arises of propagating the females of the humpless breeds so that crossbreeding can be undertaken. From this point of view, it seems essential to deliberately maintain cells of quite pure humpless cattle breeding, because policies pursued in numerous regions are not in this direction.

So one arrives at the conclusion that it is necessary to organize and control to a certain degree the large genetic flux that is taking place at present, and to underline the urgency of undertaking measures for the preservation and multiplication of certain cattle populations.

5. GENETIC IMPROVEMENT THROUGH THE INTRODUCTION OF FOREIGN BREEDS

The genetic amelioration of cattle through the introduction of foreign breeds, as adopted in certain number of African countries, has had a relatively modest impact in cases where 'exotic' breeds coming from other continents have been involved.

The most valuable example of animal movement would seem to be that of the African N'Dama cattle breed which has literally swarmed into most of the countries of the area; this phenomenon is particularly striking in Zaïre, where in 1980 approximately 250 000 N'Dama were to be found. In several other countries outside the limits of the N'Dama's native breeding area, population numbers are considerable following relatively recent introduction: Congo, Ghana, Nigeria, Gabon, Cameroon, Benin, Togo, etc.

As for breeds from other continents, their importation would seem to be best justified for the improvement of milk production. In West Africa there are some more or less successful examples of humpless cattle breeds, like the Friesians, the Jerseys, the Montbéliard, etc., being bred pure or crossed with breeds such as the Sahiwal zebu or the Red Sindhi zebu. If the breeding conditions (food, sanitary control, etc.) are satisfactory, it would indeed seem logical to take advantage of the milk potential of foreign breeds rather than to resume the long process of improving the local African breeds by means of selection. These breeds, reared in a very harsh environment, have actually suffered from the effect of a strong pressure of natural selection which is unfavourable to milk production. A selection programme would therefore have to last a long time before levels of production were obtained compatible with the economic requirements of these breeding projects.

Foreign breeds, in fairly large numbers, have been introduced for meat production. Particularly worthy of mention here are the Brahman zebu and the humpless Charolais (Lhoste, 1977). The Brahman zebu shows a valuable adaptability to difficult feeding conditions but sometimes has a problem adapting to the humid climate, revealing particularly a certain sensibility to skin complaints (dermatophilosis in Nigeria and in Cameroon).

Thus the introduction of foreign breeds is not to be rejected out of hand, especially since artificial insemination and the deep-freezing of sperm offer very valuable technical means of introduction. However, real experience in West Africa cautions prudence in this area. These projects ought not to be undertaken without precise objectives, and only under strict breeding conditions (health care, management, food) adapted to the requirements of the imported breed.

6. CONCLUSION

The bulk of West Africa bovine livestock are bred under conditions that are both extensive and traditional. The farming systems encountered are varied, and reflect very different socio-economic structures, ranging from that of the Sahelian nomad herds to that of the trypanotolerant village cattle in the humid area.

In the pastoral societies of the large Sahelian and Sahelo-Sudanian breeding area, zebu cattle principally produce milk and meat, which contributes greatly to the self-sufficiency of the herdsmen. The cattle also play an important sociological and economic role; they represent an effective means of accumulating income and a source of ready cash, as well as providing a sort of insurance. This explains the importance placed on productivity.

Throughout the humid zone the humpless cattle are often owned by ethnic groups of farmers who lack a tradition of animal farming; traditionally their animals are bred for socioreligious reasons or to serve in ritual events: for dowry, for funerals, for family celebrations, etc.

In the intermediary Sudanian area, there is particular progressive development linked to the evolution of production systems that has resulted from the

Chapter 4 references, p. 88

demands placed on animal breeders by the needs of crop cultivation systems. Apart from the standard production of meat and milk, cattle now play a more and more important role in agricultural production methods as providers of energy (animal traction) and of manure.

Possibilities do exist to increase the productivity of West African cattle, but from a practical point of view, real possibilities of improvement are limited by difficult natural conditions and by the very traditional farming methods practised, especially in the Sahelian area.

Without doubt it is in the agropastoral area and in the humid area that the biggest margins for improvement exist in terms of increasing cattle numbers, productivity and farming systems (ranching, breeding in the palm plantations, work related to crop production, etc.). In this humid zone, humpless trypanotolerant livestock are to be found in very differing densities. Considered at one time as relics whose trypanotolerance was just an additional point of curiosity, these same animals now find themselves the object of an increasing interest shown by governments and international organizations. The breeders on the other hand, naturally tend to crossbreed these small-sized humpless cattle with the larger sized zebu, thus in certain cases putting at risk the genetic 'speciality' of their cattle herds.

In the case of certain genetic groups, such as the humpless shorthorns (lagune breed), numbers are diminishing so rapidly that, taking into account the poor means available for intervention, one wonders if it is not already too late to effectively safeguard certain breeds (the humpless Dwarf).

The N'Dama, humpless West African longhorns, constitute a large genetic pool, and would seem to be much less under threat, especially now that new herds are developing in different countries.

The problems related to the development of cattle farming in Africa are not overridingly problems of genetic amelioration. Certainly, for some types, priority should be given to conservation and genetic management. For the dominant groups (zebus, zebus × humpless crossbreeds) it is more important to control the genetic flux in relation to production objectives, and to develop, with an overall organization, the exploitation of the resources by crop and animal farmers. Relevant planning should be seen in terms which take into account the genetic characteristics of the animals concerned, but which nevertheless keep the overall aim of taking maximum advantage of resources, and of reproducing the various resources of the ecosystem and of creating a balance between the activities of the people involved; the problem certainly does involve the maintenance and development of certain cattle populations, but also in some cases involves the survival of pastoral societies.

7. REFERENCES

CIPEA/ILCA, 1979. Trypanotolerant Livestock in West and Central Africa, Vol. 1, General Study and Vol. 2, Country Studies. International Livestock Center for Africa, Addis Ababa. (Also published as Report No. 20/1–2 (1980), Food and Agriculture Organization, Rome.)

Doutressoulle, G., 1947. L'Elevage en Afrique Occidentale Française. Larose, Paris, 298 pp.

Epstein, H., 1971. The Origin of the Domestic Animals of Africa, Vols 1 and 2. Africana, New York, 1292 pp.

Epstein, H., 1983. Indigenous domesticated animals of Asia and Africa and their uses. In: Domestication, Conservation and Use of Animal Resources, World Animal Science, Vol. A1, Chapter 4. Elsevier, Amsterdam, pp 63–92.

Joshi, N.R., 1957. Les Bovins d'Afrique — Types et Races. Food and Agriculture Organization, Rome.

Landais, E., 1983. Analyse des systèmes d'elevage bovin sédentaire du nord de la Côte d'Ivoire Thèse d'Etat Université de Paris Sud, Paris, 758 pp.

Leclercq P., 1976. Principales races d'animaux domestiques des zones tropicales. Institut d'Elevage et de Médecine Vétérinaire des Pays Tropicaux, Maisons-Alfort, France, 97 pp.

Lhoste, Ph., 1977. L'amélioration génétique des zébus de l'Adamaoua (Cameroun) pour la production de viande. Bouaké - Colloque Recherches sur l'Élevage en Zone Tropicale Humide, pp. 449–459.

Lhoste, Ph. and Cloe, L., 1982. Comparaison des aptitudes à la production de viande de quatre types génétiques bovins de Côte d'Ivoire. Rev. d'Elev. Vet. Pays Trop., 35(4); 381–390.

Mason, I.L., 1951. The classification of West African livestock. Technical Communication 7, Bureau of Animal Breeding and Genetics, Edinburgh.

Chapter 5

Special Regional Problems of Breeding Resources — Latin American and Caribbean Examples

JOHN V. WILKINS

1. INTRODUCTION

The immense land area of Latin America extends through 87 degrees of latitude. The large number of ecological zones that may be expected in an area that includes so many parallels of latitude is increased by a mountain chain that runs its entire length and in which may be found temperate, fertile uplands and cold, semi-arid plateaux. The area is rich in cattle genetic resources because of a long history of importation from many parts of the world and the main problem is to fit these resources to the climatic, social and economic environments of each zone.

The data shown in Table 5.1 suggest that the area including all the islands of the Caribbean contains some 22% of the world's cattle and that while meat and milk production is inferior to the world average it is superior to that of the other developing areas of Africa and Asia. The same source suggests that the area produces 18% of the world's meat and 8% of its milk. (FAO, 1979). It must be stated, however, that livestock census and production data of many countries in the area must be viewed with some caution as accuracy must be doubted in many cases. As an example, a 20% discrepancy exists between the size of cattle population in one country in the FAO Production Yearbook just cited and that given by the country's government for the same year. This necessary lack of confidence justifies the absence of national cattle breed cen-

TABLE 5.1

Cattle populations and mean production in Latin America, The Caribbean and the world

Zone	Cattle population ('000 head)	Meat production per year per head of cattle population (kg)	Mean yield of milk per milking cow per year (kg)
Central America	41 005	23.7	763
South America	215 593	32.7	1 046
Caribbean	9 801	25.3	1 334
Latin America and islands	266 399	31.1	977
World	1 213 092	38.6	1 964
Africa	168 864	15.4	478
Asia	362 259	10.3	689

Source: Derived from FAO Production Yearbook, Vol. 32 (1979).

Chapter 5 references, p. 111

sus and production data in this study. This lack of data, particularly that of cattle performance on private farms is a major limitation to genetic studies in the area. Several countries in the zone have excellent livestock recording programmes, at least in part of their territories, but it would be invidious to indicate the others.

In order to describe the current situation it is necessary to discuss briefly the history of cattle in Latin America. There are no indigenous cattle of the Americas but the criollo has been reasonably called 'native' to the area as it is the direct descendant of cattle imported during colonial times. The first were landed in the Americas on Columbus's second voyage, 127 years before the settlement of the Pilgrim Fathers, and the great majority of importations occurred in the 16th century (Rouse, 1977). The animals thrived and multiplied in what has been described as a biological wonder (De Alba, 1978). Management was extensive and artificial selection virtually non-existent. Hides, tallow and meat were important products as was farm-made cheese, and the extensive dual-purpose system continues in many areas of Latin America today both on a small and large scale. The cows and calves graze together during the day, are separated in the evening and the cows are milked in the morning at the end of the period of separation. Bulls were rarely bought but reared within the herd and in large herds natural selection doubtless ensured that any ill-effects of increasing consanguinity were eliminated. In this way subpopulations of criollo cattle became adapted to a wide range of environments from tropical flood plain to cold semi-arid Andean plateau of 4000 m altitude. Nevertheless, in small herds and isolated communities inbreeding must have had some damaging effect and criollos have been referred to as 'degenerados'.

With the knowledge of improvements made in breeding elsewhere in the world, wealthy cattlemen commenced large-scale importations in the last quarter of the 19th century with the object of improving their criollo cattle by up-crossing or stocking the newly developed lands with imported animals. A variety of European breeds were imported to the more temperate zones of the higher latitudes or altitudes and the British beef breeds were imported in great numbers to the southern area of Latin America. The virtues of zebu cattle in the tropics were understood very early on and there were two main directions of importation. Brahman cattle were imported into Mexico and Central America and then into South America reaching Argentina in the 1940's. These were followed by the Santa Gertrudis in smaller numbers. At the same time Brazil was importing zebu cattle directly from India from a variety of breeds of which the Nellore (or Ongole), Gir and Guzerat (or Kanrej) have proved to be the most successful. The zebu has been described as the spearhead of the development of Brazil towards its western borders. This population and the crossbreeds derived from it are, like the criollo, a unique resource which will be discussed later.

Having established that zebus were admirably suited to the extreme climate of the tropics and that the northwestern European breeds flourished equally well in the temperate zones of Latin America, the search began for the ideal genotype for the intermediate zones. The probing for the ideal cattle for the semi-tropics can be clearly seen in the history of hot, humid north-eastern Argentina of latitude 27°. Hereford cattle that had been very successfully bred on the temperate humid pampas of latitude 33° were gradually moved northward into this semi-tropical zone, replacing the criollo. In the late 1940's Brahman cattle were first introduced into this area followed by many other importations leading to the formation of a breed society in 1954 and the commencement of weight recording in 1962. The 1960's was the decade when the herds of the northeast were said to be 'whitened' by zebu introductions. The zebu flood continued southward and zebu crossbreds can now be found as far as latitude 37° in the semi-arid pampas (Eng. Agr. Juan Pedro Torroba, personal communication). However, recent work has suggested that reciprocal crossbreeding between Hereford and Brahman results in optimum fertility and weaning weight in the northeastern zone (Mezzedra et al., 1983a,b) so conflicting tides of zebus from the north and European breeds from the south finally merge in equilibrium.

While this has been the pattern of development throughout Latin America on commercial farms it must be noted that though Chile, Argentina, Uruguay and the southern half of Brazil are largely occupied by such properties, much of the remainder of Latin America presents a startling contrast between neighbouring modern livestock operations and very underdeveloped farms using the centuries old cattle production system already described. The cattle on such farms are usually the results of the crossing of zebus and criollos and the indiscriminate mating of their progeny. Most of these traditionally managed farms are small but some are large and, while lack of capital and education may be partially responsible, it can be caused by a history of low prices due to state control or to great distances from a market coupled with the need to conserve capital in the form of land and cattle during politically and financially unstable times. In this case the owners of both the small and large herds have other employment either as labourers or professionals. Whole areas may be locked into the system by continuing low prices and the zone may be very unproductive for no insurmountable technical reasons. As an example of such productivity, a cattle census in the Bolivian lowlands showed that there were 2.7 times more cows than calves under one year of age.

This review of Latin American cattle genetic problems will only concentrate on those unique to Latin America. Thus the criollo will be discussed at length while the enormously important beef and dairy industries of the temperate zones will be virtually ignored on the grounds that their success, their problems and their solutions are similar if not identical to those of cattle industries elsewhere in the temperate latitudes of the world. The improvement programme for the Argentine Holstein is an example of this (Musi, 1989).

2. CRIOLLO CATTLE OF LATIN AMERICA

Criollo cattle are here defined as those that are only descended from animals imported from the Iberian peninsula and their history and current situation have been exhaustively described (for example Rouse, 1977; FAO, 1981; Wilkins, 1984). They are not a breed and while possessing a distinctive curling twisting horn shape, every coat colour that has been identified in *Bos taurus* cattle is represented in the population (Rabasa et al., 1976). Although a similarity to the Retinta Andaluza of Spain has been reported, the unselected criollo more closely resembles the indigenous breeds of northern Portugal and northwestern Spain. The inheritance of coat colour has been studied and it has been demonstrated that it is different from that of the breeds of northwestern Europe. For example, the white face is not dominant in criollo cattle (Rabasa et al., 1976). The similar origins of criollo cattle throughout Latin America have been demonstrated by Quintero (1976) who compared genetic markers in Argentine criollos with those shown by Miller (1966) to exist in the Texas Longhorn, a criollo breed. The criollo has been greatly reduced in numbers by crossing with other breeds and now only remains in very large numbers in the Andes. Elsewhere it has been conserved in small numbers in selected breeds for beef, milk or dual-purpose production.

Chapter 5 references, p. 111

3. CRIOLLO CATTLE AND MILK PRODUCTION

Systematic improvement of criollo cattle for milk production is being undertaken in Mexico, Dominican Republic and Venezuela (de Alba, 1978) and in Bolivia (Wilkins et al., 1984; Wilkins and Rojas, 1989).

Colombia has two breeds of dairy or dual-purpose criollo cattle, the Costeño con Cuernos and Blanco Orejinegro. Both their performance and that of the Colombian criollo beef breeds are described in a handbook published by ICA (1976). With the exception of the Blanco Orejinegro (the black-eared white) all the selected criollo breeds are red or Jersey coloured.

Many studies have been made on the performance of criollo cattle and FAO has published an extensive bibliography on the subject (Müller Haye, 1977). However, caution is needed in interpreting some results in this field and, as Dr Dieter Plasse observed, the bibliography would have had added value if there had been a note showing if each study listed was of scientific or folkloric interest (FAO, 1981). As with literature on zebu cattle elsewhere, the problem stems from the fact that the cows may or may not be milked with the calf at foot. If they are milked with the calf at foot, corrections may arbitrarily be made for the supposed calf milk consumption. Where the cows are not milked with the calf at foot, some heifers have very short lactations because of an inability to let down their milk without the stimulus of the presence of the calf. Such lactations may be excluded from the study (Lemka et al., 1973).

The Venezuelan herd at Carrasquero has the highest mean lactation yield of 1897 kg when milked in the absence of the calf and the long established herd at Turrialba, Costa Rica under similar management has an overall long-term average of 1382 kg which is assumed to include heifer lactations (Muñoz and Deaton, 1981). The Costeño con Cuernos when milked with and without the calf has been shown to yield 996 kg and 768 kg respectively, thus demonstrating the milk letdown problem in that breed. The Blanco Orejinegro has been variously reported to yield between 220 and 656 kg of milk when suckling the calf (Gonzalez, 1976). High variation exists for milk production in all these breeds and the possibilities for improvement by selection are good. However, the main importance of the dairy criollo in the future will be in crossbreeding and Table 5.2 shows that in Colombia F_1 Holstein × criollo cows were more productive than either parent breed (Hernandez, 1976). A similar superiority was shown by F_1 Jersey × criollo cows in Costa Rica (Muñoz and Deaton, 1981).

While the breeding of relatively high-yielding criollos is feasible because outstanding individuals already exist, this might lead to a decline in the characteristics required for a crossbreeding programme with European dairy cattle—high fertility, heat tolerance and disease and parasite resistance. As will be discussed later, the low digestibility of pastures in the humid tropics limits milk production and the desirable target yield for crossbreds may be less than 3000 kg of milk per cow per year. In this case, it might be argued that the mean lactation milk yields of the improved criollo breeds of Costa Rica and Venezuela are already sufficiently high and that selection should concentrate on fertility and disease and parasite resistance.

The largest privately owned criollo herd in Latin America is that of the 1100-cow herd of the Caracú Caldeana breed maintained on the Fazenda Recreio near Poços de Caldas, M.G., Brazil. The herd is for dual-purpose production and mean lactation milk yield is reported to be 1767.4 kg in 303.6 days (Campas Pereira, private communication). The body weight is higher than is usual in criollo breeds and the mean weights reported by Hill (1967) of 800–1020 kg and 500–600 kg for males and females respectively are some 25% greater than in dairy criollos and are only rivalled by Cuban criollos (Rouse, 1977). A breed society exists with 6200 registered cows.

TABLE 5.2

Lactation performance of criollo, Holstein and Jersey and Holstein × criollo and Jersey × criollo cows in Colombia and Costa Rica

	No. of lactations	Lactation milk yield (kg)	Calving interval (days)	Yield per cow per year (kg)
Criollo[a]	652	396	453	319
Holstein[a]	162	1950	505	1409
Holstein × criollo (F_1)[a]	187	2000	426	1714
Criollo[b]	1117	1382	384	1316
Jersey[b]	433	2180	387	2060
Jersey × criollo (F_1)[b]	397	2221	378	2150

[a] Source: Hernandez (1976).
[b] Source: Alvarez (1977).

4. CRIOLLO CATTLE FOR BEEF PRODUCTION

A study in Paraná, Brazil, in which Caracú and Charolais cows were mated with Charolais semen showed that the Caracú cows were more fertile and that the crossbred calves had lower mortality and the same weaning weight as the Charolais (Peroto et al., 1983). In a trial evaluating different breeds of bull on Nellore cows the Caracú was demonstrated to be superior to the Nellore, Santa Gertrudis, Holstein and Brown Swiss (Razook et al., 1986). In feedlot, pure Caracú bulls were demonstrated to have superior live weight gain to Guzerat, Nellore and Girbulls (Teixeira Primo, 1986) and male puberty in the Caracú was shown to be earlier than in those zebu breeds (Valvasori et al., 1986).

A 600-cow criollo herd is maintained for beef production in the flood plain of the Beni, Bolivia with a herd of Brahmans and criollo × Brahman crossbreds. A similar three-genotype herd is maintained on the research station at Calabozo, Venzuela, and data from these two herds have demonstrated that criollo cattle tend to be more fertile and have higher birth weights than Brahmans but have lower weaning weights and a higher first calving age. The F_1 Brahman × criollo is superior in all these characteristics to either parent breed (Plasse, 1981). Gonzalez (1976) reported a similar result when crossing Brahmans with the Colombian criollo beef breed, the Martinero, and he found that weaning weights were highest when the mother was criollo and sire Brahman. Willis and Preston (1968) showed that Cuban criollos had higher birth weights, lower calf mortality, and faster pre- and post-weaning growth rates than Brahmans and had a similar performance to Santa Gertrudis cattle in Cuba. In the semi-arid Chaco of Argentina, Sal Paz (1977) demonstrated that pure criollo cows mated to bulls of the same breed produced a greater weight of weaner calf per hectare than zebus, British beef breeds or their crosses.

5. CRIOLLO CATTLE IN THE ANDES

In the more temperate and humid parts of the Andes the Holstein and Brown Swiss, with the Normandy and Red Poll in Colombia, have replaced the criollo to considerable altitudes. Outside these areas the criollo exists in uncounted hundreds of thousands from the semi-arid lower slopes to the cold high

Chapter 5 references, p. 111

plateau at 4000 m above sea level. Despite the Andean criollo's numerical importance, FAO (1981) was unable to cite a single study on these animals and their importance to the farmers of the area relative to sheep, llamas and alpacas.

Andean criollos are small. Rouse (1977) suggests that the males and females weigh 350 kg and 295 kg respectively but they are triple-purpose being used for work and beef and also for milk production for very short periods of the year in this extremely harsh, cold semi-arid environment. There is some evidence that calf mortality and growth rate have been adversely affected by inbreeding, and that improvement can be made in these characteristics by using bulls from other areas (Wilkins et al., 1984). A high degree of consanguinity probably exists as breeding bulls are reared rather than bought. If this observation is correct, improvements in production might be made at low cost by encouraging the exchange of bulls between isolated communities without reducing the breed's ability to survive.

6. SPECIAL PROBLEMS ASSOCIATED WITH BREEDING FOR MILK PRODUCTION IN THE ANDES

Pearson de Vaccaro (1974) states that while Brown Swiss and Holstein-Friesians are both numerous in the Andes, the former is supposed to be more resistant to altitude sickness. She observed that this problem is not serious if Holsteins are well fed and managed and reported of a successful Holstein-Friesian herd at 4000 m in Peru. A large Holstein herd is also successfully maintained at this altitude in Bolivia. The same author mentions a Holstein and Brown Swiss herd at 3200 m with an average daily yield of 10 litres and a stocking density of 5 per ha.

Negron and Terán (1978) studied a Holstein herd at 3910 m in Peru with a mean annual temperature of 6.7°C. Mean adult lactations were 2122 kg in 292 days. The authors estimated a heritability of milk yield of 0.31 and concluded that genetic improvement by selection would produce similar results to those in other zones. The lower western slopes of the Andes in Peru benefit from the cooling effect of the Humbolt current and though the area is arid, irrigation permits the cultivation of alfalfa. Holstein cattle kept intensively on such land have been reported to have a mean lactation yield of 4931 kg (Pallete, 1974). A population of 400 000 Normandy cattle exists in the Andes of Colombia and while information is scarce, their popularity must indicate successful production.

It would appear that there are special problems of management rather than breeding for intensive milk production in the Andes if rainfall or irrigation permit the production of adequate quantities of high-quality forages.

7. MILK PRODUCTION IN THE SEMI-TROPICAL AND TROPICAL ZONES

Specialized milk producers have tended to modify the environment of their properties to make them more suitable for the type of cattle that they wish to keep while beef breeders have tended to select their cattle genotypes to fit the environment of their ranches. Thus pure Holstein-Friesian cattle that are the most numerous dairy breed of Latin America can be found in much greater numbers at low latitudes than pure European beef breeds. For example there were 87 000 Holstein-Friesian herd book registrations in Brazil in 1979 and only 5613 Chianina, 4637 Hereford and 1459 Charolais.

McDowell et al. (1976a) in a study of Holsteins in Mexico between latitudes 19° and 23° showed that mean lactation yield was 4750 litres and that the progeny of American AI bulls were superior to the progeny of imported sires and that the progeny of Mexican-bred Holsteins were inferior to both groups. Another study of the same population (McDowell et al. 1976b) concluded that the total variation for milk yield appears sufficient to select for it in the Mexican environment and that, as in temperate zones, lactation length and reproductive efficiency seem largely influenced by decisions of owners. There is evidence from Venezuela that appears to give support to the belief that Holsteins can yield satisfactorily at even lower latitudes. Garroni and Verde (1976) described a 385-cow Holstein herd maintained at 450 m above sea level with a mean 305-day adjusted lactation yield of 4223 kg, and Combellas (1980) reported on the performance of Holstein kept on the farm of the Instituto de Producción Animal at Maracay at the same altitude at latitude 10° over the period 1970–80. Some of the animals studied were imported from New York State in 1967 and lactation performance is shown in Table 5.3. The author notes that 10% of the cows are culled for infertility.

The same animals were studied by Pearson de Vaccaro and Vaccaro (1981) for the same period observing involuntary losses from the herd, these being classified as caused by death, sickness, accident, poor physical condition and infertility. Losses of females from birth to 12 months of age were 13%, 12 months to first calving 5%, first to second calving 11% and second to third calving 6.5%. Of females born, 21.2% were lost involuntarily before calving once and 54.8% before calving three times. The survival rate of 252 American Holstein and 150 Dutch Friesian cattle imported into Venezuela at ages ranging from 5 to 18 months during the period 1967–72 was studied by Pearson de Vaccaro et al. (1983). Of these cattle, 68.1% did not survive until their third calving and, of the progeny of the imported animals, 8.5% died at birth and 13.7% died before one year of age. The survivors to one year of age had a mean number of calvings per lifetime of 2.3 ± 0.11 compared to 1.8 ± 0.7 for the imported females. Of the losses of the Venezuelan-born cattle between one year of age and third calving, 86% were described as involuntary. The study concludes, 'The fact that losses of the magnitude reported were obtained in herds supervised by professionals suggests the urgent need to revise carefully the economic aspects of dairy enterprises using similar animals in tropical regions.' It is clear that high yields can be achieved from Holstein cattle in the tropics. Nevertheless, it is equally certain that the feeding ration must be of high nutritive density to be within the reduced appetite of high-yielding cows in a hot humid environment and high management levels are needed to prevent or minimize other stress factors of the tropics such as parasites and diseases.

TABLE 5.3

Performance of imported and local born Holstein cows in Maracay, Venezuela

	Imported	Local
Body weight (kg)	606	517
Lactation yield (kg)	4731	4213
Lactation length (days)	323	326
Calving interval (days)	434	440

Source: Combellas (1980).

Chapter 5 references, p. 111

Should such intensive feeding levels prove to be uneconomic and it is desired to base the feeding regime on grazing, very high yields become extremely difficult to achieve because of the relatively low digestibility of pastures of the humid tropics (Minson, 1980). The feasible yields drop to that which may be obtained by crossbred cattle and these then become more profitable than European dairy breeds because they have lower calf mortality, higher fertility and similar lactation milk yields (Wilkins et al., 1979). In that study, profitability of Holstein herds observed in the Bolivian lowlands was so low because of these factors that four herds that were imported during the study have gone into liquidation and two state-owned herds have commenced crossbreeding. While the advantages of crossbreeding for milk production are clear (Pearson de Vaccaro and Vaccaro, 1981) no unanimity exists on the best or the most practicable way of maintaining a crossbred population nor which breeds are the most suitable for this purpose. A large-scale trial is underway in Brazil in which lactation performance, fertility, mortality and parasite resistance will be compared in various methods of crossbreeding Holsteins with the zebu breed, the Guzerat. The methods being compared are simple reciprocal crossing, reciprocal crossing but repeating the Holstein generation, breeding a new breed of half Holstein half Guzerat and breeding a new breed of five-eighths Holstein three-eighths Guzerat cattle (Madalena, 1981).

The Gir is the most numerous zebu dairy breed in Latin America and although mean herd yields of 2215 kg have been reported in Brazil (Alves Netto et al., 1967) herd book registrations declined 37% between 1974 and 1979. However, a substantial gene pool remains and it is a logical base for crossbreeding. The other alternative is the criollo that has been discussed already. While there may be a higher degree of heterosis in, say, F_1 Holstein × Gir than in F_1 Holstein × criollo cattle it may be that the criollo crossbreed is the more docile and manageable and a comparison between these two genotypes under the same environment and management would be of great interest. The Eurpean dairy breed that is most suitable for crossbreeding with zebu or criollo cattle is still debated although Pearson de Vaccaro (1984) has demonstrated that the Holstein is superior to the Brown Swiss for this purpose. One school of thought favours the Jersey which is a parent breed of the Jamaica Hope that will be discussed later.

Programmes for the formation of new 'breeds' of cattle derived from zebu and European dairy breeds are being initiated in many countries with very limited populations perhaps with little appreciation of the difficulties that will be met and the size of population that is necessary to permit progeny testing and the elimination of undesirable characteristics that will occur when the uniformity of the F_1 disappears in the subsequent generations. There is evidence to support the theory that the new breeds will be inferior in performance to the parent cross. This is due to a decline in hybrid vigour and the fact that crossbreeds can be obtained from purebred bulls that have been selected by progeny testing in large populations while animals of the new breeds have sires from the small new populations where selection cannot be so intense and indeed where progeny testing often cannot be practised because of small numbers. Results obtained with the Pitangueiras breed may illustrate this. This breed was formed from five-eighths Red Poll and three-eighths zebu cattle in Brazil at latitude 21° at 503 m altitude. The area has a mean average temperature and rainfall of 24°C and 1346 mm. Mean lactation yield is reported to be 2780 kg in 281 days (Lobo et al., 1984). The performance of this breed was compared with that of five-eighths Red Poll three-eighths zebu cows produced by mating three-quarters zebu one-quarter Red Poll cows with pure Red Poll bulls. The cows with Red Poll sires yielded 15% more milk and had shorter calving intervals (Lobo, 1976). However, despite the probable inferior performance of the new breeds compared to that of the original crosses and the difficulties and length of time required to create a new breed, these disadvantages are outweighed in the opinion of many by the practical difficulties of maintaining a continuous crossbreeding programme. It has been observed that many new 'breeds' fail to meet the admirable definition of a breed as 'a group of animals that has been selected by man to possess a uniform appearance that is heritable and distinguishes it from other groups of animals within the same species' (Clutton-Brock, 1987).

The creation of the Jamaica Hope breed has been asserted to be one of only three successful attempts in the world to produce a tropical dairy breed from a crossbreed *Bos taurus* and zebu foundation. The Jamaica Hope was established by the Jamaica government from the progeny of Sahiwal bulls and cows of various European dairy breeds. The progeny were subsequently mated with Jersey bulls and the present breed is said to be stabilized with 80% Jersey, 15% Sahiwal and 5% Holstein-Friesian inheritance and to be resistant to anaplasmosis and babesiosis. The breeding has remained largely in the hands of the government which has proved to be both its strength and weakness. It has given continuity to the work during 70 years and has probably given more emphasis to selection for production and fertility than for uniformity of colour and conformation than would have been the case had the breed had a powerful breed society. The breed is less uniform in these latter characteristics than many photographs would indicate. A breed society of 50 owners does exist but apparently little enthusiasm has been expressed by them to use semen of young unproven bulls in their private herds in order to progeny test, as they prefer to use mature, supposedly proven bulls. The government herd is too small to test the necessary 10–25 bulls per year which could only be done using AI and recording in the private farms. Bull mothers are selected from cows with a lactation yield of over 4545 kg and the government herd mean lactation yield is 3218 kg. A study of private herds graded as having good, mediocre or poor management obtained mean yields of 2905, 2000 and 1623 kg respectively (Wellington and Mahadevan, 1975). The authors of this study suggest that two lessons may be learnt from the experiences gained with the Jamaica Hope for new breed development elsewhere. The first is that investigations to decide the best breeds for crossing in order to form the new breed must be tested in more than one experimental herd as it would normally be inadequate. The second is that breed development 'except perhaps in its formative stages' should not be confined to one herd. As large a population as possible should be incorporated in the programme through AI and milk recording and these must be efficiently managed to permit progeny testing. They conclude that without the active participation of private breeders, 'a relatively small nucleus of cattle of a new breed is unlikely to have a significant impact' on a national cattle population. Davidson (1970) gave the data shown in Table 5.4, indicating the superior productivity of Holstein over Jamaica Hope cows. He noted that the Jamaica Hope cattle included 'commercial cows' presumably suggesting that they were substandard for the breed. Despite the apparently good fertility of

TABLE 5.4

Comparative lactation data of Holstein and Jamaica Hope cattle on a commercial farm in Jamaica

Breed	No. of cows	Yield (kg)	Lactation length (days)	Calving interval (days)
Holsteins	42	3334	306	401
Jamaica Hope	64	2653	290	393

Chapter 5 references, p. 111

the Holsteins in the table, the author stated that the absence of oestrus after calving caused problems in rebreeding the Holstein cows. A new breed of 5/8 Holstein 3/8 Zebu and another in 3/4 Holstein 1/4 Zebu are being developed in Cuba and look very promising because of the large populations involved and the support of an AI and recording programme (Lopez, 1989).

Of the programmes to develop new dairy breeds in Latin America, that of Cuba, in which a new breed is being formed from 3/8 Holstein 5/8 Gir cattle, looks particularly promising because of the large number of animals involved and the support of an AI and recording programme.

Some programmes appear to modify their objectives as the programme develops. The Carora breed of Venezuela, which was produced from crossing Brown Swiss and indeterminate criollo × zebu cattle, is gradually increasing its percentage of Brown Swiss blood with the use of pure Brown Swiss bulls. This highlights another risk in the formation of a new breed for a specific environment. The programme must be long term but the environment does not remain constant. An area that is unsuited to Holstein cattle today may support such animals profitably in the future because of improvements in veterinary care, the discovery of new pasture species or an increase in the price of milk permitting improved nutrition.

The limit of the zone that is suited to intensive milk production with Holstein cattle is debatable although its position, as has already been suggested, has more to do with the prices of milk and concentrates and the availability of a veterinary and advisory service than with mean annual temperature and humidity and is therefore not absolute nor permanent. In the Caribbean islands, Puerto Rico has an intensive dairy industry where the DHIA herds were reported to have a mean lactation yield of 3800 kg (McDowell et al., 1976,a,b) and the whole island has a mean annual yield per cow of 2137 kg which is the highest national average for Latin America and the Caribbean (FAO, 1979). In Jamaica, the Jamaica Hope already referred to is threatened by the increasing popularity of imported Holstein cattle, but in Cuba the large crossbreeding programme mentioned above has commenced in recent years indicating that in an environment very similar to that of Jamaica and Puerto Rico, lower cost milk production may necessitate Holstein × zebu matings.

In the Dominican Republic there are many apparently successful Holstein herds but a recording scheme is only in its infancy. It was observed that mean yields reported by Holstein breeders in that country are high when selling cows but low when demanding higher milk prices and protection from imported dairy products. Whatever is the unverifiable truth in that situation, a need was expressed by many for a crossbreeding programme and a criollo improvement project was initiated in 1978 by a non-profit making group of business men with government support. The object of the project is to provide progeny-tested criollo bulls for use in reciprocal crossbreeding programmes with Holstein semen imported from the U.S.A. Consultants have urged the need for an expansion in herd size to permit progeny testing and to concentrate on the selection for fertility, parasite resistance, good temperament and persistent lactations of high repeatability rather than high milk yield which might be negatively associated with some of the desired characteristics and which would be provided for in the crossbreeding programme by the Holstein breed. A simple method of overcoming some of the difficulties implicit in reciprocal crossing using AI has been suggested for this programme. At commencement all the cows on the farm are inspected and those that are believed to have more than 75% blood of European dairy breeds are marked in the left ear and the others in the right. Cattle marked in the left ear are always inseminated with criollo semen and the others with Holstein. Female progeny are marked at birth in the opposite ear to their mothers (Wilkins, 1979).

An apparently successful reciprocal crossbreeding programme has been observed by the writer in the hot humid lowlands of Zulia, Venezuela in which American Holstein and Brahman semen is used in alternate generations. The cows are machine milked in the absence of the calf. Data does not appear to have been published or, where it has the crossbreds are referred to as of uncertain origin.

In those countries where a substantial number of Holstein-Friesian inseminations are performed annually, a controversy exists regarding the desirability of relying on the importation of semen of proven bulls from the developed countries compared to the alternative of establishing progeny testing schemes within the country. As McDowell et al. (1974a) have shown, the risk of genotype–environment interaction is not great and bulls with superior progeny in the United States are likely to have superior progeny in Latin America. An economic evaluation of the advisability of the initiation of a local AI programme would have to consider:

(1) the number of recorded cows in the population;
(2) the relative efficiency of the AI and recording service;
(3) the cost of proven imported semen;
(4) the willingness of farmers to use the semen of young unproven bulls on their cows; and
(5) the total number of inseminations required for the breed per year.

A difficult situation exists in those settlements where forests are being cleared at the foot of the eastern slopes of the Andes. Here land is being settled by peasants who often possess no cattle and plans are being developed to provide loans to purchase breeding females. In Bolivia plans existed to import Holstein-Friesian cattle to stock the land. Model calculations in this latter case indicated that it would be economically and practically more desirable to buy cheap zebu × criollo ranch heifers in the country and mate them to Holstein bulls for two generations and then subsequently with criollo and Holstein bulls in reciprocal crossing (Wilkins et al., 1979). Bulls would be owned communally until AI becomes feasible in the area. Cattle development projects have taken place in which the financial situation of a percentage of participating farmers was worsened. Genetic and economic aspects should be carefully examined before commencement of such programmes to ensure that this risk is minimal considering the quality and availability of the advisory and animal health services that exist in the area.

In those areas where milk is to be obtained from cows that graze pasture unsupplemented by concentrates, the nutritive limits of the available forage ensure that the lactation yield of crossbred cows is not superior to that of improved criollo or Gir cattle. In this management system the improved criollo or Gir cattle would be equally productive but would have lower veterinary costs, particularly for parasite control, and would be more profitable and easier to manage than crossbreds (Wilkins, 1986).

8. BEEF BREEDING IN SEMI-TROPICAL AND TROPICAL ZONES

Madalena's comprehensive review 'Crossbreeding systems for beef production in Latin America' (1977) clearly shows that breeding principles from elsewhere are being adopted with the expected results in temperate and semi-tropical Latin America. In the temperate zones various European breeds are being utilized in crossbreeding programmes complementing each other in such characteristics as fertility, mothering ability, post-weaning speed of growth and carcase quality. In the semi-tropics the tendency has been to improve the performance of the European breeds that existed in the area by the introduction of zebu blood, while in the tropical areas the reverse has tended to take

Chapter 5 references, p. 111

place and the performance of the existing zebu when maintained on improved pastures has been improved by crossing with European breeds. However, an excessive enthusiasm may have existed for performance testing of bulls in the tropical zone without sufficient consideration for the characteristics required for weaner production which often takes place on unimproved pastures and with little control of parasites. Some lands in the tropics are extremely acid with a high bauxite content and very low fertility and are unlikely to be used for breeding high-potential crossbred cattle in the foreseeable future. In the case of other areas, there is technical knowledge available for the development of improved pastures but economic constraints do not permit this. On the Cerrado of Mato Grosso, it has been calculated that it is only economically advisable to establish improved pastures on 5–10% of the ranch (Monteiro et al., 1981). A breeding programme in this type of environment has to cater for the probably conflicting needs of high weaner numbers and fast growing, good quality steers. Economic and genetic assessments have to be made together when designing a programme for such an environment in order to maximize profit for the two linked operations—the production of weaners and the production of fattened cattle. Good fertility and mothering ability and low calf mortality are essential for the former and high speed of growth, linked to high adult weight, and good conformation are required for the latter. Unfortunately not all these characteristics are positively related when the breeding cow herd is managed extensively. For example, high birth weight is positively associated with high speed of growth but if the birth weights are so high as to result in parturitions that require assistance, this will lead to high calf (and cow) mortality where the calvings cannot be supervised. If tick control is not practicable in the breeding enterprise this too might limit the choice of breeds used in the programme, eliminating some which might be very suitable for the post-weaning stage on good pastures.

Two schools of thought exist regarding the most productive ranch cow in the humid tropics on natural grazing and browse. One group considers that it must be the pure zebu and the other believes that fertility is higher and calf mortality lower in a cross European beef breed × zebu cow. This latter belief possibly stems from numerous results in the United States (see, for example, Koger et al., 1973) where the Brahman is inferior in fertility and has a higher calf mortality than British beef breeds and the crosses between the two. The fertility of the Brahman is known not to be high though it was shown to be superior to that of the Santa Gertrudis in the Dominican Republic (Velarde, 1978). The reasons for this low fertility and high calf mortality are not clearly established although it is thought to be genetic in origin. In any event, the results achieved on experimental stations in the United States may not necessarily be repeated in a tropical environment with the added challenge of parasites and disease, although Willis and Preston (1968) showed the Brahman to have higher calf mortality than criollos, Santa Gertrudis and Charolais in Cuba.

While all zebu breeds probably have a self-protective mechanism whereby they can reduce their fertility in a stress situation in order to survive, this does not necessarily mean that they wean less progeny in a lifetime in a harsh environment than, say, a very fertile animal who succumbs to some disease under the twin stresses of lactation and pregnancy. Variation may exist in fertility and calf mortality between zebu breeds and it would be of great interest to compare the fertility and calf mortality of the Brahman with that of the other zebu breeds that exist in Latin America.

While many countries in Latin America and the Caribbean have zebu breed societies that maintain stud books and performance records, the Associacao Brasileira de Criadores de Zebú (ABCZ), based in Uberaba, Minas Gerais, Brazil, has the greatest importance due to the large population of zebu cattle that it registers and records and the efficiency of its organization, that is now supported by EMBRAPA (the Brazilian Institute of Agriculture). This latter organization analyses the cattle growth data recorded by the breeders' society. The ABCZ maintains a milk recording scheme for Gir and Guzerat (Kanrej) cattle and growth performance testing for these and the Nellore (Ongole) Tabupua and Indu-Brasil. These two latter breeds are descended from a mixed inheritance which may include the Guzerat, Nellore, Bagnari, Krishna Valley, Hariana, Gir, Sindhi and Mysore breeds.

The breeders' society has registered nearly 3 million cattle and in 1983 was weight recording 116 921 head on 497 ranches. The combined use of AI and performance testing is resulting in steady improvement in growth characteristics but it may be that this tendency could be taken too far if it were to result in declining fertility or higher calf mortality. Indeed there is evidence that the Brazilian rancher is interested in characteristics other than high speed of growth. Post-weaning speed of growth trials both of 20 years ago (Hill, 1967) and today (Da Silva, 1983) show that the Indu-Brasil is superior in this characteristic to the Nellore, yet annual stud book registrations of the Indu-Brasil have fallen 25% to 12 441 head during the period 1974–79 while Nellore registrations rose 41% during the same period to 213 825 head. (Guzera registrations rose 12% during the period but remained less than those of the Indu-Brasil.)

The data produced by Da Silva (1983) that indicate the superiority of growth rate of the Indu-Brasil over the Nellore are shown in Table 5.5.

It has been suggested that a reason for the decline in popularity of the Indu-Brasil and the rapid multiplication of the apparently inferior Nellore is due to the high calf mortality and low mean weaning percentage of the Indu-Brazil compared to that of the Nellore (A. Ribeira, private communication). A need obviously exists to test the validity of this observation and to ensure that selection programmes are adjusted to the relative importance of high weaning rate in the ranch environment.

Another criticism in the past of otherwise excellent programmes is the exclusive stud book registration of those zebu cattle that are descended only from animals imported from the Indian subcontinent, thus excluding the possibility of any grading-up scheme. The zebu societies of Colombia are now more flexible in their rules and have thus considerably widened the genetic base of their breeding population. Such a change in rules is usually very difficult to achieve as it is against the immediate financial interest of the society members who benefit from the high prices obtained for the cattle that they sell because of their relative scarcity.

The crossbreeding of zebu and criollo cattle for beef production has already been discussed and it is of great interest in this context as hardiness or tolerance to the tropical environment is unlikely to be impaired by crossing

TABLE 5.5

Birth, 205-day and 18-month mean weights of zebu cattle on Brazilian ranches

Breed	Birth weight (kg)	205-day weight (kg)	18-month weight (kg)
Gir	23.5	126.1	226.3
Indu-Brasil	31.1	152.9	283.0
Guzerat	28.0	142.0	252.8
Tabupua	31.0	161.9	279.0
Nellore	28.5	149.6	267.2

Chapter 5 references, p. 111

two tropical breeds and Plasse (1981) has shown that this crossbred in a very unfavourable environment has superior fertility, weaning weight and post-weaning gain to either parent breed. Such crossbred cows might be mated advantageously to a large European beef breed and their progeny might be fattened on improved pastures in another area. Despite this possibility, the practical problems of operating a continuous crossbreeding programme under an extensive management system are considerable and a need exists to systematically select the available breeds in their pure form within the extreme environment.

The formation of a new breed from crossing a European beef breed with zebu cattle has been attempted several times in Latin America and the Caribbean. While at least some of these breeds have been subject to many studies, evaluations of the new breed compared to zebu or European beef breeds appear rare. For example, a useful booklet on the Canchim breed of Brazil that is derived from five-eighths Charolais three-eighths zebu crossbred cattle provides 74 abstracts of studies on that breed without any breed comparison (Motta et al., 1981). Teixara Vianna and Jondet (1978) reported the data shown in Table 5.6. The validity of the results may be challenged on the grounds that the breed of bulls may have biased the result in favour of the Canchim.

The breeding programme that led to the formation of the Canchim breed began in 1940 and a breed society was formed in 1971 that initiated its stud book in the following year with a pedigree and grading-up register. The society now has 132 registered breeders with a population of some 5000 'purebreds' and 20 000 in the grade register.

Mello de Alencar (1983) recorded the data shown in Table 5.7 without that of any other breed for comparison. The same author reviewed 49 more recent studies on the Canchim (Mello de Alenaar, 1986). Comparative studies using the Nellore as the control are being carried out in Sao Carlos.

It is argued that the Canchim may be most profitably utilized as a sire breed on zebu cows in the ranch areas to produce progeny of both sexes for fattening. In this situation, the Canchim bulls will be more vigorous than bulls of European beef breeds. Evidence already exists that shows that Canchim × Nellore crossbred cattle have superior post-weaning gain to pure Nellore cattle (C. Mello de Alencar, private communication).

Another breed being formed in Brazil is the Ibagé in the south of the country from five-eighths Aberdeen Angus and three-eighths zebu cattle. In a breed trial in Mato Grosso do Sul some 12 degrees of latitude nearer the equator than their place of origin, the Ibagé were shown to be insignificantly inferior in

TABLE 5.6

Percentage of live calves born to cows of various breeding in San Carlos, Brazil

No. of cows	Breed of cows	Breed of bull	% Live calves born
184	Charolais	Charolais	24.8
292	Indu-Brasil	Charolais	42
32	Nellore	Charolais	45.3
44	Guzerat	Charolais	31.2
168	F_1 Charolais × zebu	Charolais	64.8
164	3/4 Charolais × 1/4 zebu	Charolais	60.9
58	Canchim	Canchim	64.5

Source: Teixara Vianna and Jondet (1978).

TABLE 5.7

Mean performance of Canchim cattle of Brazil

	Males	Females
Birth weight (kg)	36.3	34.0
205-Day weight (kg)	177.5	162.7
18-Month weight (kg)	305.8	260.6
30-Month weight (kg)	445.0	371.9
First calving age (days)	—	1022.5
Calving interval (days)	—	405.2

TABLE 5.8

Performance of Jamaica Red, Jamaica Black, zebu and crossbred cattle in Jamaica

Breed or cross	210-day weaner weight (kg)	Calving interval (months)	Live weight production per month (kg)
Pure Jamaica Red or Black	167.2	13.65	12.2
Pure zebu	166.0	13.5	12.2
Jamaica R or B dam, zebu sire	181.1	14.1	12.8
Zebu dam, Jamaica R or B sire	175.5	13.92	12.8
Zebu × Jamaica R or B dam, Jamaica R or B sire	182.6	12.88	14.2
3/4 Jamaica R or B dam, Jamaica R or B sire	172.8	14.07	12.3

Source: Creek (1967).

post-weaning growth on improved pastures to pure Nellore cattle and significantly inferior to F_1 Chianina × Nellore crossbreds (Mariante, 1983). The Ibagé cattle used in this trial may not have been truly representative of this breed (J. Freitas-Trovo, private communication).

Two new breeds have been formed in Jamaica. The Jamaica Black is derived from crossing Aberdeen Angus and zebu cattle and is thus similar to the Ibagé but it is longer established, a breed society having been formed in 1954. A herd book and grading-up register exist for the breed. The Jamaica Red, that is also known as the Jamaica Red Poll and Good Hope Red, is bred from Red Poll and zebu cattle and a breed society was formed in 1952. The society's herd book was closed in 1960.

The performance of the Jamaica Red and Jamaica Black was studied in comparison with that of zebu and zebu × Jamaica Red or Black cattle (Creek, 1967). The data on the Red and Black cattle were pooled to provide the information shown in Table. 5.8. No difference in efficiency of production between zebu and pure Jamaica Red or Jamaica Black cattle could be detected in the study. The study indicated that half-bred dams with Jamaica Red or Jamaica Black sires were the most efficient cows by 15.6% but the breeding of the half-bred dams reduced improvement to 9% and the author observed that the gains made by crossbreeding can be counter-balanced in part in some large herds by the alternative of having one single large population under pedigree breeding and selection. The same author provided the data shown in Table 5.9 in which the performance of a zebu and a pure Jamaica Red herd were compared when

Chapter 5 references, p. 111

TABLE 5.9

Comparative performance of a pure zebu and pure Jamaica Red herd maintained under optimum conditions in Jamaica

	Zebu	Jamaica Red
Percentage cows in calf	96.5	93.5
Percentage calves weaned to cows exposed	92	92
Adjusted male 210-day weight (kg)	209.6	221.4
Adjusted female 210-day weight (kg)	194.1	197.3

Source: Creek (1967).

both were maintained under optimum conditions. Under these conditions both breeds had the same high weaning percentage of 92% but the mean Jamaica Red weaner weight was 4% greater than that of the zebus.

In summary, very little evidence exists to suggest that the new breeds produced in Latin America and the Caribbean for beef production are more efficient than zebu cattle when maintained under ranch conditions. Continuous crossbreeding programmes do result in increased efficiency of production but produce considerable management problems of which the maintenance of bulls of European beef breeds in the ranch situation is not the least. While not insurmountable, these will ensure the continuing paramount importance of pure zebu breeding for beef production for many years.

N'Dama cattle from West Africa were imported into Martinique and Guadeloupe in 1825 and to the Virgin Islands between 1870 and 1914. They were imported into Antigua in 1945. They were crossed with Red Poll cattle and the resulting progeny are known as Nelthrop or Senepol cattle. They have only local minor importance but a herd exists in an experimental station on St Croix.

9. CATTLE FOR WORK

Cattle are still widely used for both draught and traction in the area but little selection takes place currently for this purpose. The cattle now registered by the Jamaica Brahman and Ongole Breed Societies owe their origins to cattle imported for work in the sugar industry and in the Dominican Republic draught oxen are still of fundamental importance in the sugar harvest in taking the cane short distances from the field to the network of light railway lines on which the cane is then transported to the factory. The multinational company Gulf and Western developed its own breed, the Romana Red, from a cross of zebu and criollo cattle specifically for this purpose on its plantations. Selected bulls are maintained at the company's AI station.

Criollo oxen are still commonly used for traction in the Andean republics where they are preferred to zebu cattle because of their docility. Should continuing recession make farm mechanization even more uneconomic for the small-scale farmer, the selection of improved heavier oxen with greater traction would have considerable benefits for this sector, especially if it were complemented by the introduction of better harness and tools.

In summary, the following cattle genetic problems need to be investigated with some urgency:

(1) If milk is to be produced from grazing crossbred cattle in the humid

tropics, the most suitable breeds to form this cross should be identified and the most practicable system of producing and maintaining this crossbred must be determined. The Holstein has been frequently mentioned as the obvious European dairy breed for this cross but a school of thought exists with a persuasive argument in favour of the smaller Jersey. The relative merits of the Gir and criollo for the programme need to be investigated. If the latter is to be used for this purpose, the selection aims for the criollo must be clarified in order to ensure that the required characteristics for crossing with a European dairy breed are retained and improved.

(2) The continuing importance of dual-purpose beef and milk production must not be ignored. Improvements in the traditional system are now being tested and a suitable genotype for the modified system must be developed that will respond to improved nutritional levels. These cattle must be produced in a breeding programme that is feasible for the small-scale farmer.

(3) The relative fertility and calf mortality of the available zebu breeds and crossbreds needs to be determined under extensive management on natural grazing in the humid tropics in order to provide fundamental information for the planning of breeding programmes for a stratified beef industry in which weaners are produced under harsh conditions and finished on improved pastures.

10. BUFFALOES IN LATIN AMERICA AND THE CARIBBEAN

It is possible that the first buffaloes landed in Latin America were swamp buffaloes from Indo-China imported by the penitentiary administration of French Guiana as work animals. From there animals were taken to the Amazon delta of Brazil and to Surinam in 1895. Swamp buffaloes from Surinam were subsequently taken to Guyana for work on the sugar plantations. The buffalo no longer has any economic importance in French Guiana, Surinam or Guyana. Importations of buffaloes by state or private institutions to the hot humid lowlands of Colombia, Peru and Venezuela have demonstrated their considerable potential in that environment but the respective populations are too small to have had any impact on the livestock industry of those areas.

The source of the Venezuelan and Colombian buffalo populations was Trinidad, where there are now over 8000 head, the population having doubled in size since 1947 despite the export of females. Examples of various buffalo breeds of the Indian subcontinent — Murrah, Jafarabadi, Nagpuri, Surti, Ravi, Bhadawari and Nili — were imported from 1905 onwards for work on the sugar plantations. A belief apparently existed that they were immune to TB which at that time was endemic in the zebu cattle of the Caribbean. Buffaloes are still used for haulage but they have a steadily increasing importance as beef producers on the island. They are rarely if ever milked. They are commonly kept without wallows and it would seem that these are not necessary even after work because of equable temperatures and very frequent rain. Buffalo meat has a ready market in the country. The beef-type buffalo developed in Trinidad from mating many of the breeds mentioned above is known as the buffalypso and is, ideally, stocky, straight-backed, short-horned and brown in colour. Experimental evidence of comparative performance of cattle and buffaloes in Trinidad is scarce. Mahadevan (1974) cites an unpublished thesis in which buffaloes were reported to grow faster than cattle when grazing and without wallows. The same thesis reported mean daily live weight gains of buffaloes grazing pangola grass to be 658 g between 227 and 409 kg live weight and 477 g between 409 and 545 kg. Fertility has been reported of 75% (Rastogi et al., 1978). Both meat and milk products are imported into Trinidad and in

Chapter 5 references, p. 111

order to meet this potential demand the buffalo population must continue to grow rapidly. Mean female slaughter ages should rise and exports be restricted in order to maximize population growth.

Several countries have imported buffaloes with little success either due to lack of acceptance by the farmers and their employees or to insufficient numbers being imported for the establishment of this livestock sector. In Bolivia the feral survivors of one importation were hunted to extinction. As Ross Cockrill (1974) put it, 'The moral of this brief sad history would seem to be that it is not sufficient to import water buffaloes into new areas and to hope for success with the management methods which have been applied to local cattle. It is advisable to introduce also some of the particular management skills which are applicable to water buffaloes.'

Brazil appears to have followed this advice with conspicuous success and now possesses an estimated population of over 400 000 head. Individual breed numbers cannot be determined but in 1979 the buffalo breeders' herd society with 292 members registered 615 Murrah, 890 Jafarabadi, 121 Mediterranean and 4 Carabao. It should be noted that buffaloes originating from southern Europe are classified as the Mediterranean breed in Brazil. Although Carabao or swamp buffalo were the first imported into Brazil, it is probable that their popularity is reduced by their unsuitability to extensive ranching systems as they become feral much more rapidly than river buffalo. Perhaps 25% of the population is maintained in areas such as São Paulo state, where their efficiency of production compared to that of cattle in the traditional dual-purpose system is debatable. Official milk records of 194 buffaloes during 614 lactations in São Paulo showed a mean lactation yield of 1616.1 kg of milk and 113.1 kg butterfat in 221.4 days (Villares et al., 1979). Languidey and Pereira (1971) described the management of a herd of Murrah-type buffaloes in São Paulo that were milked twice a day leaving one teat for the calf. The cows were fed *Pennisetum purpureum* and a concentrate and were reported to have a mean yield of 1921.1 kg of milk at 6.96% butterfat in 234 days.

Although the majority of registered breeders of buffaloes are found to the south of Amazonia, some 75% of the animals are maintained on the banks and islands of the lower Amazon and its estuary and it is in this area of high rainfall and temperature and natural pastures of high yield but low protein and digestibility that the buffalo has been demonstrated to be superior to cattle. The relative efficiency of digestion of buffaloes compared to zebu cattle when receiving rations of high fibre and low protein was demonstrated by Bose et al. (1979), confirming findings in Asia. Nascimento and Moreira (1974) showed that buffaloes grazed more at night than zebu cattle and spent more time during the 24 hours grazing and ruminating. Canto (1975) studied the rate of growth of zebus and buffaloes grazing Echinochloa pyramidalis and obtained mean live weight gains per day of 335 g and 545 g respectively for the zebus

TABLE 5.10

Zebu and buffalo performance on an Amazonian ranch

	Zebus	Buffaloes
Weight at one year (kg)	120	173
Age at slaughter weight of 330 kg (months)	46	24
Age at first calving (years)	3^+	2^+
Calving interval (months)	18.5	14.5
Calf mortality (%)	12	4

Source: Ross Cockrill (1974).

and buffaloes. Ross Cockrill (1974) obtained the data shown in Table 5.10 from an Amazonian property that maintained zebus and buffaloes.

Milk composition of Red Sindhi and Mediterranean buffaloes was studied at Belém on the Amazon (Huhn et al., 1978) and the results are shown in Table 5.11.

In Amazonia, buffaloes are rarely owned by peasant farmers but are kept in very large herds for extensive milk production. This traditional system (under which zebu cattle are also kept in the area) produces milk products for the river towns by once per day hand milking with the calf at foot. Milking frequently has to take place on elevated platforms as the area may be flooded. Ross Cockrill (1974) reported mean daily yields of 3.5 kg of milk during a lactation of 270 days. He found 85% fertility on one farm and stated that fertility was generally reported to be higher than in other parts of the world. Positive responses to internal parasite control have been reported but fascioliasis which is a major buffalo scourge in many parts of the tropics apparently does not exist in this area.

The frequent handling of cows and calves that is necessary in this dual-purpose system permits the management of buffaloes in very large herds with few reverting to a feral state even though milking may have to be abandoned on some properties during times of excessive flooding. Good fencing is required for extensive buffalo management and fence damage by buffaloes is reported to be greater than that by zebus. Dehorning reduces this problem and the practice is increasing in popularity.

Buffaloes are commonly used for transport on the ranches and are frequently ridden. The 48 000 km^2 Amazonian island of Marajó is a major buffalo area. Here Nascimento et al. (1978a) recorded growth rates of small numbers of swamp, Jafarabi and Mediterranean buffaloes and recorded mean female 24-month weights of 288.5, 292.5 and 343.3 kg respectively. A profounder study by Villares et al. (1979) found food conversion efficiency of Jafarabis to be superior to that of Mediterranean buffaloes and the latter to be superior to Murrahs in this characteristic.

Interbreed comparisons for milk production have not been encountered but the potential for milk production by buffaloes on inundated pasture in Amazonia is shown in Table 5.12. The half Murrah, half Mediterranean cows were maintained on *Echinochloa pyramidalis* on an experimental station near Belém in the period 1970–79 (Carvalho et al., 1980).

Costa et al. (1981) reported on a herd of Mediterranean buffaloes kept extensively on an experimental station near Monte Alegre with a mean temperature of 26°C and on annual rainfall of 2100 mm. Mean performance data are shown in Table 5.13. The authors reasonably conclude that 'these data indicate that buffaloes have the capacity to produce well under the

TABLE 5.11

Milk composition of Sindhi cattle and Mediterranean buffaloes in Belém, Brazil

	Red Sindhis (%)	Buffaloes (%)
Dry matter	11.6	16.4
Fat	4.19	7.9
Solids not fat	7.41	8.47
Casein	2.43	3.59
Lactose	3.61	3.60

Source: Huhn et al. (1978).

Chapter 5 references, p. 111

TABLE 5.12

Performances of Murrah × Mediterranean crossbred cows on flooded *Echinochloa pyramidalis* pasture near Belém, Brazil

	Weight at calving (kg)	Lactation milk yield (kg)	Days in lactation (days)
First calving	462.9	1626.1	299
Second calving	497.6	1847.2	281
Third calving	506.4	2027.3	297

TABLE 5.13

Performance of a herd of Mediterranean buffaloes kept on an experimental station near Monte Alegre, Amazonia, Brazil

Calving interval (days)	387
Mean male 180-day weight (kg)	133.0
Mean female 180-day weight (kg)	128.3
Mean male 360-day weight (kg)	215.5
Mean female 360-day weight (kg)	204.5

Source: Costa et al. (1981).

adverse conditions of flooded lands on the middle and lower Amazon'. This potential is well-understood in Brazil and in order to further multiply the species as rapidly as possible to stock the huge areas that are suited to them, export restrictions were enforced which, while understandable, had an unfortunate effect on Peru where buffaloes have been demonstrated to be very productive on the university farm at Iquitos in the Peruvian Amazon and where hopes had existed to import them in large numbers up the Amazon from Brazil. Export restrictions on buffaloes from Brazil were lifted in 1986.

In Venezuela it has been observed that considerable areas of low-lying land are covered with *Paspalum fasciculatum* of which only the young shoots are eaten by cattle. This grass has been shown to be readily eaten by buffaloes at all stages of growth and to produce reasonable live weight gains. The logical source of buffaloes for Venezuela is Trinidad whose total population has already been stated to be only about 8000 head. The problem of Venezuela and Peru is shared by Colombia and Bolivia; in both of these countries there is some evidence of buffaloes thriving in environments where cattle performance is modest. These four countries, like others with environments suited to buffaloes, have to determine the following:

(1) Have the investigations already completed in these countries convinced farmers and developing agencies of the desirability of buffaloes?

(2) Will farmers manage them in a manner that is likely to be successful? Traditional extensive cattle-keeping systems that do not involve milking are unlikely to have a felicitous result.

(3) Is the superiority of performance of buffaloes over cattle in the area sufficient to justify the loss of foreign exchange in importing a population that is big enough to be self-sustaining?

(4) Can health and quarantine regulations be such that the considerable risks of importing diseases with the animals are minimized?

11. REFERENCES

Alvarez, J., Deaton O. and Muñoz, H., 1978. Veinticinco años de selección de un hato lechero del trópico húmedo. ALPA Memoria, 13: 149.

Alves Netto, F., Fang, I., de Mello Telles, J.D., Gubrotti Fonzari, W.M. and Kvarnstrom, O.R., 1967. Comportamento medio das vacas e rebanhos controlados pelo servicio de Controle Leitero de Asociacao Paulista de Criadores de Bovinos 1945–66. Rivista das Criadores, 38: 18–108.

Bose, M.L., Barbin, D. and Demetrio, C.B.G., 1979. Habilidade digestiva de bovinos e bubalinos. In: Encontrol Sobre Bubalinos. ANAIS, Araçatuba SBZ, pp. 162–171.

Botero, F.M., 1976. Ganado blanco orejinegro. Manual de Asistencia Técnica 21 ICA, Bogotá, pp. 17–61.

Canto, A. do C., 1975. Pesquisas zootéchnicas e agrostológicas na amazonia brasileira. IPEAADO-EMBRAPA, Manaus, 15 pp.

Carvalho, L.O.D. de M., Batista, H.A.M., Lourenco Junior, J. de B., Nascimento, C.N.B., Kass, M.L. and Costa, N.A., 1980. Eficiencia productiva de bubalinos mesticos 1/2 Murrah–1/2 Mediterraneo. In: Reuniao Anual de Sociedade Brasileira de Zootecnia, Vol. 17, Ceará. Resumo.

Clutton-Brock, J., 1987. A natural history of domesticated mammals. Cambridge University Press, Cambridge.

Combellas, I., 1980. Información obtenida durante diez años (1970–1980) con un rebaño de ganado Holstein en Maracay, Venezuela. Informe Anual, Instituto de Producción Animal, Maracay, pp. 87–100.

Costa, N.A., Nascimento, C.N.B., Lourenco Junior, J., Carvalho, L.O.D. and Batista, H.A.M., 1981. Comportamento productivo de búfalos mediterráneos de corte em pastagem nativa. In: Reuniao Anual da Sociedade Brasileira de Zootecnia, Vol. 18, Guiania. Resumo.

Creek, M.J., 1967. A study of the effects of some husbandry practices on the productivity of beef cattle and of land grazed by beef cattle in Jamaica. Doctoral thesis, University of London, 212 pp.

Da Silva, L.O., 1983. An analysis of beef recording data of zebu cattle in Brazil. Preliminary results. Proc. Reunión de Especialistas en Mejoramiento Genético de Razas Subtropicales. EMBRAPA, Campo Grande, mimeo, 14 pp.

Davidson, K.B., 1970. Alcan Jamaica Ltd. Agricultural Report, 1969, mimeo, 85 pp.

De Alba, J., 1978. Progress in the selection of the Latin American Criollo. World Anim. Rev. (FAO), 28: 26–30.

FAO, 1979. FAO Production Yearbook, Vol. 32. Food and Agriculture Organization, Rome, 287 pp.

FAO, 1981. Recursos genéticos animales en américa latina. Estudio FAO: Producción y Sanidad Animal 22, 168 pp.

Garroni, J. and Verde, O., 1976. Producciones parciales y total en ganado Holstein puro. ALPA Memoria, 11: 171–179.

Gonzalez, F., 1976. Ganado San Martinero. Manual de Asistencia Técnica 21, ICA, Bogotá, pp. 63–81.

Hernandez, G., 1976. Ganado Romosinuano. Manual de Asistencia Técnica 21, ICA, Bogotá pp. 1–16.

Hill, D.H., 1967. Cattle breeding in Brasil. Anim. Breeding Abstr., 35(4): 545–564.

Huhn, S., Guimaraes, M.C.F., Nascimento C.N.B., Carvalho, L.O.D., Moreira, E.D. and Lourenco Junior, J., 1978. Estudio comparitivo da composicao do leite de zebuinos e bubalinos. In: Reuniao Anual da Sociedade Brasileira da Zootecnia, Vol. 15, Belém. ANAIS, Belém SBZ. Resumo.

ICA, 1976. Razas criollas colombianas. Manual de Asistencia Técnica 21, ICA, Bogotá, 106 pp.

Koger, M., Cunha, T.J. and Warnick A.C., 1973. Crossbreeding beef cattle, Series 2. University of Florida, Gainesville, 459 pp.

Languidey, P.M. and Pereira, P.A.S., 1971. Consideracoes preliminares sobre o comportamento de bubalinos na regiao Leste. Revista das Criadores, São Paulo, 42(503): 32–34.

Lemka, L., McDowell, R.E., Van Vleck, L.D., Gaha, H. and Salazar, J.J., 1973. Reproductive efficiency and viability in two *Bos indicus* and two *Bos taurus* breeds in the tropics of India and Colombia. J. Anim. Sci., 36: 644–652.

Lobo, R.B., 1976. Estudio genético da performance produtiva e reprodutiva de bovinas pitangueiras. Ribeirao Preto, Faculdade de Medecina U.S.P. (Thesis), 171 pp.

Lobo, R.R., Duarte, F.A.M., Goncalves, A.A.M., Oliveira, J.A. and Wilcox, C.J., 1984. Genetic and environmental effects on milk yield of Pitangueiras cattle. Anim. Prod., 39: 157–163.

Lopez, D., 1989. New dairy breeds in Cuba. Rev. Brasil, Genet. 12,3 — Supplement 231–239.

Madalena, F.E., 1977. Crossbreeding systems for beef production in Latin America. World Anim. Rev. (FAO), 22: 27–33.

Madalena, F.E., 1981. Crossbreeding strategies for dairy cattle in Brazil. World Anim. Rev. (FAO), 38: 23–30.

Mahadevan, P., 1974. The buffaloes of Trinidad and Tobago. In: W. Ross Cockrill (Editor), The Husbandry and Health of the Domestic Buffalo. Food and Agriculture Organization, Rome, 993 pp.
Mariante, A., 1983. Programa de melhoramento animal do Centro Nacional de Pesquisa de Gado de Corte. EMBRAPA. Presented at Reunión de Especialistas en Mejoramiento Genético de Razas Subtropicales. EMBRAPA, Campo Grande, mimeo.
McDowell, R.E., Wiggans, G.R., Camoens, J.K., Van Vleck, L.D. and St. Louis, D.G., 1976a. Sire comparisons for Holsteins in Mexico versus the United States and Canadá. J. Dairy Sci., 59(2): 298–304.
McDowell, R.E., Camoens, J.K., Van Vleck, L.D., Christensen, E. and Cabello Frias, E., 1976b. Factors affecting performance of Holsteins in subtropical regions of Mexico. J. Dairy Sci., 59: 722–729.
Mello de Alencar, M., 1983. Canchim study at EMBRAPA. Proc. Reunión de Especialistas en Mejoramiento Genético de Razas Subtropicales. EMBRAPA, Campo Grande, mimeo.
Mello de Alencar, M. 1986. Bovino-Raca Canchim: Origem y Desenvolvimento. EMBRAPA, Sao Carlos. Doc. 4, 102 pp.
Mezzadra, C., Miguel M.C., Molinuevo, H., Kraemer, S. and Melucci, L., 1983a. Evaluación de caracteres de crecimiento en cruzamiento alternado Brahman–Hereford. Rev. Arg. Prod. Anim., 4(9): 909–922.
Mezzadra, C., Miguel, M.C., Molinuevo, H., Kraemer, S. and Melucci, L., 1983b. Evaluación de caracteres de fertilidad en un cruzamiento alternado Brahman–Hereford. Rev. Arg. Prod. Anim., 4(3): 289–296.
Miller, W.J., 1966. Blood groups in Longhorn cattle. Genetics, 54(2): 391.
Minson, D.J., 1980. Nutritional differences between tropical and temperate pastures. In: F.H.W. Morley (Editor), Grazing Animals. Elsevier, Amsterdam. pp. 143–157.
Monteiro, L.A., Gardner, A.L. and Chudlergh, P.D., 1981. Beef production in the Cerrado region of Brazil. World Anim. Rev. (FAO), 37: 37–44.
Motta, C.A., Naves, A.C. and Da Silva, D.A., 1981. Canchim: Resumes informativos. EMBRAPA, Brasilia, 92 pp.
Müller Haye, B.D., 1977. Bibliografía del ganado vacuno criollo en Las Américas. Estudio FAO: Producción y Sanidad Animal 5, 67 pp.
Muñoz. H. and Deaton, O.W., 1981. Producción de leche en cruzamientos con ganado criollo. Estudio FAO: Producción y Sanidad Animal 5, pp. 40–47.
Musi, D.O., 1989. The genetic improvement programme of Argentine Holsteins. Rev. Brasil, Genet. 12,3 — Supplement 321–330.
Nascimento, C.N.B. and Moreira, E.D., 1974. Estudio comparativo sobre hábitos de novilhas bubalinas e zebuinas em pastagen de terra firme. Boletín Técnico 58, IPEAN Belém, pp. 43–53.
Nascimento, C.N.B., Salinos, E.P., Carvalho, L.O.D. and Lourenco Junior, J.B., 1978. Peso ao nascer e desenvolvimento ponderal de bufalos de raca carabao em pastagen nativa. In: Reuniao Anual de Sociedade Brasileira de Zootecnia, Vol. 15, Belém. ANAIS, Belém SBZ. Resumo.
Nascimento, C.N.B., Salinos, E.P., Carvalho, L.OD. and Lourenco Junior, J.B., 1978a. Peso ao nascer e desenvolvimento ponderal de buffalos da jafarabadi em pastagen nativa. In: Reuniao Anual de Sociedade Brasileira de Zootecnia, Vol 15, Belém. ANAIS, Belém SBZ. Resumo.
Nascimento, C.N.B., Salinos, E.P., Carvalho, L.O.D. and Lourenco Junior, J.B., 1978b. Peso ao nascer e desenvolvimento ponderal de bufalos de raca mediterráneo em pastagem nativa. In: Reuniao Anual de Sociedade Brasileira de Zootecnia, Vol. 15, Belem. ANAIS, Belém SBZ. Resumo.
Negron, A. and Terán, B., 1978. Producción de leche en el Altiplano Peruano. ALPA Memoria, 13: 150.
Pallete, A., 1974. Servicio de control de productividad lechera: Resultados oficiales 1963–73. UNA, Lima, 17 pp.
Pearson de Vaccaro, L., 1974. Dairy cattle breeding in Tropical South America. World Anim. Rev. (FAO), 12: 8–13.
Pearson de Vaccaro, L., 1979. El papel del mestizaje en la producción de leche en el trópico. ALPA Memoria, 14: 169–177.
Pearson de Vaccaro, L. and Vaccaro, R., 1981. Duración de vida y causas de salida de hembras Holstein del rebaño del Informe Anual, Instituto de Producción Animal, Maracay, 37–38.
Pearson de Vaccaro, L., Vaccaro, R., Cardozo, R. and Benezra, M.A., 1983. Survival of imported Holstein and Friesian cattle and their locally born progeny in Venezuela. Trop. Anim. Prod., 8(2): 87–98.
Pearson de Vaccaro, L., 1984. The comparative performance of Holstein Friesian and Brown Swiss breeds in crosses with tropical cattle: A review of the literature. Trop. Anim. Prod., 9(2): 86–93.
Perroto, D., Cubas, A.C., Mancio, A.B. and Lesskin, C., 1983. Resultados preliminares de avaliacao dos cruzamentos Charolais × Caracú e Aberdeen Angus × Canchim pure producao de carne na regiao Centro-Sul do estado de Paraná. Presented at Reunión de Especialistas en Mejoramiento Genético de Razas Subtropicales. EMBRAPA, Campo Grande, mimeo, 7 pp.
Plasse, D., 1981. El uso de ganado criollo en programas de cruzamiento para la producción de carne en América Latina. Estudio FAO: Producción y Sanidad Animal 22 pp. 77–107.

Prada Niurka, 1979. Programa de cruzamiento lechero en Cuba. ALPA Memoria, 14: 163–167.
Quintero, I.R., 1976. Estudio racial comparativo de marcadores genéticos en bovinos criollos. Mendeliana 1: 9–16.
Rabasa, C., Sal Paz, A., Sal Paz, F., Bergman, F. and Rabasa, S.L., 1976. Genética de pelajes en bovinos criollos. Mendeliana 1(2): 81–90.
Rastogi, R., Youssef, F.G. and Gonzalez, F.O., 1978. Beef type water buffalo of Trinidad. World Rev. Anim. Prod. 14(2): 49–56.
Razook, A.G., Leme, P.R., Packer, I.U., Luchiari Filho, A., Nardon, R.F., Trovo, I.B., Capelozza, C.N.Z., Pires, F.L., Nascimiento, J., Barbosa, C., Coutinho, J.L.B., and Oliveira, W.J., 1986. Evaluation of Nellore, Canchim, Santa Gertrudis, Holstein, Brown Swiss and Caracu as sire breeds in mating with Nellore cows. Effects on progency growth, carcass traits and crossbred productivity. In: Proc. 3rd World Congress on Genetics Applied to Livestock Production, Lincoln, Nebraska, 1986.
Ross Cockrill, W. (Editor), 1974. The Husbandry and Health of the Domestic Buffalo. Food and Agriculture Organization, Rome, 993 pp.
Rouse, J.E., 1977. The Criollo: Spanish Cattle in the Americas. University of Oklahoma Press, Norman, Oklahoma, 303 pp.
Sal Paz, F., 1977. Experiencia con ganado bovino criollo. Ciencia e investigación, 33: 157–161.
Teixara Vianna, A. and Jondet, R., 1978. The Canchim breed of Brazil. World Anim. Rev. (FAO), 26: 34–41.
Teixeira Primo, A., 1986. Conservation of animal genetic resources: Brazil's national programme. CENARGEN, EMBRAPA, Brasilia, mimeo, 15 pp.
Valvasori, E., Trovo, J.B., Procknor, M. and Razook, A.G., 1985. Biometria testicular em tourenhos Gir, Guzera, Nellore y Caracú. B. Industr. Anim., Nova Odessa, S.P. (Brazil), 42(2): 155–166.
Velarde, C.R., 1978. Comportamiento reproductivo de Brahman, Charollais y Santa Gertrudis en un hato en la República Dominicana. ALPA Memoria, 13: 174.
Villares, J.B., Battiston, W.C. and Santiago, A.A., 1979. Efecto da ordem e a duracao da lactacao sobre a producao leitera de bufalos. In: Bubalinos. Campinas, Universidade Estadual, pp. 217–234.
Villares, J.B., Silveira, A.C. and Ramos, A.A., 1979. Conversao de alimentos de bubalinos mediterranao, Jaffarabadi e Murrah. In: Bubalinos. Campinas, Universidade Estadual.
Wellington, K.E. and Mahadevan, P., 1975. Development of the Jamaica Hope breed of dairy cattle. World Anim. Rev. (FAO), 15: 27–32.
Wilkins, J.V., 1979. Informe al Gobierno de la República Dominicana sobre el programa de Conservación y del Mejoramiento del Ganado Criollo en el CIMPA. Food and Agriculture Organization of the United Nations, Santo Domingo, mimeo, 35 pp.
Wilkins, J.V., 1984. Criollo cattle of the Americas. AGRI. 1: 1–19.
Wilkins, J.V., 1986. Productive and reproductive performance of cattle in the tropics. In: Proc. Conference on Nuclear Techniques in Animal Production and Health Investigations, IAEA, Vienna, 1986, pp. 31–39.
Wilkins, J.V. and Rojas, F. 1989. Criollo cattle utilization for dairy production in Bolivia. Rev. Brasil, Genet. 12,3 — Supplement 221–230.
Wilkins, J.V., Pereyra, G., Alí, A. and Ayala, S., 1979. Milk production in the tropical lowlands of Bolivia. World Anim. Rev. (FAO), 32: 25–32.
Wilkins, J.V., Rojas, F. and Martínez, L., 1984. The criollo cattle project of Santa Cruz, Bolivia. AGRI. 3: 19–30.
Willis, M.B. and Preston, T.R., 1968. The performance of different breeds of beef cattle in Cuba. Anim. Prod., 10: 77–83.

Chapter 6

Utilizing Genetic Resources in Canada

HOWARD T. FREDEEN

1. INTRODUCTION

Members of the family Bovidae were widespread through all regions of the world prior to the time of domestication. Among the species still extant are several forms of bison indigenous to the great central plains of North America (bison), Europe (wisant), India (gaur) and northern Cambodia (kouprey); the buffalo and the zebu of Asia and Africa; the yak of the Himalayan region; the muskox of extreme northern latitudes; and *Bos taurus* which was indigenous to much of mainland Europe and Asia. Several of these species have been domesticated, notably *B. taurus, Bos indicus* (zebu) and yak, but the majority of present-day breeds of cattle in latitudes north of 40° derived from local strains of *B. taurus.*

These local strains evolved under a wide range of climatic and topographic extremes. Islands and western coastal regions, many lying north of latitude 60°, were of relatively low altitude, with climatic extremes muted by their proximity to ocean waters. East and south to latitude 40° in central Europe were mountainous regions where climate was greatly modified by altitude. Further east still were the arid steppes, deserts and mountain ranges of Asia where, north from Latitude 35°, the continental climate was featured by seasonal extremes of temperature, precipitation and wind.

The genetic adaption of local strains to these environmental circumstances was an inevitable consequence of natural selection. Following domestication, however, the environmental circumstances and the selection process changed. Through the use of artificial enclosures, housing and management, man sought to control both the cattle and the extremes of environment, and selection was applied to emphasize specific production objectives. As human settlements grew in population density and in emphasis on crop production, the need increased for cattle to produce milk and for draft purposes. Meat production, an obvious salvage product, probably remained paramount only in areas of sparse settlement where feral cattle were harvested as required.

All of these factors contributed to the evolution of local strains of domestic cattle. Although adequately documented breed histories rarely pre-date the 18th century, some broad generalizations of breed origins may be made from information recorded by Mason (1969) in his dictionary of livestock breeds (Table 6.1). Breeds derived from some strains (e.g., Swedish Mountain) have remained of relatively local interest. Others representing beef, dairy and dual-purpose types have achieved prominence throughout the world. In some instances, these breeds appear to be primary derivations of early feral types (e.g., Friesian, Simmental, Swiss Brown) but the majority represent combinations of local indigenous types with one or more of the major source strains (e.g., the origin of the U.S.S.R. Bestuzhev breed is described by Mason, (1969) as Frie-

Chapter 6 references, p. 135

TABLE 6.1

Origin of native cattle strains in the Northern Hemisphere which contributed prominently to present-day cattle breeds

Latitude	Region	Indigenous type	Present distribution of derivative breeds
N of 60°	Northern Norway	10th century cattle	Icelandic (dairy) cattle, local to Iceland
N of 60°	Scandinavia	Swedish Mountain	Progenitor of several Scandinavian dairy breeds including North Finnish (Finland) and Blacksided Trondheim and Nordland (Norway)
55–60°	Scotland	Aberdeen Angus	Worldwide as a meat breed. Brangus (U.S.A.) a derivative
55–60°	Baltic area	Angeln (Baltic Red)	Widespread in Europe as Danish Red, Estonian Red, Latvian Brown. Secondary derivatives include Bulgarian Red, German Red, Red Steppe, Roumanian Red
50–55°	Lowlands	Friesian	Worldwide as progenitor of Friesian dairy breeds, numerous Black and White Pied breeds of Europe and secondary derivatives (e.g., Kholmogor, Archangel, U.S.S.R.)
50–55°	England	Hereford	Worldwide as a meat breed. Brayford (U.S.A.) one derivative
50–55°	England	Shorthorn	Worldwide; a milking breed now primarily meat. Contributor to Charolais, Maine Anjou, Santa Gertrudis and other breeds
45–50°	Alpine Europe	Bernese	Progenitor of the Simmental (worldwide, milk and meat) and numerous derivatives
45–50°	Alpine Europe	Brown Mountain	Progenitor of all brown mountain breeds of Europe. Some of these, notably the Swiss Brown, are worldwide (milk, meat) and have contributed to many other breeds
45–50°	Alpine Europe	Gray Steppe (Podolian)	Progenitor of gray meat breeds of Bulgaria, Hungary, Italy (Chianina, March, Marchigiana), Romania, Ukraine, Worldwide
45–50°	Alpine Europe	Iberian	Progenitor of Albanian, Brown Atlas (North Africa), Busa (Yugoslavia) and others

From Mason (1969).

sian, Simmental and Shorthorn × local with recent additions of Kohlmogor and Oldenburg).

Many factors may have contributed to breed differences in popularity. Some (e.g., Swedish Mountain) may have been supplanted by others of equivalent (or even inferior) merit simply because of limitations imposed by population size. There may also have been genetic differences in general adaptability with demand favouring those that were most versatile. Judging from present-day breed distributions, however, it is evident from Table 6.1 that latitude of origin has not been a sufficient criterion of potential adaptability. The Friesian of lowland origin, the breeds originating from central and northern areas of Britain, and those derived from strains native to Alpine Europe have all proven adaptable to climatic conditions characterizing a wide range of latitudes.

Perhaps the most stringent environments to which they have been exposed are those associated with the central areas of the vast land masses which characterize Asia and the North American continent. Temperatures in these areas range from extreme heat in summer to frigid winters of 3–5 months duration. Precipitation is limited and summer pastures range from desert conditions to semi-forested areas in boreal and alpine regions. Feral cattle were rare under these conditions, indeed the only Bovidae species native to North America was the bison, but domesticated cattle introduced to these areas have survived and reproduced adequately if protected from extreme winter weather.

Western Canada is one of the most northerly areas of the world where intensive beef production is practised under these environmental conditions. Most of the beef production in this area is concentrated between the latitudes of 47° (boundary with the U.S.A.) and 52° with few cattle raised north of 56°.

2. INTRODUCTION OF CATTLE TO NORTH AMERICA

The first European settlers arrived on the eastern shore of North America about 450 years ago. With them came the cattle strains of their homeland communities in Britain, France, Germany, Holland and Scandinavia. The names of these strains, if ever recorded, were not long remembered but early agricultural writings indicate that they were intended to serve the triple purpose of draft, milk and meat. Sporadic attempts were made to develop new strains adapted to the new environmental circumstances but history records only one success, the Canadian breed developed in the province of Quebec (MacEwan, 1941). This dual-purpose breed, evolved from cattle introduced from Normandy and Brittany, is still raised in its province of origin.

The first importations of recognized breed types occurred in the early 1600's. Dutch immigrants brought black and white 'Holland' cattle to New York state in 1621 and settlers from Suffolk, England, brought their 'Suffolk Duns' to colonies in Vermont, Virginia and Mississippi (Vaughn, 1931). The 'Holland' cattle were few in numbers, their identity was quickly lost, and the present-day Holstein-Friesian breed in North America dates no earlier than 1857. The 'Suffolk Dun' fared better. It survived as the Red Polled breed, thus meriting recognition as the earliest recorded breed on the continent (Vaughn, 1931). The first importation of pedigreed Shorthorns was in 1783 with Herefords following in 1817, Aberdeen Angus in 1860 and Brown Swiss in 1869.

All of these breeds had been developed in countries that lay north of the St. Lawrence river, the eastern boundary between Canada and the U.S.A. Husbandry practices, too, were imported from these same countries and the breeds performed well in their new surroundings. Thus, when agriculture expanded westward during the mid-1800's, the breeds and husbandry methods

Chapter 6 references, p. 135

which accompanied the wave of settlement were those which had already proven successful.

Neither the breeds nor the management practices were adequate to accommodate the environmental challenges of western Canada. Settlers quickly learned that, under the range management appropriate to this area, more reliable production was obtained from cattle imported from the western U.S.A. These cattle, many of which had originated as far south as Texas, lacked the conformation and growth characteristics of the traditional breeds but these deficiencies were more than compensated by their extreme hardiness. These were not purebreds. Their ancestors were the survivors of many different breeds, including the Texas Longhorn which traced back to Spanish cattle imports in 1640, and their hardiness was a direct result of unprogrammed natural selection and hybrid vigour.

Although cows of these hybrid mixtures continued to dominate cattle production in western Canada into the present century their influence was gradually reduced by crossing with breeds of British origin. These crosses, particularly with the Hereford, had more acceptable conformation and growth and, if provided with modest shelter and feed during winter months, were capable of reasonable reproductive rates. As western cattle production matured, the cow herds were replaced by direct crosses among the three British breeds, Hereford, Angus and Shorthorn. Over time, a substantial purebred industry was developed in western Canada to provide bulls for commercial breeding operations. Occasional crosses were made with other breeds, notably the Galloway and Highland to improve winter hardiness and the Red Polled and Brown Swiss to improve milk production, but their influence was negligible and their popularity in Canada, particularly the west, never challenged that of the Hereford, Shorthorn and Angus (Table 6.2).

3. EARLY BREEDING RESEARCH

Given the Canadian climate, it was predictable that winter hardiness would be the first issue to attract research attention. That improved hardiness might result from bison × cattle crosses had been indicated as early as 1750 through practical experience in the south-central U.S.A. with natural crosses

TABLE 6.2

Registration statistics in 1978 for purebred beef and dairy cattle breeds registered under the auspices of the Canadian National Livestock Records

Breed [a]	Year breed incorporated	Total registrations since incorporation	Registrations in 1978	
			Total	% in western Canada
Angus	1906	493 437	15 194	86
Canadian	1895	58 159	769	0
Galloway	1882	14 200	338	70
Hereford	1890	1 812 600	69 555	85
Highland	1964	3 218	132	68
Red Poll	1905	31 859	93	65
Shorthorn	1886	1 079 000	4 776	61
Ayrshire	1898	666 319	9 228	12
Swiss Brown	1914	20 300	1 216	40
Guernsey	1905	200 000	2 079	14
Jersey	1901	603 000	5 838	17

[a] The Holstein-Friesian breed maintains its own registry system. It is the most popular of the dairy breeds with annual registrations, mainly from eastern Canada, exceeding 100 000 in 1978.

between these two species. By 1885, deliberate matings of these species were being made by ranchers in the northern states and Canada. Among the recorded successes was an Ontario breeder, Mossom Boyd, who began his crossing programme in 1894. He termed the hybrid the Cattalo. When his herd was dispersed in 1916, the Canadian government acquired 20 head, 16 females and 4 males, for experimental evaluation in the western province of Saskatchewan. In 1919, the herd was moved to Alberta and augmented by the introduction of cattle, bison and yak. According to Deakin et al. (1935), none of the original Boyd Cattalo produced offspring, and all results obtained in the experiment were from the animals introduced after 1919.

Hybridization with the yak was discontinued in 1928, their progeny having been judged as inferior in hardiness to those incorporating bison blood. As for the bison crosses, high calf mortality (77%) featured the pregnancies resulting from the mating of domestic cows with bison bulls and males of this and the reciprocal cross were invariably sterile (Deakin et al., 1935). Fertility of the F_1 females was also low but, through back-crosses with domestic sires, a Cattalo line was established. Functional males carrying more than one-eighth bison were never observed (Peters and Newbound, 1957). This established the maximum limit to the genetic contribution of this species. Subsequent studies indicated that, compared with Herefords, the Cattalo cows had superior winter hardiness but their progeny had no advantage in growth (Keller and Lawson, 1978) or carcase performance (Lawson and Peters, 1976). This research was discontinued in 1965.

To Shaw and MacEwan (1938) goes credit for the first North American experiment designed to test the adaptability of established beef breeds to the production conditions that characterized the central plains. Their experimental herd comprising 160 cows, 40 each of the Angus, Galloway, Hereford and Shorthorn breeds, was assembled in Saskatchewan in 1930 and maintained to 10 years of age under open range conditions. Their progeny, representing all reciprocal crosses and purebreds of these breeds, were confined for winter feeding then shipped to England for carcase evaluation in the Smithfield market. No breed differences were noted in cow longevity or reproductive performance. However, observations indicated a breed ranking of Galloway > Hereford = Angus > Shorthorn for winter hardiness of the cows and the same breed ranking for bull performance during the summer breeding period. Angus cows weaned the heaviest calves, and Galloway the lightest. Crossbred calves were clearly superior to purebreds in growth rate and carcase merit but all crosses were essentially equivalent in feedlot performance. These results contributed to the subsequent growth in popularity of the Hereford and Angus breeds.

National policies designed to promote purebreeding discouraged the extension of this research to evaluate the potential of heterosis for enhancement of reproductive traits. However, practical experience in the commercial industry had clearly demonstrated the reproductive superiority of crossbred females and research was begun in 1950 to evaluate the hardiness and productivity of females produced by crossing Brahman and Highland bulls with cows of the British beef breeds. These studies were carried out at Manyberries, Alberta, the same location that served for evaluation of the Cattalo herd from 1950 to 1965.

The Brahman, a breed developed in southern United States from zebu strains imported from India, was expected to be less hardy than the long haired Highland which was native to the damp, mountainous regions of northern Scotland. However, crossbred females from both sire breeds proved to be excellent range cows with the prime example of hybrid vigour provided by the Brahman × Shorthorn cross (Lawson, 1983). These females conceived easily, consistently produced heavy calves at weaning, had greater longevity, and

Chapter 6 references, p. 135

their lifetime production of weaned calf weight exceeded contemporary Herefords by 52%.

4. NEW BREEDS IN CANADA

A new era in Canadian beef production began in 1951 when some enterprising cattlemen in western Canada imported a few Charolais cattle from the United States. Commercial cattlemen, impressed with the outstanding carcase merit and growth potential of Charolais crosses, began to switch their allegiance from the traditional breeds and pressure mounted to open the door, long closed for reasons of animal health security, to importation of breeds from continental Europe. The late Senator Harry Hays, then Minister of Agriculture for Canada, responded to this pressure in 1964 by establishing quarantine facilities and rigorous health inspection procedures for cattle entering the country.

The first European imports, Charolais and Simmental, cleared quarantine in 1967. These breeds were augmented in 1968 by Limousin, Maine Anjou and Brown Swiss. By 1978, a total of 28 new European breeds had entered North America via the Canadian quarantine facilities (Fredeen, 1980). Bulls predominated in the early importations and grading-up procedures were adopted to initiate breed foundations. These procedures involved recordation of initial crosses with full registration status limited to full-bloods and to progeny from three or more back-crosses to the sire breed. Several of the imported breeds, represented by bulls only, had limited potential but others, particularly among the first imports had grown to substantial numbers by 1979 (Table 6.3). The preponderance of activity with all of these breeds was in western Canada.

5. CANADIAN RESEARCH WITH THE NEW BREEDS

Growth rate, muscular conformation and mature size were the attributes of these new breeds which first attracted the attention of western Canadian cattlemen. Thus the initial emphasis in their use was to produce F_1 calves for slaughter production with some attention given to selecting the superior F_1 females required to subtend breed propagation. It was evident, however, that the genetic dissimilarity of these breeds relative to the breed populations in Canada might confer greater heterosis for reproductive traits than had been achieved by crosses among the British breeds. Indeed, this had been the practical experience of those who had worked with Charolais crosses since the early 1950's. To provide experimental evidence on this possibility, scientists in western Canada documented a research proposal in 1967 to provide information on the lifetime reproductive performance of F_1 cows derived by crossing these new breeds with breeds of British origin. This experiment, still in progress in 1984, has been the central focus of Canadian beef breeding research since 1970. As it represents the most comprehensive documentation of the adaptability of beef cattle to western Canadian climatic conditions, its design and results merit detailed review.

5.1. Experimental design

Populations of F_1 females were produced by inseminating cows of Angus, Hereford and Shorthorn breeding in herds maintained under range conditions by cattlemen in western Canada with semen from imported Charolais, Limousin and Simmental sires. The female progeny were reared from weaning

Table 6.3

Registrations and recordations in 1978 for cattle breeds imported to Canada after 1967

Breed	Total numbers[a] registered or recorded from date of entry			Numbers[b] registered or recorded in 1978			Percentages from western Canada	
	Final year	Registered	Recorded	Registered	Recorded	Total	Registrations	Recordations
Aubrac	78	5	—					
Belgian Bhee	77	6	—					
Blonde d'A				—	—	1 230		
Charolais				—	—	11 120		
Chianina	78	1 240	18 366	259	661	—	86	90
Devon	78	172	—	14	—	—		
Flamande	77	1	—					
Gasconne	76	2	—					
Gelbvieh				—	—	516	98	98
Limousin				—	—	4 147		
Lincoln Red	77	609	275	54	36	—	35	56
Luing	78	135	121	52	13	—	100	100
Maine Anjou				—	—	4 092	93	93
Marchigiana	75	3	35				100	100
Meuse-Rhine-Ijssel	78	95	208	10	46	—	100	100
Murray Gray	78	1 035	4 754	327	478	—	90	97
Normande	78	29	576	4	38	—	100	100
Parthenay	77	3	25				100	100
Pinzgauer				—	—	600		
Romagnola	78	135	639	59	18	—	100	100
Romagnola-Marchigiana				—	—	170	100	100
Salers	78	241	3 191	82	460	—	96	96
Santa Gertrudis	75	360	—	2	—	—		
Simmental				—	—	17 928	99	99
South Devon	78	240	124	48	42	—	85	100
Tarentaise	78	121	3 040	36	179	—	100	100
Welsh Black				—	—	1 177		

[a] Entries represent the totals processed during the time period the breed records were processed under the auspices of Canadian National Livestock Records.
[b] Totals only for those breeds which provided their own registration systems from the date of importation to Canada.

Chapter 6 references, p. 135

to 12 months of age at the research facilities at Brandon (Manitoba) and Lacombe (Alberta), then transferred to two locations, Brandon and Manyberries (Alberta) for evaluation of lifetime reproductive performance. Transfers from each rearing environment were equally at random within each breed cross to each recipient location. The crossing programme produced 1000 F_1 females and this number was augmented by purchase of 150 range-bred Hereford × Angus females to serve as a control population. The breed cross composition was essentially identical for each herd (Table 6.4).

The two locations designated for maintenance of these breeding herds were deliberately chosen to represent the extremes of environment and management most characteristic of western Canada. Brandon provided the semi-intensive management and climatic conditions typical of the cultivated pasture areas of the central prairies in Canada and north-central U.S.A. The climate of this area features seasonal extremes of temperature with moderate to heavy snow cover during winters averaging 4–5 months in duration. Manyberries provided the extensive range management employed throughout the semi-arid short-grass plains which occupy much of the western portion of Canada and the U.S.A. This treeless area lies in the rain-shadow of the western mountain ranges and is subject to a wide variation in winter temperatures, snow conditions and wind. While this variation breaks the winters sufficiently to permit year-round grazing management of cow herds, emergency feed and the natural shelter provided by topography are essential.

The data recorded for each cross included conception rates, number of services to conceive, birth weight and calving ease for each gestation, cow weights at calving, breeding and weaning, causes of cow and/or calf mortality, calf weaning weight, and feedlot and carcase evaluation of the progeny. Matings

TABLE 6.4

Number of hybrid females of each birth year entering the project

Breed cross[a]		Brandon				Manyberries				
		Year born				Year born				Overall
Sire	Dam	1970	1971	1972	Total	1970	1971	1972	Total	total
H	A	30	45	–	75	30	45	–	75	150
C	H	18	22	14	54	21	24	8	53	107
	A	17	18	16	51	16	21	15	52	103
	N	6	31	8	45	7	30	6	43	88
C		41	71	38	150	44	75	29	148	298
S	H	25	36	–	61	25	39	–	64	125
	A	29	31	–	60	27	33	–	60	120
	N	19	36	7	62	18	36	8	62	124
S		73	103	7	183	70	108	8	186	369
L	H	10	25	13	48	9	25	15	49	97
	A	8	21	22	51	7	20	23	50	101
	N	21	44	–	65	20	50	–	70	135
L		39	90	35	164	36	95	38	169	333
	H	53	83	27	163	55	88	23	166	329
	A	54	70	38	162	50	74	38	162	324
	N	46	111	15	172	45	116	14	175	347
Total		183	309	80	572	180	323	75	578	1150

[a] Sire breeds: H = Hereford; C = Charolais; S = Simmental.
Dam breeds: H = Hereford; A = Angus; N = Shorthorn.

were by artificial inseminations during a 9-week period commencing mid-June. All calves produced were three-breed crosses. Yearling heifers were bred to Red Angus and Beefmaster sires with subsequent progeny produced by Charolais, Chianina, Limousin and Simmental sires (Lawson et al., 1980; Fredeen et al., 1981a).

The initial input of females was completed in 1973 and the cow herds were maintained without replacement to the completion of the study. Females that proved barren in their heifer production year were culled only if examination (rectal palpation) revealed anatomical defects. Subsequently, females were culled if barren in two consecutive years. In the last years of the study, cows exhibiting extreme physical deterioration were also culled.

Lifetime reproductive performance was evaluated when the first input females (born 1970) were 8 years of age. At this time, the data represented 4930 progeny living at birth. After 1978, the surviving cows were assigned to other research uses where a substantial number have continued to reproduce regularly to the present time.

5.1.1. Cow growth patterns

Initial weights for females of the three input age groups (born 1970, 1971 and 1972) were identical at the two locations, as were the mature cow weights taken at weaning in 1979 (Fredeen et al., 1981a) but there were substantial location differences in growth patterns during the intervening years. The F_1 females at Brandon grew in accordance with expectations. Rapid weight gains to 30 months of age were followed by a gradual deceleration of growth with animal weight changes featured by gestation gains (winter and nursing losses (summer). Maximum weights were recorded at 6–7 years of age (Fig. 6.1). In contrast, the growth patterns at Manyberries featured wide annual fluctuations with large gestation losses and nursing gains (Fig. 6.2). Winter weight losses were particularly large in 1973 and 1974 with the result that cow

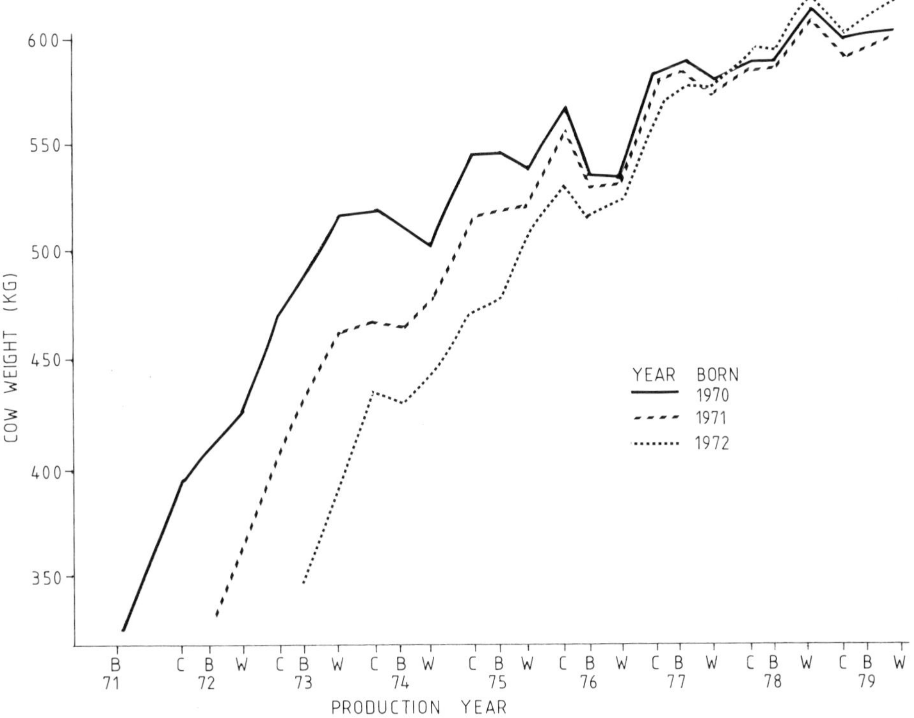

Fig. 6.1. Annual cow weights at calving (C), breeding (B) and weaning (W) for three cow age groups at Brandon.

Chapter 6 references, p. 135

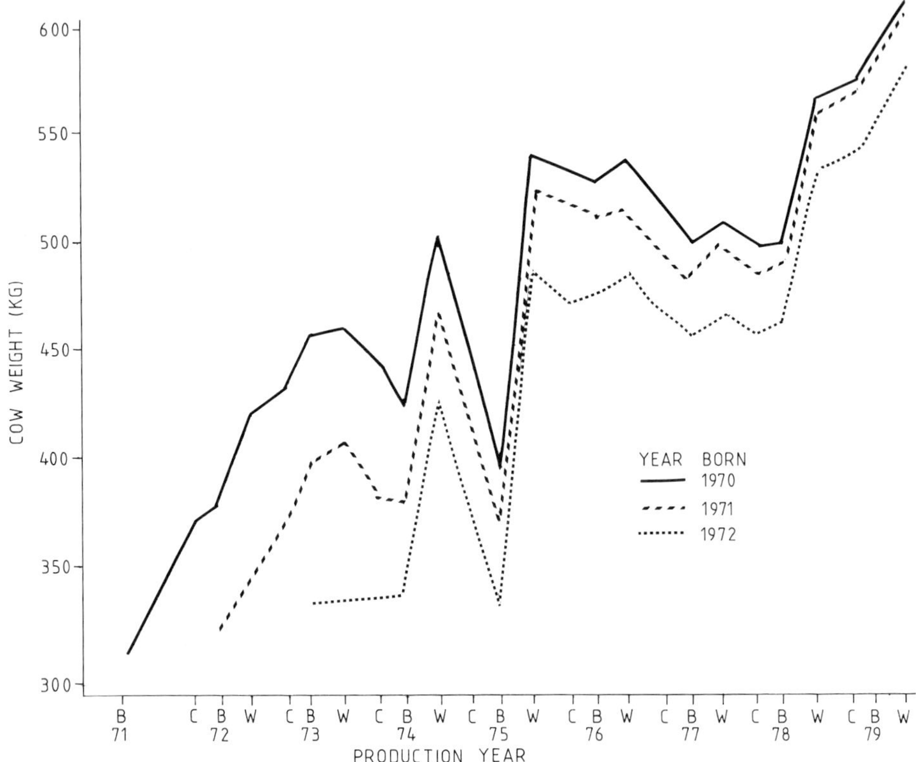

Fig. 6.2. Annual cow weights at calving (C), breeding (B) and weaning (W) for three cow age groups at Manyberries.

weights at breeding in 1975 averaged 86, 93 and 99% of those taken 24 months previously for females born in 1970, 1971 and 1972. Indeed, the June 1975 weights of cows born in 1972 did not differ from those recorded when they were 14 months of age. Weights stabilized after this date but weight equivalence with Brandon females did not occur until after 1977 when the practice of winter grazing at Manyberries was replaced by the confinement system employed from the outset at Brandon.

The average cow weights at calving, breeding and weaning (Figs 6.1 and 6.2) included all cows, whether nursing, dry or barren, present at each weighing period. However, nursing status had a profound effect on weights and weight changes and conception rates were influenced by weight when exposed to breeding (Table 6.5). For cows nursing when bred in year n, the average breeding weight of those that conceived and reared a calf in year $n+1$ (NN status) were almost invariably heavier at breeding than those which failed to conceive (ND status). The weight advantage generally persisted through the summer and winter following breeding with the ND cows exhibiting large gains during their subsequent non-nursing summer. Thus cows which were dry in the breeding season when they conceived (DN status) were substantially heavier when exposed than either the NN or ND cows and maintained this weight advantage through to the time the resulting calf was born. They also averaged heavier than the NN cows when the calf was weaned but weighed less than ND cows at this time.

These patterns of weight changes in relation to cow nursing status were observed at both locations but they were most pronounced under the environmental conditions provided by Manyberries (Fig. 6.3).

Breed crosses differed in absolute weights within and between locations but they did not differ in the characteristics of their growth patterns. In terms of

TABLE 6.5

Influence of nursing status[a] on cow weights at breeding (B) in year n and calving (C) and weaning (W) the subsequent year during each production cycle for cows born in 1971

			Brandon				Manyberries			
Nursing status:			NN		(ND–NN)	(DN–NN)	NN		(ND–NN)	(DN–NN)
Production cycle	Breeding year	Weight period	Average (kg)	SE	(kg)	(kg)	Average(kg)	SE	(kg)	(kg)
1	1972	B	326	1.8			320	2.3		
		C	410	2.7			374	1.8		
		W	456	3.2			398	3.2		
2	1973	B	412	3.6	−17*	15*	396	2.7	−14*	28*
		C	468	3.6	−40*	44*	371	2.7	34*	40*
		W	460	4.1	62*	37*	448	4.1	107*	26*
3	1974	B	468	4.1	−28*	4	381	4.1	−23*	16*
		C	508	4.1	−22*	45*	391	4.5	3	48*
		W	510	4.5	38*	35*	493	5.9	77*	33*
4	1975	B	522	4.5	−3	−10	380	4.1	−30*	10
		C	553	4.1	−2	27*	523	5.0	−72*	17*
		W	520	4.5	88*	9*	509	4.5	45*	2
5	1976	B	527	4.1	−5	34*	515	4.1	−16	14
		C	578	4.1	−46*	46*	491	4.1	−3	18
		W	568	4.5	39*	25*	493	3.6	49*	9
6	1977	B	582	7.7	20	1	490	4.5	−25*	1
		C	583	4.1	10	35*	480	5.0	12	34*
		W	600	5.0	67*	18	546	5.0	59*	18
7	1978	B	578	5.0	10	41*	501	5.4	−26*	−4
		C	582	5.4	8	59*	557	5.4	−30*	47*
		W	590	5.4	50*	34*	585	5.9	63*	18

[a] Nursing status defined as NN = nursing when bred, conceived and nursed; ND = nursing when bred, dry in subsequent year; DN = dry when bred, conceived and nursed.
[b] Data for the production cycle initiated in 1971 by breeding of the first input heifers are not presented. Production cycle 1 thus represents matings of females born in 1970 and 1971 with subsequent cycles representing all three input groups.
* Weight differences significant ($P < 0.05$).

Chapter 6 references, p. 135

average annual weaning weights for cows of NN status, those sired by Charolais weighed 17–23% more than the Hereford × Angus while cows by Simmental and Limousin sires averaged approximately 10% more than the HA control (Fig. 6.4). Ranking of weaning weight based on dam breed of the F_1 females was Hereford > Shorthorn > Angus > HA control. These rankings for breed of sire and breed of dam applied to both locations and were constant for cows of NN, ND and DN nursing status.

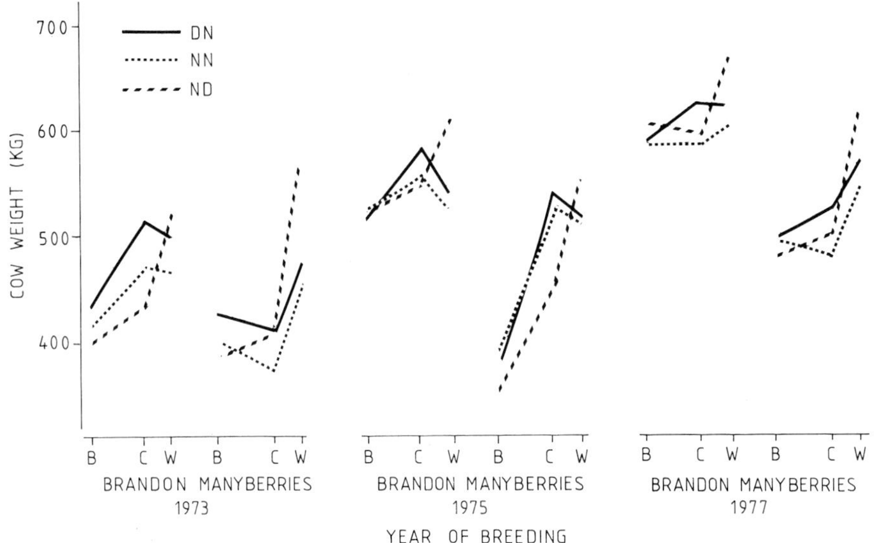

Fig. 6.3. Influence of cow nursing status on patterns of weight change from breeding (B) in year n to calving (C) and weaning (W) in year $n+1$ for cows born in 1971.

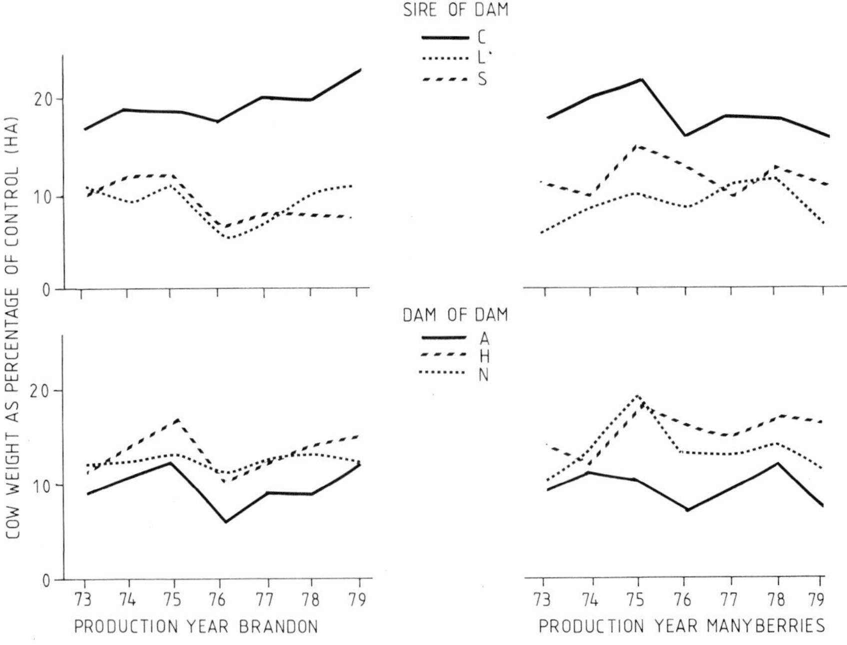

Fig. 6.4. Percentage deviations from contemporary control (Hereford × Angus) females in annual cow weaning weights in relation to sire breed and dam breed of the F_1 females.

5.1.2. Cow attrition

Total cow losses during the experiment were greater at Manyberries (32%) than at Brandon (27%). Most of the losses were due to breeding failure with 21% at Manyberries and 18% at Brandon culled as barren for two consecutive years. At both locations the lowest attrition rates were recorded for F_1 females sired by Charolais or out of Angus dams. The highest attrition rates were for females by Limousin sires or out of Shorthorn dams (Table 6.6.). Attrition was particularly high for the Limousin × Shorthorn cross, 46.2% at Brandon and 41.4% at Manyberries (Fredeen et al., 1981b). This specific cross also recorded the highest incidence of breeding failures.

TABLE 6.6

Percentage attrition due to culling for barren status vs. non-barren losses for all input females of each breed of sire and breed of dam group at each location

Culling cause: Breed cross[a]		Brandon			Manyberries		
		Barren	Other	Total	Barren	Other	Total
Sire	Dam						
H	A	17.3	5.4	22.7	21.3	9.4	30.7
C	H,A,N	16.0	4.0	20.0	14.9	11.4	26.3
S	H,A,N	18.6	9.8	28.4	20.4	14.5	34.9
L	H,A,N	20.1	13.4	33.5	26.6	7.7	34.3
C,S,L	H	19.6	9.2	28.8	21.1	12.6	33.7
C,S,L	A	14.8	6.8	21.6	15.4	8.7	24.1
C,S,L	N	20.3	11.7	32.0	25.7	12.6	38.3
Total		18.2	8.7	26.9	20.9	11.1	32.0

[a] Breed crosses defined in Table 6.4.

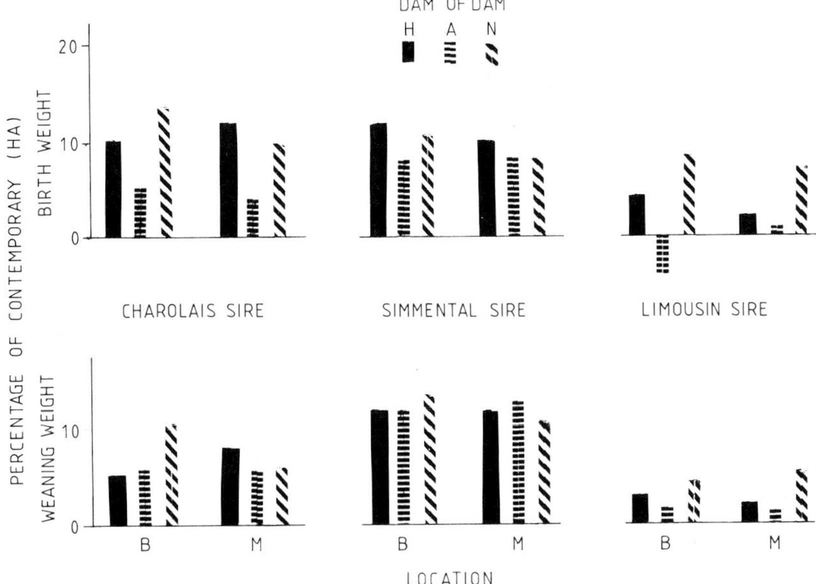

Fig. 6.5. Average weights at birth and weaning for progeny of each breed cross of dam expressed as percentage deviations from progeny weights for the contemporary control (Hereford × Angus) populations at Brandon (B) and Manyberries (M).

Chapter 6 references, p. 135

5.1.3. Calving ease and mortality

Sex of calf was the most important determinant of calving ease. Females at both locations averaged 6% less than males in birth weight and 9% of females required assistance compared with 22% for males. Hereford × Angus and Limousin × Angus produced calves with the lightest birth weights (Fig. 6.5) and required less calving assistance than progeny from other dam crosses. Location differences in calf weight at birth was negligible (Brandon greater by 1.2%) but there were no location differences in calving ease. However, the Brandon cows were substantially heavier at calving and the weight of calves born unassisted at this location averaged 8% of their dam's weight compared with 10–11% at Manyberries. Obviously the lighter weights of cows at Manyberries did not compromise calving ease.

Calf mortality at birth averaged 2.5% with no differences associated with location, sex of calf or breed cross. However, total pre-weaning mortality was greater for males than females (9.5 vs. 5.5%), greater at Manyberries than at Brandon (9.5 vs. 5.7%) and higher for progeny from dams sired by Limousin than for progeny from the other crosses (Fredeen et al., 1982a). This adverse result for the Limousin cross dams was not associated with calving difficulty as these dams required the least calving assistance.

One observation from the data was that for each breed cross of dam, greater calving difficulty was recorded from dams that had been dry the previous year than from those which had produced calves.

5.1.4. Pre-weaning growth

Average weaning weights of all progeny groups produced by dam crosses sired by Charolais, Limousin and Simmental sires exceeded those from the Hereford × Angus control (Fig. 6.5). Simmental cross cows weaned the heaviest calves at both locations with the greatest advantage over the Hereford × Angus (13.5%) recorded for the Simmental × Shorthorn dams at Brandon.

In terms of average daily gains to weaning, the progeny from the Limousin crosses were approximately equivalent to those from the Hereford × Angus and their differences in weaning weight (Fig. 6.5) represented little more than their average differences in birth weight (Fredeen et al. 1982b).

Pre-weaning growth rate was 10–13% greater at Brandon than at Manyberries and genotype–environment interactions were evident for this trait. Thus the ranking of cow crosses by their breed of dam for progeny growth rate and weaning weight was Shorthorn > Angus > Hereford > Hereford × Angus at Brandon and Hereford = Angus > Shorthorn > Hereford × Angus at Manyberries (Table 6.7).

These results suggest that the superior milk production expected of F_1 female progeny by Simmental sires or out of Shorthorn dams was more fully expressed under the Brandon than under the Manyberries environment.

5.1.5. Lifetime productivity

The 1150 F_1 females which entered the programme had a total of 1150 mating opportunities in their initial mating year with mating opportunities in each subsequent year diminished by cow attrition. The total number of mating opportunities recorded in the period 1971–78 was 6245. These resulted in 5053 pregnancies for a conception rate of 80.9% and 4640 calves weaned for a weaning rate of 74.5%.

Location differences in the incidence of barren matings (22% at Manyberries vs 16% at Brandon) and in total calf mortality (approximately 5% greater at Manyberries) resulted in a difference in weaning rates of 8.7% in favour of Brandon (Table 6.8). This difference, coupled with the Brandon advantage in pre-weaning growth rate, produced a location difference of 25% in the average

TABLE 6.7

Progeny performance averages and standard errors (SE) at Brandon (B) and Manyberries (MB) for dams sired by Charolais, Simmental and Limousin with probability levels (P) for dam differences (Dm) and location × dam (Lo–Dm) interaction

Breed cross[a]		Performance trait								
		Weaning age (days)			Adjusted weaning Weight (200 days) (kg)			Average daily gain to weaning (g)		
Terminal sires	Dam cross	B		MB	B		MB	B		MB
S,L,Chi	HA	196.0		191.6	211.1		190.4	855		752
	CH	194.5		190.5	222.4		203.6	890		794
	CA	194.0		189.7	224.8		201.5	912		798
	CN	196.5		193.1	232.4		200.8	935		783
		1.2		1.2	2.0		2.2	8		9
	P (Dm)		0.12			0.0001			0.0001	
	P (Lo–Dm)		—			0.005			0.01	
C,L,Chi	HA	196.3		192.1	211.2		190.3	856		751
	CH	193.4		190.4	238.1		213.9	966		850
	CA	192.5		188.9	238.6		213.6	973		849
	CN	195.3		190.5	239.9		211.6	976		837
		1.1		1.2	1.7		1.8	8		8
	P (Dm)		0.03			0.0001			0.0001	
	P (Lo–Dm)		—			—			—	
C,S,Chi	HA	196.3		190.9	215.0		192.8	868		761
	CH	194.2		191.1	221.8		195.5	888		767
	CA	193.3		190.7	220.6		193.5	897		761
	CN	195.5		191.2	227.5		203.2	915		798
		1.3		1.5	2.1		2.3	9		10
	P (Dm)		—			0.0001			0.0002	
	P /Lo-Dm)		—			—			—	

[a] Terminal sire breeds and dam crosses as defined for Table 6.4.

Chapter 6 references, p. 135

TABLE 6.8

Location differences in the primary factors associated with cow productivity

	Brandon	Manyberries	Total
Mating opportunities (MO)	3 186	3 077	6 245
Pregnancies (P)	2 653	2 400	5 053
Calves weaned (W)	2 489	2 151	4 640
Conception rate (% P of MO)	83.7	78.0	80.9
Weaning rate (% W of MO)	78.6	69.9	74.5
Barren rate (% B of MO)	16.3	22.0	19.1
Calf loss (% W of P)	6.2	10.4	8.2
Average weight of calf weaned per MO(kg)	170.0	135.4	153.0

weaned weight of calf produced per mating opportunity.

For each of these components of lifetime productivity there was evidence of genotype–environment interactions (Table 6.9). The highest conception rates were recorded for the Charolais × Angus at Brandon and Charolais × Shorthorn at Manyberries with the lowest rates given by Limousin × Angus at Brandon and Limousin × Shorthorn at Manyberries. The same breed cross rankings for weaning rates were observed at Brandon but at Manyberries the Charolais × Angus had the highest and the Limousin × Hereford the lowest rank.

Cow performance, summarized by breed of sire and breed of dam (Table 6.10), showed that the most durable females at both locations were those sired by Charolais or out of Angus dams. They had the least attrition and thus completed the highest percentages of potential breeding years in the project. Charolais-sired females also had the highest conception rates and highest weaning rates at both locations with breed of sire differences substantially greater at Manyberries than at Brandon. Smaller differences in these traits were associated with dam breed of the F_1 females but females out of Angus cows gave the highest weaning rate at Manyberries. For net productivity of each cross, estimated as the weight of calf weaned per mating opportunity, the females by Simmental sires or out of Shorthorn dams ranked highest at Brandon while those from Charolais sires or out of Angus dams were superior at Manyberries.

5.2. Integration of evidence

Long experience, both applied and experimental, has confirmed the importance of hybrid vigour to cattle production in western Canada. Purebred cattle of all breeds survive and reproduce well if suitably protected from environmental extremes but only through the exploitation of hybrid vigour is it possible to successfully raise cattle under the practical management conditions prevailing in the commercial industry.

The important contribution of heterosis to hardiness, specifically as expressed in the durability and reproductive performance of females, has been recognized and exploited by western Canadian cattlemen since the very beginning of cattle production in this area. Through experience, they learned that the best female cross among the breeds available to them was the Hereford × Angus. No one anticipated that the superiority of this cross, derived as it was from breeds of proven capabilities in Canada and continuously updated by the use of bulls from herds with long histories of acclimatization to the area, would be seriously challenged by crosses with any of the European breeds imported after 1950.

TABLE 6.9

Location differences among F^1 females born in 1971 for percentage conception, percentage weaned and average weight of calf weaned per mating opportunity

Breed cross[a]		Brandon			Manyberries		
Sire	Dam	% Conception	% weaned	Average weaning weight (kg)	% conception	% weaned	Average weaning weight (kg)
H	A	82.5	77.0	154	79.0	72.1	124
C	H	85.6	79.7	169	80.4	72.9	140
	A	87.6	81.4	175	82.0	76.9	144
	N	85.9	79.6	180	87.2	75.0	144
S	H	82.2	79.6	178	77.0	67.4	138
	A	85.5	80.8	182	77.3	73.3	145
	N	84.5	78.8	181	76.1	66.7	136
L	H	80.7	75.9	163	69.8	64.3	120
	A	79.2	72.8	150	78.8	66.3	121
	N	84.7	77.0	167	75.7	67.5	129
Total		83.8	78.2	170	78.2	70.1	138

[a] Breed crosses defined for Table 6.4.

Chapter 6 references, p. 135

TABLE 6.10

Average performance of first-cross females, summarized by their breed of sire and breed of dam, for components of lifetime reproduction

Breed cross[a]	Brandon					Manyberries				
	Total cow losses (%)	Years in herd as a percentage of potential years	Conceptions per mating opportunity (%)	Calves weaned per mating opportunity (%)	Weight of calf weaned per mating opportunity (kg)	Total cow losses (%)	Years in herd as a percentage of potential years	Conceptions per mating opportunity (%)	Calves weaned per mating opportunity (%)	Weight of calf weaned per mating opportunity (kg)
HA	22.7	88	82.5	77.0	154	30.7	84	79.0	72.1	124
C	20.0	91	86.2	80.1	176	26.3	88	83.6	74.9	143
S	28.4	89	84.0	79.9	181	34.9	84	76.8	69.0	139
L	33.5	86	82.1	75.8	161	34.3	81	74.8	66.4	125
H	28.8	89	82.6	78.6	171	33.7	84	76.1	68.2	133
A	21.6	92	84.0	78.4	172	24.1	88	79.1	72.5	139
N	32.0	84	84.9	78.4	176	38.3	81	79.0	69.3	135

[a] Breed crosses as defined in Table 6.4.

Interest in these breeds derived solely from their attributes of growth and carcase, attributes which gave promise of their potential value as terminal sires. Winter hardiness and reproductive performance were not considered relevant since they and their top-cross progeny would be reared under management and housing practices that provided protection against climatic extremes.

Canadian research experience with these breeds has confirmed the expectation of their potential for enhancing growth and carcase merit of their crossbred progeny (e.g., Rahnefeld et al., 1983). More important, however, is the detailed evidence it has provided on the superior lifetime reproductive performance of their crossbred females relative to the traditional Hereford × Angus cross and the interplay between genetics and environment in the expression of reproductive traits.

This Canadian research has encompassed few of the many new breeds now available in this country. These few breeds, however, were chosen deliberately to represent a wide range of mature size and milking potential. Thus the significance of the results obtained rests not in the specific breeds compared but rather in the generalizations they subtend regarding the nature of genotype–environment interactions.

Central to these generalizations is the biological fact that reproduction, while a regular occurrence in the normal life cycle of a beef cow, imposes certain stresses on the female. Further, the degree of stress will be directly related to productivity. Thus cows with the greatest potential for milk production will be more heavily stressed during the lactation period than those of low milking potential and this stress will be accentuated by any environmental adversities that may occur.

The female's genetic potential for milk production will be modified in some degree by the environment but, in general, she will tend to maintain lactation under adverse environments by drawing on her own energy reserves. Prolonged anoestrus thus becomes her only defence against the body depletion that accompanies this sacrifice to the milk demands of her calf. The direct economic benefits of rapid pre-weaning growth are self-evident but they can be more than nullified by the economic losses associated with reduced conception rates.

In their choice of breeds for production of hybrid females, cattlemen must seek to match the genetic potential for lactation with the environment they are prepared to provide. Failure to achieve the proper balance will compromise attainment of maximum productivity.

An extensive body of research information has been developed on the relationship between nutritional status and reproductive performance of the bovine female (e.g., Lamond, 1970). This literature has subtended general recommendations on nutritional standards (e.g., Anon., 1965; 1976). Unfortunately, these recommendations lack the precision required for meaningful extension to the variety of environmental conditions encountered in beef production. Experience with the F_1 cow herd maintained under the Manyberries environment has indicated that backfat thickness at weaning time, which serves as both an insulator and as a source of energy for the cow, is a crucial indicator of her potential for winter survival and/or successful conception the following summer (Lawson, 1984). Problems arise when average fat, measured ultrasonically at weaning time, is less than 5 mm. Such measurements have characterized all F_1 crosses at Manyberries (0–5 mm) except the Hereford × Angus (8–9 mm) and the daily energy intake required to restore fat levels to 5 mm have ranged from 30 to 50% higher than the intakes recommended (Anon, 1965; 1976). These same data have demonstrated that, even with these increased levels, it may prove impossible to save very thin cows, particularly when they are exposed to severe winter wind chill.

Chapter 6 references, p. 135

6. FUTURE RESEARCH

Since completion of this study on lifetime reproductive performance, the F_1 cow herds at the two locations have been employed in a study of breed cross differences in feed energy requirements for winter maintenance and summer lactation. Data collected have included all the items recorded during the preceding reproductive studies plus daily feed intake, milk production and composition, and frequent ultrasonic measurements of backfat on all cows to provide a comprehensive evaluation of the rate of fat depletion and restoration during each reproductive cycle. Data analyses, when completed, may provide more meaningful guidelines for establishing energy intake levels.

The study was broadened in 1979 to evaluate the lifetime reproductive performance under the same environments of back-cross females produced by mating between the F_1 cows and sires of their parental breeds. The back-cross herds, totalling approximately 1200 breeding females, will complete their reproductive cycles in 1987. At that time they will be replaced by multidisciplinary studies of genetic differences in various components of the reproductive cycle.

The breeding herds for these studies will represent the direct descendants of the F_1 females which recorded above-average lifetime reproductive performance in the period 1972–79. Matings for this study have been in progress for 3 years. The cow herds projected after 1987 will range between 500 and 800 breeding females at each location (Brandon and Manyberries). Exchanges of females between the two locations after that date will add additional information on genotype–environment interactions.

Eight elements of the western Canadian research programme initiated with these new breeds in the late 1960's have been crucial to its success:

(1) Inclusion of a substantial control population (Hereford × Angus) of proven adaptability, performance and acceptabilty to the cattle industry.

(2) Designation of two locations which provided a clear contrast among the environments which feature conventional cattle production practices.

(3) Choice of breeds to represent a range of biological types.

(4) Solid pre-planning of the statistical design, of the comprehensive performance data requirements, and of the management and recording systems to be employed.

(5) Large animal populations.

(6) Project design, operation and interpretation by Canadian scientists with solid backgrounds of practical and research experience in western beef cattle production.

(7) Unbroken continuity of project involvement by these scientists.

(8) Their direct and continuous 'hands on' approach to all operational procedures and data recordations.

These elements have been incorporated in the western Canadian research now planned and/or in progress and they represent the basic principles which should characterize any research intended to evaluate the genetic resources present in the world's livestock populations. The purposes they serve are, for the most part, self-evident. Genetic research with the bovine, the species of farm livestock with the lowest reproductive rate and the longest generation interval, involves large annual investments which must be continued over long periods of time. To justify these expenditures, animal breeding research programmes must be designed to maximize the yield of statistically valid data covering the entire spectrum of performance traits. The requisites of such experimental designs are large animal populations, appropriate controls, thorough pre-planning, and comprehensive recording of performance data.

Less evident, perhaps, is the relevance of those elements relating to the qualifications and dedication of the scientists involved. Suffice it to say that an adequate understanding of the livestock and the livestock husbandry practices appropriate to any given country is not provided by the written word. It comes from hands-on experience in that country. Advanced scientific training and experience in statistics, genetics and other relevant disciplines are obviously essential but the trained scientist who lacks appropriate and thorough hands-on experience is ill-equipped to plan, let alone supervise, research of the magnitude required to evaluate livestock genetic resources.

7. REFERENCES

Anon., 1965. The Nutrient Requirements of Farm Livestock, No. 2, Ruminants. Agricultural Research Council. London.

Anon., 1976. Nutrient Requirements of Beef Cattle (5th Edition revised). U.S. National Research Council, National Academy of Sciences, Washington, D.C.

Deakin, A., Muir, G.W. and Smith, A.G., 1935. Hybridization of domestic cattle, bison and yak. Publication 479, Canadian Department of Agriculture.

Fredeen, H.T., 1980. The Canadian beef industry. Can. Vet. J., 21: 39–46.

Fredeen, H.T., Weiss, G.M., Rahnefeld, G.W., Lawson, J.E. and Newman, J.A., 1981a. Growth patterns of first-cross cows under two environments. Can. J. Anim. Sci., 61: 243–259.

Fredeen, H.T., Weiss, G.M., Lawson, J.E., Newman, J.A. and Rahnefeld, G.W., 1981b. Lifetime reproductive efficiency of first-cross beef cows under contrasting environments. Can. J. Anim. Sci., 61: 539–554.

Fredeen, H.T., Weiss, G.M., Rahnefeld, G.W., Lawson, J.E. and Newman, J.A., 1982a. Environmental and genetic effects on pre-weaning performance of calves from first-cross cows. 1. Calving ease and pre-weaning mortality. Can. J. Anim. Sci., 62: 35–49.

Fredeen, H.T., Weiss, G.M., Rahnefeld, G.W., Lawson, J.E. and Newman, J.A., 1982b. Environmental and genetic effects on pre-weaning performance of calves from first-cross. II. Growth traits. Can. J. Anim. Sci., 62: 51–68.

Keller, D.G. and Lawson, J.E., 1978. Influence of bison percentage on pre- and post-weaning traits of cattalo calves. Can. J. Anim. Sci., 58: 537–545.

Lamond, D.R., 1970. The influence of undernutrition in reproduction in the cow. Anim. Breeding Abstr. 38: 359–372.

Lawson, J.E., 1983. Canadian Government beef breeding research. Proc. Western Region Coord. Comm., Beef Breeding Research, Havre, Mont. (unpubl.), 6 pp.

Lawson, J.E., 1984. Selection of range cattle: A Canadian viewpoint. Lethbridge Research Station, Mimeo, 10 pp.

Lawson,J.E. and Peters, H.F., 1976. Growth and carcass traits of Cattalo, Hereford and 1/4 Brahman bull calves. Can.J. Anim. Sci., 56: 193–199.

Lawson,J.E., Fredeen, H.T., Newman, J.A. and Rahnefeld G.W., 1980. Crosses of three exotic and three British breeds: Performance in two environments of two-year old cows and their calves. Can. J. Anim. Sci., 60: 811–824.

MacEwan, J.W.G., 1941. The Breeds of Livestock in Canada. Thomas Nelson, Toronto, 526 pp.

Mason,I.L., 1969. A dictionary of livestock breeds. Technical Communication 8, Commonwealth Agricultural Bureaux, Farnham Royal, U.K.

Peters, H.F. and Newbound, K.B., 1957. Intra-testicular temperature and fertility of bison, cattalo and Hereford yearling bulls. Can. J. Anim. Sci., 37: 14–20.

Rahnefeld, G.W., Fredeen, H.T., Weiss, G.M., Lawson, J.E. and Newman, J.A., 1983. Breed of terminal sire effects on carcass characteristics of three-way cross cattle reared at two locations. Can. J. Anim. Sci., 63: 523–549.

Shaw, A.M. and MacEwan, J.W.G., 1938. An experiment in beef production in western Canada. Sci. Agric., 19(4): 177–198.

Vaughn, H.W., 1931. Breeds of Livestock in America. R.G. Adams, Columbus, Ohio, 780 pp.

Chapter 7

Genetic Resource Problems: Temperate North America

T.G. MARTIN

1. INTRODUCTION

Cattle genetic resources of temperate North America have been utilized in the development of two highly specialized industries. One emphasizes genetic potential for milk production while the other develops cattle particularly adapted for meat production. In the beef industry, some farm and ranch units concentrate on maintenance of cow herds and production of feeder calves while others specialize in feeding cattle prior to slaughter. The management of available genetic resources is unique for each industry.

Four species *(Bos taurus, Bos indicus, Bos bubalis* and *Bison bison)* contribute to production of meat and milk. The latter two are present in small numbers and their limited contribution is to the meat production industry.

Characteristics of the cattle population, beef industry and dairy industry (U.S. Department of Agriculture, 1983; B.W. Kennedy, personal communication, 1984) are shown in Table 7.1.

2. PRESENT AND FUTURE STATUS OF CATTLE POPULATIONS

2.1. The dairy industry

North Americans consume 69.9 million tonnes of milk annually which is produced by 12.8 million lactating cows. The total number of dairy cows has remained stable since 1976 but has declined by almost 50% since 1945. In that period, total milk production has remained constant. Constant total supply coupled with increased population has resulted in reduced per capita consumption with the current rate at 112 litres of fluid milk and 186 kg of whole milk equivalent as other dairy products.

Production levels have increased almost 100% since 1945 due to improved selection techniques and high levels of grain feeding. The average cow in U.S.A. and Canada, respectively, consumes 2445 and 2006 kg concentrates to produce 5598 and 4496 kg milk. Average numbers of cows per herd are 37 and 32, respectively, in U.S.A. and Canada. In both countries, more than 40% of the cows are on milk recording programmes. Herds following performance testing programmes have almost twice as many cows per herd and herd average milk yields 25% higher than the national averages. Income from milk sales represents approximately 20% of total farm income.

2.2. The beef industry

North Americans consume 11.5 million tonnes of beef and veal derived from

Chapter 7 references, p. 150

TABLE 7.1

Characteristics of the cattle population, beef industry and dairy industry in temperate North America

Item	U.S.	Canada	Combined
No. of cattle[a] (millions)	115.6	12.1	127.7[b]
No. of dairy cows 2 years or older (millions)	11.1	1.87	13.0[b]
Milk production (million tonnes)	61.6	7.8	69.4[b]
Liquid milk consumption (litres per person)	111.8	109.3	111.6[c]
Milk production (kg per dairy cow)	5,598	4,496	5,452[c]
Milk processing, fluid/factory (%/%)	38/62	34/66	37.5/62.5[c]
Dairy cows on performance test (%)	43	49	43.8[c]
No. of beef cows 2 years or older (millions)	38.1	3.5	41.6[b]
Beef and veal production, carcase (million tonnes)	10.5	1.0	11.5[b]
Beef and veal consumption (kg per person)	45.4	41.6	45.0[c]
Carcase production (kg per cow)	213.4	192.3	211.4[c]

[a] Beef cows + dairy cows
[b] Total.
[c] Weighted average based on population, number of cows, or number of dairy cows.

54.4 million cows. Specialized beef cows represent 76% (41.6 million) of the total cow herd. The number of beef cows has declined from a maximum of 49 million in 1975. Current consumption rate is 45 kg of carcase beef per person. Carcase beef production per cow is currently 211 kg. This high level of production is attributable to heavy slaughter weight, moderately high birth rate and low death rate. Only 8% of the slaughter cattle are calves while 65% are young cattle (< 2 years of age) which have been fed on grain. Only 28% are cows, bulls and young grass-fed cattle. Average carcase weight is more than 270 kg. Annual calf crop varies from 85 to 90% of the number of cows present on farms and average annual death rate is less than 5%. The most unique characteristic of the North American beef industry is the proportion of young cattle finished on feed grains. The beef industry produces 20–25% of total farm cash receipts.

2.3. Geographic distribution of cattle

Large numbers of cattle are found in all regions of North America. The variation is associated with types of cattle rather than with population density of cattle. Northeast and eastern/north-central regions have 56% of the dairy cows and 45% of the population of U.S.A. Eastern Canada is the home of 72% of the people and 77% of the dairy cows in Canada.

Western/north-central and south-central regions contain 53% of the beef cattle of U.S.A. In the two regions, there are 8.98 beef cows per km^2 which is more than 10 times the concentration of dairy cows in the same regions. Western Canada has 70% of the beef cows in Canada. Beef cattle population is most dense in areas of lower population density having moderate to high rainfall and sufficient soil fertility to support high production levels of forage and/or grain. The regions having the greatest numbers of beef cattle are also regions which produce large amounts of feed grains and have lower human populations.

2.4. Buffalo in North America

The University of Florida at Gainesville maintained a research herd of approximately 100 buffalo for several years. Hentges et al. (1978) reported a comparison of *B. bubalis* (Buffalo), *B. indicus* (Brahman) and *B. taurus* (Angus). Buffalo were observed to be more heat tolerant than Angus cattle in the summer and more tolerant of cold and wind in the winter than Brahman cattle. Growth rate of buffalo calves was comparable to that of Angus and Brahman calves on improved pasture. However, lower reproductive rate and longer gestation periods resulted in lower levels of total productivity for buffalo. Buffalo readily consumed forage of low quality aquatic and semi-aquatic plants when confined to a lakeside ecosystem. Their conclusions were that buffalo may offer an economically viable means of utilizing swamp and marshland which will not support cattle and that buffalo are not likely to replace beef cattle on improved pastures. The Florida herd is now privately owned and there is at least one other sizeable herd located in southern California. The buffalo population does not currently constitute an economically important segment of North American cattle and buffalo genetic resources.

2.5. Bison in North America (Fig. 7.1)

Hudson and Bunnell (1981) reported that there are more than 40000 plains bison and small numbers of wood bison located in parks and reserves and on private ranches in North America. Bison are cross-fertile with cattle (Peters, 1958) and, when present, compete with cattle for feed resources. As a result, they must be considered to be part of the genetic resources available to the beef industry.

2.6. Future of the cattle industry

In the various regions of the world, future development of cattle populations will require different population structures, market balances and selection goals. In North America, the total of 127.7 million cattle, a few hundred buffalo and 40000 bison will change in response to changes in both local and world demand for the various food sources.

Dairy cattle numbers have stabilized and are meeting market demands by increasing level of production per cow. Increased proportion of Holstein cattle

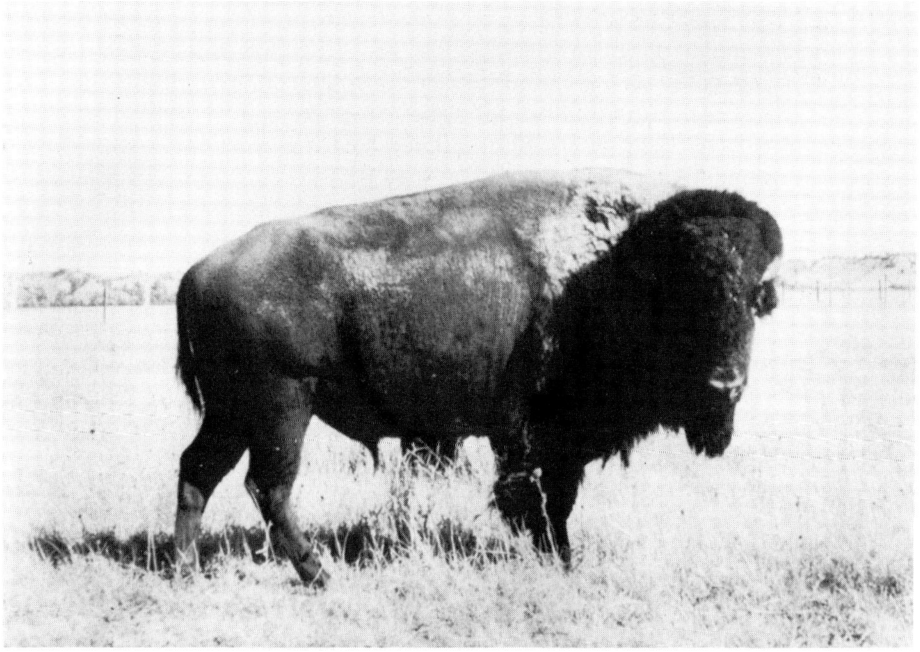

Fig. 7.1. American bison, *Bison bison*. Courtesy of Department of Animal Sciences, Purdue University, West Lafayette, Indiana.

Chapter 7 references, p. 150

(86% in U.S.A. according to Sechrist, 1980), increased levels of grain feeding and larger specialized dairy herds have contributed to higher cow productivity. Numbers should remain relatively constant, but either high cost or reduced supply of feed grains could lead to increased numbers of dairy cows.

Beef cattle numbers have been sensitive to changes in price of beef, weather patterns and declining numbers of sheep and dairy cattle. Greater world demand for grain crops would reduce meat production per cow, but increased beef production and number of beef cattle could be associated with improved forage crop technology and utilization of grain crop residues such as stalks and straw. The number of beef cattle should increase slightly in the future.

Buffalo numbers are likely to increase only if meat demand requires increased interest in exploiting marginal wetlands which will not support cattle. There is no reason to expect bison numbers to increase.

3. BREEDING PROGRAMMES

The two major methods of improving genetic capacity for production are selection, which implies that a performance testing programme exists, and crossbreeding. Selection leads to increased frequency of desirable characteristics which are transmissible from parent to offspring while crossbreeding leads to increased frequency of non-transmissible effects associated with the heterozygous genetic state. Since cattle breeding is directed toward specialized objectives in North America, the beef and dairy cattle breeding programmes are each structured to meet the needs of a specific industry. Differences in the programmes may be traced to heritability and mode of expression of principal characteristics, characteristics of and variation among available breeds and degree of acceptance of artificial insemination (AI).

3.1. Dairy cattle programmes

3.1.1. Selection

Genetic improvement of dairy cattle has been primarily based on selection favouring high milk yield. The pricing structure of most milk markets has made this one trait inordinately high in economic importance. Early efforts to measure milk yield of individual cows eventually led to establishment of centralized dairy herd improvement (DHI) programmes in both U.S.A. and Canada. Currently, more than 40% of all cows are enrolled in DHI.

These data have been used to estimate breeding values (EBV) of sires for more than 40 years. AI was fully accepted in the dairy industry shortly after it became available. More accurate estimation of breeding values, based on progeny test (daughter performance), became possible due to increased numbers of daughters and due to usage of sires in multiple herds. Development of methods for freezing semen and the advent of the computer allowed even wider usage of sires and accumulation of records from all states or provinces. Contemporary comparison and mixed model analysis techniques (Henderson, 1973) are now used to estimate EBV of sires.

Attainable annual genetic change in milk yield associated with single-trait selection was estimated by Specht and McGilliard (1960) to be 1.0–2.3%. However, genetic improvement actually achieved was only 0.7–1.3%. The slippage presumably was largely due to selection for traits other than milk yield. The problem posed by these results is that of the appropriateness of selection actually being practised by dairymen.

Freeman (1976) and Skjervold (1963) estimated that approximately 45, 28, 21 and 6%, respectively, of attainable genetic progress occurs through selection of sires of bulls, dams of bulls, sires of cows and dams of cows. As a result, considerable effort is now exerted in identifying dams of bulls to be entered into progeny test. EBV's of high producing cows are now calculated using the same data and techniques as are used to identify high EBV sires.

Accuracy of the sire evaluation programmes was tested by Croak-Brossman et al. (1982) using the design proposed by Hickman and Freeman (1969). High EBV (+487 kg milk) and average EBV (+3 kg milk) groups of sires produced daughters which differed by 670 kg milk yield. Expected difference was 484 kg milk yield. This study also indicated that daughters of high genetic potential sires were more subject to mastitis, disease and injury than daughters of average genetic potential sires. High genetic potential plus high levels of grain feeding place considerable stress on cows. As a result the average life of a dairy cow is less than four lactations in North America.

3.1.2. Corrective mating

Phenotypic assortative mating systems have been advocated since Bakewell set forth the principle of 'mating the best to the best' more than 200 years ago. Various organizations in North America are currently advocating systems of 'corrective mating' which is a form of negative assortative mating. Inordinate attention to correcting type or conformation traits could easily lead to reduced selection differential for milk yield, while use of sires high in EBV milk yield whose daughters are unsound could easily reduce average herd life.

Lush (1945) described the effects of assortative mating as influencing the variance rather than the mean of populations. McGilliard and Clay (1983) described a system of defining herd breeding goals, selecting a group of sires which will attain those goals and using those sires in a practical manner to avoid excessive inbreeding and to mate cows with serious faults to bulls with strength in those traits. The emphasis should be on the bulls selected rather than on how they are mated.

3.1.3. Crossbreeding

Young (1984) reviewed crossbreeding in dairy cattle and concluded that it offers potential improvement of genetic merit through two avenues. As the mating system pairing mates which are least alike, it offers the opportunity to create genotypes with a high degree of heterozygosity and consequent heterosis. Secondly, it is a means of transferring genes from one population to another or of forming a new breed by combining genes from two or more existing breeds.

Crossbreeding has not been adopted by the dairy industry in North America. The Holstein average milk yield is 15–20% higher than that of any other breed present in North America. Milk payment systems emphasize milk yield or volume and do not adequately reward higher solids production. The estimates of heterosis for individual traits tend to be low. Touchberry (1970) and McDowell (1976) suggested that accumulation of heterosis over several traits creates an economic situation such that crossbreeding could be used to advantage under present and past circumstances. A summary by Martin (1978) concludes that some crosses have been shown to equal, but not exceed, the Holstein with regard to economic return.

Crossbreeding has generally produced a genetic buffering system which results in greater relative advantage where environment is not optimum or where management is marginal. The commercial dairyman who has experienced problems concerning calf mortality, difficult breeding and cow longevity might well benefit by using an occasional outstanding sire from a breed other than the Holstein. Irregular usage of sires from other breeds would also alleviate problems which might be associated with inbreeding.

The use of crossbreeding as a means of improving a breed or forming a new

Chapter 7 references, p. 150

breed was discussed by Martin (1978). Two principles must be followed if crossbreeding is to be a major breeding system in North America. The two or more breeds must each be superior and their genetic backgrounds must be different. If two breeds are to be used, the second breed must be brought to approximately 90% of the level of the Holstein in terms of milk yield and/or economic return.

Two research projects in North America have used crossbreeding to form an improved breed or line. The A line in the Agriculture Canada project (McAllister et al., 1978) was initiated using Ayrshire from Canada, Finland and U.S.A., Brown Swiss from U.S.A. and Norwegian Red breeds. C.W. Young (personal communication, 1984) formed a red and white breed based on the Milking Shorthorn from U.S.A. and New Zealand, Illawara Shorthorn from Australia, Ayrshire from U.S.A. and Canada and Norwegian Red breeds. Production levels have not equalled the Holstein levels. However, both groups report regular and consistent progress relative to milk yield, milk composition and fitness characteristics.

3.1.4. Herd stratification

Lush (1945) described a pyramidal breeding structure of a breed which is composed of three segments: (1) elite breeders who produce most of the purebred sires, (2) propagators who buy sires from elite breeders and sell sires to commercial producers and (3) commercial producers. The genetic time lag was two generations from the elite to the commercial segments.

Artificial insemination more or less relegated the propagators to the role of commercial producers. Frozen semen and computer processing of records have further altered the structure of the dairy breeds. AI organizations have combined and the sire selection committees now use a list of high EBV cows to select mothers of bulls to be progeny tested. The elite cow herd consists of the top 5% of cows with little regard for location of the herds in segments of the pyramid. The elite sires consist of the AI sires having the highest EBV's. Services of the elite sires are equally available to all herds. In effect, the AI organizations are now the elite breeders and virtually all herds are commercial producers. However, a few high producing herds contain a significantly higher proportion of mothers of bulls than would be expected based on chance alone.

Burnside et al. (1982) suggested that a global strategy for dairy cattle breeding should be considered. They indicated that this strategy should consider population sizes, breeding goals, exchange of semen between populations, inbreeding, heterosis and development of new breeds by crossbreeding existing breeds.

3.2. Beef cattle programmes

3.2.1. Selection

Performance testing programmes for beef cattle were initiated in the 1940's and emphasized growth rate initially. Weaning (205-day) and yearling (365-day) weights along with post-weaning gain were the basic characteristics included in the early programmes. Each state and breed developed its own programme and, while there are common traits, the programmes have not been completely standardized.

The number of traits which must be considered in developing a profitable beef industry include growth rate, carcase characteristics, feed conversion of growing animals and cows and maternal characteristics. In the cow–calf phase of the industry, such factors as calving ease (dystocia), fertility, calf viability and milking ability (progeny weaning weight) influence cow productivity and enterprise profitability. In the feedlot industry, growth rate, feed conversion, carcase composition and carcase quality grade affect profitability.

There has been considerable diversity of opinion concerning the overall description of the animal or family of animals which will best meet the needs of processors, retailers and consumers. Changing price structures favouring heavier or lighter carcases and changing standards for the various grades of carcases have made it difficult to establish selection goals. In some cases, the desired combination has involved changing genetically antagonistic traits. The most notable example involves the dual grading system of carcase evaluation where the desired product should contain a low proportion of fat to produce a high yield of lean cuts and a moderately high degree of intramuscular fat (marbling) to produce the U.S. Department of Agriculture choice quality grade which has been used as a measure of tenderness and palatability (Fig. 7.2).

Based on the breed promotion advertising, each breed would like to be recognized as the one breed which will best meet all needs of the industry. Therefore, many breeds have developed performance testing programmes which include growth traits, maternal traits and carcase traits. Willham (1982a,b) described the performance programmes of ten breed associations, the use of reference sires to obtain between-herd estimates of breeding value (EBV) and the methods of computation of EBV.

Because of the large number of traits influencing either biological or economic efficiency of production, the definition of desired selection goals for beef cattle is not a simple problem. Dickerson (1982) states that 'clear definition of breeding objectives is essential if livestock breeding programs are to have maximum impact upon the efficiency of animal production.' He defines biological efficiency as feed energy (or protein) input per unit of output and states that this measure of efficiency is largely independent of variability in prices of input and output units. He defines economic efficiency as the total enterprise costs per unit of animal product.

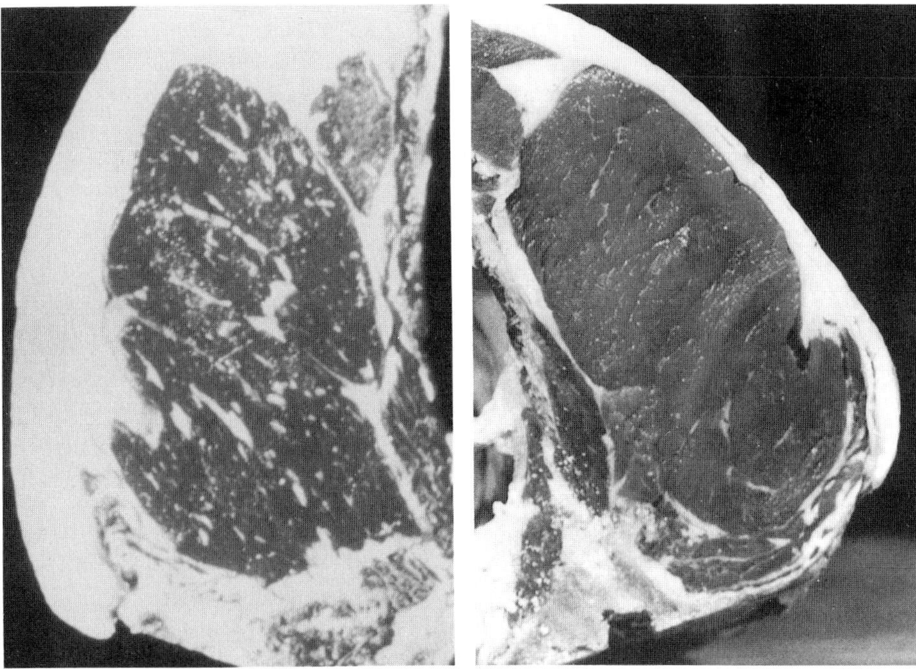

Fig. 7.2. American Quality and Yield grading systems represent antagonistic selection objectives. The highly marbled USDA Prime carcase (left) represents the highest quality grade while the USDA Standard carcase (right) is three grades lower. Yield grades are USDA No. 4 (left) and USDA No. 1 (right).

Chapter 7 references, p. 150

Breeders of beef cattle have made less than optimal changes in production efficiency because their selection goals have been based on fashionable conformation or easily measured traits such as growth rate. The effects of single-trait selection may be evaluated by considering the study reported by Martin and Alenda (1982). Annual genetic increase of 4.06 kg weight (at 365 days of age) was accompanied by a reduction in carcase fat percentage and an increase in carcase lean percentage. A later analysis of the cow productivity traits in the same herd (Leusakul-Reodecha, 1983) revealed that increased 365-day weight was associated with delayed age at sexual maturity and reduced cow longevity. Excessive emphasis on a single trait led to negative effects on other components of the efficiency equation.

Wilton (1979) discussed the use of mathematical modelling in defining selection goals and concluded that statement of the economic objective in terms of maximizing return per breeding female or return per herd or of minimizing cost per unit of product may lead to very different optima for the component characteristics. He also suggested that use of more complex selection indices may be necessary to properly consider traits which are quadratically related to the efficiency function and to restrict change in certain traits to a specific amount.

Quadratic response of economic efficiency indices to changes in growth and milk production were demonstrated by Cartwright (1979). This type of response dictates that, at some level of milk production or growth rate, selection methods must be directed toward minimizing change.

The combination of component traits (growth, mature body size, reproductive rate, milking ability, etc.) which will produce optimal economic response may be different for each set of environmental factors (climate, available feed, etc.). The development of optimal selection strategy for beef cattle will require that research workers estimate both direct and correlated response to selection favouring the major traits. Cartwright (1979) stated that reproduction, growth rate (body size), maturity rate and milk production differences accounted for most of the differences in economic efficiency.

Wilton (1979) stated that selection objectives in the purebreds would not be the same for breeds contributing to commercial production as purebreds, breeds used in a rotational cross, breeds used to produce crossbred commercial cows (maternal breeds) or breeds used to sire commercial calves (paternal breeds).

The resources provided by computer simulation, analyses of field data and applied breeding experiments are all needed to answer the complex problems involved in a complete selection programme for beef cattle.

3.2.2. Crossbreeding and breed comparison

Prior to 1950, there were only a few British-origin breeds plus Brahman *(B. indicus)* cattle in temperate North America and the general pattern of production was to rely on purebreds to produce beef in the U.S.A. and Canada. Importation of Charolais was followed by importation of continental European breeds such as Simmental, Limousin, Chianina, Pinzgauer, Gelbvieh and many others.

New breeds were formed as early as the 1930's in southern U.S.A. Fusion of one or more British breed(s) with Brahman provided the basis for breeds such as Santa Gertrudis (Shorthorn and Brahman), Brangus (Angus and Brahman) and Braford (Hereford and Brahman) (see Figs 7.3, 7.4 and 7.5). In recent years, several other new breeds have been established. There are presently more than 50 breeds of beef cattle in North America. Comparison of these breeds and evaluation of crossbreeding was the major topic of investigations conducted in the 1960's and 1970's.

Cundiff (1982) described the systems of utilizing crossbreeding as:

(1) rotational crossing produces relatively high amounts of heterosis, but additive genetic differences among breeds may cause considerable variation from one generation to the next;
(2) static-terminal-sire systems maximize the use of additive breed differences and complementarity between breeds but, since about 50% of the cows and 25% of the calves are purebreds, maximum heterosis is produced in only 50% of the progeny;

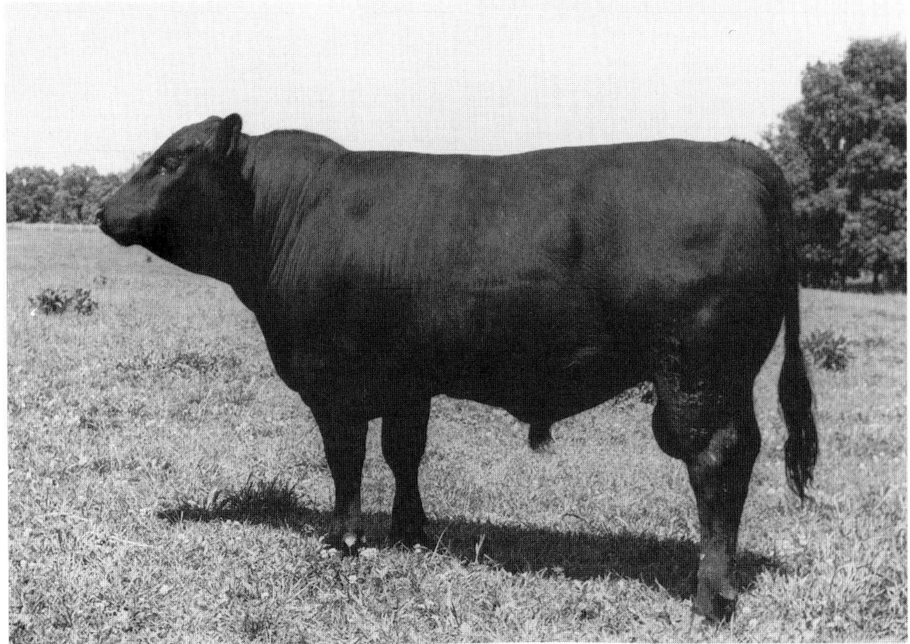

Fig. 7.3. American Angus bull representative of the *Bos taurus* species.

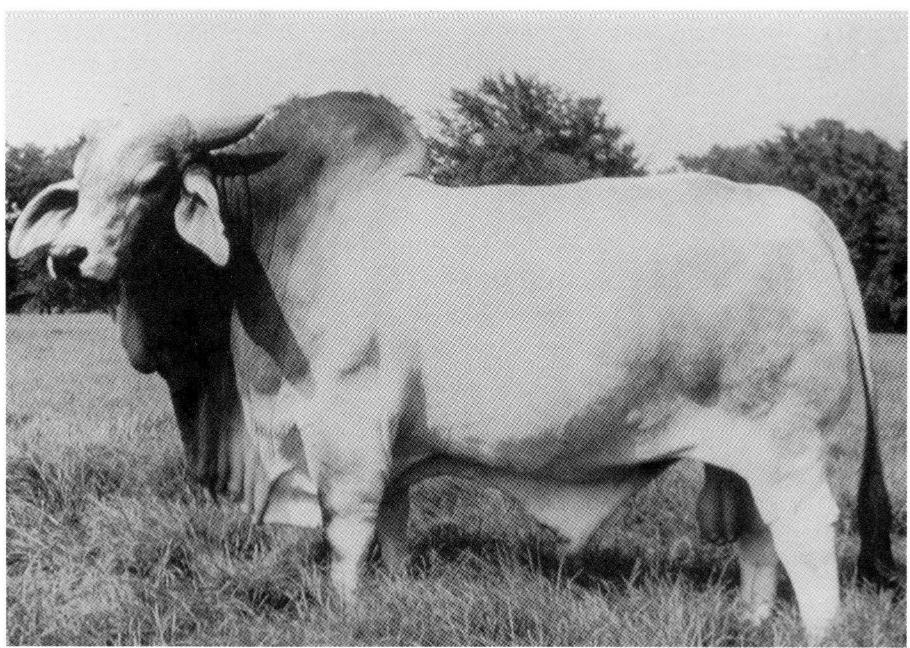

Fig. 7.4. American Brahman bull representative of the *Bos indicus* species. (Photo courtesy of the American Brahman Breeders' Association, Houston, Texas.)

Chapter 7 references, p. 150

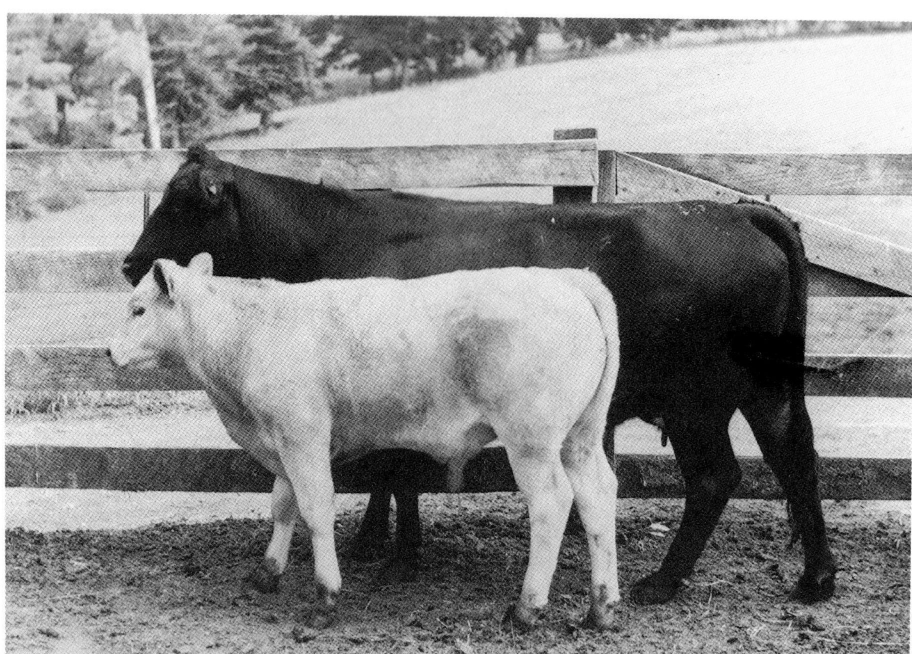

Fig. 7.5. Angus × Milking Shorthorn F_1 cow with calf sired by a Charolais bull.

(3) rotational-terminal-sire systems produce maternal and individual heterosis through rotational crossing of maternal breeds to produce commercial females and also utilize additive breed differences and complementarity by using large, lean breeds as terminal sires to produce about 50% of the calves; and
(4) composite breed formation utilizes both additive and non-additive effects to degrees intermediate to those of the rotational and static-terminal-sire systems.

Dickerson (1973) expressed additive genetic effects, heterosis effects and recombination loss associated with the individual, the dam and the sire as deviations from the mean of purebreds entered in the crossbreeding system. Alenda et al. (1980) estimated these effects through linear contrasts of breed means while Dillard et al. (1980) obtained these estimates by regression techniques. Estimates of these effects are needed in order to make intelligent choices of breeds for specific crossbreeding systems.

Breed evaluation or comparison may be approached by comparing straightbreds, conducting a diallele cross or comparing top-cross individuals. Comparison of straightbreds estimates the breed additive differences but does not provide a good estimate of comparison of breeds in specific crosses.

The diallel cross coupled with a generation of back-crosses or three-breed crosses can be used to derive accurate estimates of the individual and maternal additive and heterosis effects. However, the number of classes of breed combinations required to complete the experiment is quite large and diallel designs involving more than three or four breeds are rarely used with cattle. Alenda et al. (1980) reported means for 27 breed classes including straightbreds, F_1's, three-breed crosses and back-crosses with only three breeds.

Large numbers of breeds may be compared using top-cross evaluations where all breeds of sires are mated to one or two well-adapted native breeds. Two-breed rotational crosses plus F_2 and F_3 matings made in subsequent generations will provide estimates of the maternal and genetic effects. Cundiff

(1982) gives a brief report of a top-cross evaluation of 16 sire breeds conducted at the U.S. Meat Animal Research Center. More detailed reports of these studies may be found in the series of progress reports (e.g., Cundiff et al., 1984).

Numerous other crossbreeding studies have been conducted in Canada and U.S.A. In general, the conclusions have shown:

(1) Sire breed influences rate of growth of calves with a strong positive correlation between mature size and growth rate.
(2) Carcase traits are influenced by sire breed. Large breeds generally produce leaner carcases with less marbling than those from small breeds.
(3) Females from smaller breeds reach puberty at earlier ages and lighter weights than those from large breeds.
(4) Crossbred cows produce a higher percentage calf crop than purebred cows.
(5) Crossbred calves grow faster than purebred calves.
(6) In general, a small to medium-sized cow with high milk production mated to a large-breed sire will be, economically and biologically, the most efficient cow–calf unit.

The choice of a crossbreeding programme for a given economic unit must be influenced by several considerations such as:

(1) The advantage of a high milk producing breed is much more clearly defined in a region where feed supply is plentiful than in the more arid regions of western North America.
(2) Market discrimination against either very large or very small carcases will influence the profitability of certain breeds.
(3) Climatic and parasitic influences differ among breeds and use of *B. indicus* breeding may be very important in certain regions.
(4) Ease of managing the system varies from the easily managed production of straightbreds or composite breeds to the relatively complex management of the rotational-terminal-sire systems.

As in selection, there is a need for computer simulation work and the results of designed experiments to provide the basis for the decision-making process relative to crossbreeding.

3.2.3. Herd statification

The pyramidal structure is much more evident in the beef breeds than in the dairy breeds. Elite breeders, propagators and commercial producers interact in the manner described by Lush (1945). Artificial insemination and ova transplant programmes have reduced the time distance between elite breeders and commercial producers.

The management of beef herds in North America generally involves the use of pastures or ranges and the labour involved in AI is much greater than the labour associated with natural service. The use of AI will increase above the current level, but not greatly.

3.2.4. Interaction between genotype and environment

The research evidence generally indicates that the interaction between breeds and environments or strains and environments is of small magnitude. However, at least two studies have shown these effects to be of significant magnitude. In Australia, Hearnshaw and Barlow (1982) compared straightbred Hereford (H) and F_1's by Simmental (S), Brahman (B) and Friesian (F) sires and out of Hereford cows. Under good pasture conditions, SH and FH grew faster than BH and HH while, under poor pasture conditions, BH grew faster than SH, FH and HH. Interaction between two lines of Hereford cattle and two widely differing climatic locations (Florida and Montana) was observed by Burns et al. (1979). Reciprocal exchange of cattle native to each location and subsequent performance data showed that, at each location, the

Chapter 7 references, p. 150

native cattle were superior to the introduced cattle.

Interaction does exist when the environments and/or strains or breeds differ widely. Therefore, in the planning of breeding programmes, we should consider which breeds are adapted to the particular environment.

4. CONTROL OF REPRODUCTION

4.1. Artificial insemination

The ability to breed several thousand cows annually to each genetically superior bull has provided the means to greatly increase the selection differential in males and, consequently, to increase the rate of genetic change in cattle for milk and meat production. The ability to produce many offspring in several herds has enhanced the accuracy of estimating breeding value of bulls. Freeman (1976) estimated that 45, 28 and 21% of the total genetic progress is due to sires of bulls, dams of bulls and sires of cows.

The use of frozen semen and rapid transport has made it possible to develop national and international strategies for improvement of cattle. Furthermore, current techniques have made the use of artificial insemination economically and practically feasible.

4.2. Super ovulation and embryo transfer

Collection of multiple fertilized ova from a single female and long-term storage of the embryos in the frozen state has reduced the cost of using embryo transfer and has made possible the consideration of this technique as an economically feasible means of increasing rates of genetic improvement. Nicholas and Smith (1983) estimated that embryo transfer could be used to improve rate of annual genetic change by about 30% with much of the improvement due to increasing the probability of obtaining son(s) of high performing cows. This rate of change is, however, dependent on an accurate and comprehensive usage of performance data on relatives to increase the accuracy of estimating breeding value of both females and males.

Embryo transfer and storage of embryos may also be used to improve the rate of increasing numerical size of small populations of cattle, for international movement of cattle and as a means of preserving rare genotypes (Land, 1982). Land (1982) also suggests that, in most cases, embryo transfer would result in 10% or less improvement of selection response.

4.3. Embryo splitting and cloning

The ability to split embryos into two, four or more identical individuals offers the possibility of improving the accuracy of estimating breeding values of individuals, but does not greatly improve the probability of increasing selection differentials (Nicholas and Smith, 1983).

Cloning, defined as the ability to continue the splitting process indefinitely, is not currently possible in mammals. However, if it should become possible, the propagation of cattle would become similar to the vegetative propagation of plants and genetic improvement would be based on the location of new zygotes which are superior to those currently in use. The commercial marketing of zygotes by commercial concerns would be the norm. The annual genetic change would be 30% or more above that possible with progeny testing and artificial insemination (Nicholas and Smith, 1983).

4.4. Sex determination

Expression of an antigen on the surface of male embryos may provide a way to separate male and female embryos (Land, 1982). The ability to choose the sex of the offspring would have a great impact on husbandry techniques, but would probably have little effect on annual genetic progress.

4.5. Genetic improvement of reproductive rate

Little is known about the physiological basis for differences in ovulation rate or fertility in cattle. Estimates of heritability of the primary trait are low and it is known that temperature, body condition and other major environmental factors influence reproduction. One possibility for alteration of reproductive rate is to define and measure the hormonal causes of differences in reproduction and select directly for the correlated trait.

4.6. Conclusion

Any increase in reproductive rate can be used to improve annual genetic change in the economically important production traits. The selection objectives must be clearly defined and selection of sperm and ova donors must be chosen on the basis of superiority based on performance tests.

5. EXCHANGE OF GENETIC MATERIAL

Gene migration from one population to another results in continuous change in breeds and in national herds of cattle. Importation of European stock into North America was virtually at a standstill until Canada established a quarantine station. Continued supervision of importations must be maintained in order to protect against disease. However, the rate of genetic change in the cattle populations of North America could be accelerated by a more liberal importation policy. The search for promising new genetic material should be broadened to include Asia and new species. One possibility would be the mithan *(Bos frontalis)* of India and Bhutan described by Hickman (1982). The mithan is a large animal which produces milk with an extremely high solids content (10.6% butterfat).

6. MANAGEMENT CONSIDERATIONS

Nutritional levels and management procedures have been shown to influence the productivity of beef cows (Lemenager and Martin, 1982). Examples include a later negative effect of supplemental feed for suckling replacement heifers on number of calves weaned over lifetime and average progeny weaning weight; low nutritional levels for heifers result in delayed puberty and lowered pregnancy rates while exceptionally high nutritional levels for heifers result in reduced longevity and impaired milking ability. The conclusion is that fertility and milking ability of the cow can be influenced by her nutritional status as a calf and growing heifer. Nutritional levels should be adequate for growth and development but low enough to avoid excessive fatness.

Management levels must be high enough to allow expression of the inherent ability to grow, lactate or reproduce. In low management level herds, heritabilities of the economically important traits have frequently been found to be low. Accuracy of estimated breeding values and magnitude of selection differentials may be reduced under lower management levels.

Chapter 7 references, p. 150

In deciding which breeding techniques to use, one must consider herd size, cost of the procedure, requirements for labour and confinement and probable genetic gain. Artificial insemination has costs associated with heat detection, breeding fees and physically inseminating the cow while producing benefits derived from use of a superior sire and not being required to purchase, maintain and manage a bull.

Choice of a crossbreeding system also involves management decisions. The least effort is required to straightbreed or use a composite breed. Strict adherence to a three-breed rotational system will require maintenance of sires of all three breeds or use of artificial insemination, while any relaxation of strict adherence will result in lower levels of heterosis.

Use of crossbreeding without selection will gain the heterosis advantages but will not change the additive genetic merit. High performance bulls and cows are important in the commercial operation as well as in the nucleus herd.

Group breeding schemes have not and do not appear to be likely to become an important factor in North American cattle breeding. This is not because the advantages have not been recognized but, rather, because the cattle breeders are independent and choose not to become part of an organization.

7. ACKNOWLEDGEMENTS

The author greatly appreciates the contributions of Dr J.F. Hentges, University of Florida, concerning buffalo numbers and research on utilization of buffalo in North America, and Dr B.W. Kennedy, University of Guelph, concerning the cattle industry of Canada.

8. REFERENCES

Alenda, R., Martin, T.G., Lasley, J.F. and Ellersieck, M.R., 1980. Estimation of genetic and maternal effects in crossbred cattle of Angus, Charolais and Hereford parentage. 1. Birth and weaning weights. J. Anim. Sci., 50: 226.

Burns, W.C., Koger, M., Butts, W.T., Pahnish, O.F. and Blackwell, R.L., 1979. Genotype by environment interaction in Hereford cattle. II. Birth and weaning traits. J. Anim. Sci., 49: 403.

Burnside, E.B., Schaeffer, L.R. and Kennedy, B.W., 1982. Design, structure and economics of a national dairy cattle improvement scheme. In: Proc. 2nd World Congress on Genetics Applied to Livestock Production, Madrid, Vol. 5, p. 357.

Cartwright, T.C., 1979. The use of systems analysis in animal science with emphasis on animal breeding. J. Anim. Sci., 49: 817.

Croak-Brossman, S.J., Martin, T.G. and Dillon, W.M., 1982. Performance of daughters of high and average predicted difference sires. J. Dairy Sci., 65: 1357.

Cundiff, L.V., 1982. Exploitation and experimental evaluation of breed differences. In: Proc. World Congress on Sheep and Beef Cattle Breeding, Vol. 1, p. 71.

Cundiff, L.V., Gregory, K.E. and Koch, R.M., 1984. Germ Plasm Evaluation Program Progress Report No. 11. ARS-1, U.S. Department of Agriculture, Agricultural Research Service.

Dickerson, G.E., 1973. Inbreeding and heterosis in animals. In: Proc. Animal Breeding and Genetics Symposium in Honor of Dr J.L. Lush. American Society of Animal Science and American Dairy Science Association, Champaign, IL.

Dickerson, G.E., 1982. Principles in establishing breeding objectives in livestock. In: Proc. World Congress on Sheep and Beef Cattle Breeding, New Zealand, Vol. 1, p. 9.

Dillard, E.V., Rodriguez, O. and Robison, O.W., 1980. Estimation of additive and nonadditive direct and maternal effects from crossbreeding beef cattle. J. Anim. Sci., 50: 653.

Freeman, A.E., 1976. Genetic progress. Proc. National Workshop on Genetic Improvement Dairy Cattle, St Louis, MO, U.S.A.

Hearnshaw, H. and Barlow, R., 1982. Genotype × environment interactions in crosses among beef cattle. In: Proc. World Congress on Sheep and Beef Cattle Breeding, Vol. 1, p. 469.

Henderson, C.R., 1973. Sire evaluation and genetic trends. In: Proc. Animal Breeding and Genetics Symposium in Honor of Dr J.L.Lush. American Society of Animal Science and American Dairy Science Association, Champaign, IL.

Hentges, J.F. Jr., Collins, S.E. and Robey, C.A. Jr., 1978. Comparison of cattle and water buffalo

in Florida. Florida Beef Cattle Research Report for 1978. University of Florida, Gainesville, pp. 40–46.
Hickman, C.G., 1982. Cattle breeding in Bhutan, In: Proc. 2nd World Congress on Genetics Applied to Livestock Production, Vol. 8, p. 148.
Hickman, C.G. and Freeman, A.E., 1969. New approach to experimental designs for selection studies in dairy cattle and other species. J. Dairy Sci., 52: 1044.
Hudson, R.J. and Bunnell, F.L., 1981. Grazing in tundra and northern boreal environments. In: F.H.W. Morley (Editor), World Animal Science, Vo. B1, Grazing Animals. Elsevier, Amsterdam.
Land, R.B., 1982. Genetic implications of the control of reproduction. In: Proc. World Congress on Sheep and Beef Cattle Breeding, Vol. 1, p. 387.
Lemenager, R.P. and Martin, T.G., 1982. Production systems and productivity in the beef cow herd. In: Proc. Symposium on Management of Food Production Animals, West Lafayette, IN, Vol. 2, p. 709.
Leusakul-Reodecha, C., 1983. Effects of selection for 365-day weight on maternal performance of beef cows. PhD thesis, Purdue University Library, West Lafayette, IN.
Lush, J.L., 1945. Animal Breeding Plans (3rd Edition). Iowa State University Press, Ames, Iowa.
McAllister, A.J., Batra, T.R., Chesnais, J.P., Darisse, J.P.F., Emsley, J.A.B., Lee, A.J., Nagai, J., Roy, G.L., Vesely, J.A. and Winter, K.A., 1978. The National Cooperative Dairy Cattle Breeding Project. Technical Bulletin 1, Agricultural Research Institute.
McDowell, R.E., 1976. Will crossbreeding pay in dairy production? Animal Science Mimeo Series No. 30, Cornell University, Ithaca, NY.
McGilliard, L.D. and Clay, J.S., 1983. Selecting groups of sires by computer to maximize herd breeding goals. J. Dairy Sci., 66: 647.
Martin, T.G., 1978. Crossbreeding and introduction of new genetic material. In: C.J. Wilcox and H.H. Van Horn (Editors), Large Dairy Herd Management. University of Florida Press, Gainesville.
Martin, T.G. and Alenda, R., 1982. Genetic trends in a herd of Angus cattle selected for 365-day weight over 21 years. In: Proc. World Congress on Sheep and Beef Cattle Breeding, New Zealand, Vol. 1, p. 249.
Nicholas, F.W. and Smith, C., 1983. Increased rates of genetic change in dairy cattle by embryo transfer and splitting. Anim. Prod., 36: 341.
Peters, H.F., 1958. Hybridization of domestic beef cattle and American bison. In: Proc. 10th International Congress of Genetics, Vol. 2, p. 216.
Sechrist, R., 1980. National Dairy Herd Improvement Association Newsletter dated March 1980. U.S. Department of Agriculture, Washington, DC.
Skjervold, H., 1963. The optimum size of progeny groups and optimum use of young bulls in A.I. breeding. Acta Agric. Scand., 13: 131.
Specht, L.W. and McGilliard, L.D., 1960. Rates of improvement by progeny testing in dairy herds of various sizes. J. Dairy Sci., 43: 63.
Touchberry, R.W., 1970. A comparison of the general merits of purebred and crossbred dairy cattle resulting from twenty years (four generations) of crossbreeding. In: Proc. 19th Annual Session, National Poultry Breeders' Roundtable, Kansas City, MO, pp. 18–58.
U.S. Department of Agriculture 1983. Agricultural Statistics 1983. U.S. Govt Printing Office, Washington, DC.
Willham, R.L., 1982a. Predicting breeding values of beef cattle. In: Proc. World Congress on Sheep and Beef Cattle Breeding, New Zealand, Vol. 1, p. 209.
Willham, R.L., 1982b. Use of records in beef cattle selection in the United States of America. In: Proc. World Congress on Sheep and Beef Cattle Breeding, New Zealand, Vol. 2, p. 41.
Wilton, J.W., 1979. The use of production systems analysis in developing mating plans and selection goals. J. Anim. Sci., 49: 809.
Young, C.W., 1984. Systems of mating, problems and opportunities. Proc. National Invitational Workshop on Genetic Improvements in Dairy Cattle. Cornell University Ithaca, NY.

Chapter 8

Draught Cattle World Resources, Systems of Utilization and Potential for Improvement

PAUL STARKEY

1. INTRODUCTION

Draught animals play an extremely important role in the agriculture of the world. To give an idea of the order of magnitude of the use of animal energy for work, Ramaswamy (1984) estimated that there are up to 400 million draught animals in developing countries, directly or indirectly serving 2000 million people. They are used to cultivate up to half of the total area cropped in developing countries, and they haul 25 million carts. Their overall capital value is around $\$100 \times 10^9$. To replace their 150 000 MW of power with mechanical power would require $\$280 \times 10^9$ in capital machinery, plus $\$5 \times 10^9$ a year in annual fuel costs. In India alone there are 80 million draught animals, and together these provide more power than the hydroelectric and fossil fuel power stations in that country.

The vast majority of the world's draught animals are found in developing countries, where they represent an efficient and appropriate technology, that makes use of renewable sources of energy. Draught animals are generally part of highly adapted, integrated, smallholder farming systems, where they have a variety of different technical, economic and social functions, that reduce the drudgery of the farming family, and improve the efficiency of their operations.

However, despite their worldwide use, draught animals have been neglected, in recent decades, by governments, research workers and development agencies. The extent of this neglect has been highlighted by FAO (1982) and by many of the authors cited here, including Smith (1981), Goe (1983) and Ramaswamy (1984). It will become apparent in this chapter, that, despite the very widespread use of draught animals, there is a lack of published knowledge concerning the actual extent of draught animal usage, optimum systems for their utilization, and the potential to improve the animal's performance through breeding or management.

Reasons for the neglect of draught animals in recent years are many and complex. However, two general points stand out. First, in developed countries during the past 60 years there has been a dramatic change from draught animal power to mechanized agriculture and road transport. For example, in the United States between 1910 and 1960, the number of draught animals fell from 22 million to 3 million, while the number of tractors rose from 10 000 to 5 million and the number of farm trucks rose from zero to 3 million (Binswanger, 1984). Prior to this revolution in agricultural power, significant resources, most often in the private sector, had been put into the breeding of draught animals, and the development of more efficient designs of equipment and systems of utilization. However, with the development of mechanization, resources in the more developed countries were naturally concentrated on improving the efficiency of mechanized agriculture. In terms of research and

Chapter 8 references, p. 196

development, draught animal power was considered outmoded and was consequently neglected.

Sadly this attitude was transmitted to the developing countries, both through the preconceptions of expatriates in agriculture and education and in particular through the training of indigenous staff at institutions in developed countries where animal traction was considered outmoded. This led to a whole generation of influential staff in the ministries, universities and research institutions in developing countries, that were under the impression that draught animal power was mainly of historical interest and that it would rapidly be replaced by mechanical power. This attitude was perpetuated and reinforced through the agricultural curricula of schools and universities in these countries. As a consequence of this attitude, many countries in Africa, Asia and Latin America devoted scarce public resources in an attempt to speed up the process of mechanization, and the ruins of such programmes are clearly visible today. In a study on mechanization in developed and developing countries, Binswanger (1984) argues, with many examples, that the pace of mechanization throughout the world has been largely determined by a wide range of agricultural, social and economic conditions, and not by direct government interventions or mechanization subsidies. Any such interventions have often had adverse social and economic effects. However, in many developing countries, policy makers are still reluctant to accept that the universal aspiration of mechanized agriculture cannot be achieved in a short time. Such individuals are often in key positions, and can effectively inhibit the appropriate development and improvement of the draught animal sectors in their countries. Nevertheless there is now a growing awareness that draught animal power will continue to be important for decades, if not centuries, to come, and such awareness is beginning to be reflected in government policies towards research, education and mechanization.

The second major reason for the neglect of draught animal power is that the millions of draught animals in the world are generally owned by the smallholder or subsistence sectors of the economy and these comprise people without great purchasing power. Thus there is not a great financial incentive for commercial enterprises to invest in large-scale, privately funded improvement work. This is in contrast to the milk and beef sectors of the cattle industry and to the pig, poultry, and wool/fibre/fur industries which are generally producing for the more affluent sectors of the economies. In these other animal production sectors there is seen to be significant scope for profit through the development and promotion of improved genotypes and management systems. In these other fields, the commercial sector has carried out, or funded, its own research and development work, and has encouraged governments, universities and research institutes to study and invest in these areas also. There is an inevitable tendency for research biases to become self-perpetuating. Once national research programmes are established, the personnel naturally publicize and promote their own fields of interest, and so subjects such as draught animal power, neglected in early planning, may remain excluded, particularly when budgetary constraints necessitate restriction and cutbacks.

An example of the problem of the self-perpetuating neglect of draught animal power may be seen in the field of commercial scientific publishing. Scientific publishers naturally have to follow market trends, and publish in those fields where there is a clear demand. In this present comprehensive series on World Animal Science, Elsevier has tried to meet the needs of a wide range of animal scientists in the world. For example, in their analyses of market demand, it has been considered that the commercially important field of fur production requires a separate volume. In contrast the worldwide topic of draught animal power is not given such resources or prominence. This does not suggest any valued judgements by the series editors or publishers relating to draught animal power, but simply that to date there has been little research interest or market demand by animal scientists in this subject. Such an example illustrates that an area of historical neglect will remain neglected until there is sufficient interest among scientists, institutions and governments to stimulate a change.

As a result of neglect, during a century that has seen amazing changes in the technology of transport, communications, aerospace and weapons, that of the draught animal continues largely unchanged. This would suggest either that the technology is perfectly adapted to its situation, or that the scope for improving the technology is enormous. FAO (1982) is adamant in its assertion that there is both the potential and the need for major qualitative and quantitative improvements in draught animal power systems to meet the increasing demands for agricultural power in developing countries. There is great scope for improving almost all aspects of draught animal power. The animals themselves can be improved through selection, breeding and improved systems of feeding, management and health care. Commonly employed harnessing systems have been condemned as both cruel and inefficient (Smith, 1981; Goe 1983; Ramaswamy, 1984). Implements used with draught animals, ploughs, cultivation equipment, carts and stationary machinery often use materials and designs that have been used for generations. The potential for introducing new materials or design improvements is therefore vast.

However, the animals, harnessing systems and implements should not be studied in isolation. Draught animals form part of complex socio-economic systems. Commonly, draught animals are maintained for many reasons, and they may provide milk, meat, dung or important social status, in addition to their work. Thus the observed apparent inefficiencies in utilization may not be simple technical constraints, but may relate to the complex social and economic conditions in the various countries. Thus while certainly not technically perfect, the present system may be the best compromise in the prevailing ecological and socio-economic environments. Technological improvements must be appropriate to the whole agricultural and social system.

It would therefore seem apparent that research and development activities relating to draught animals must be carried out in full recognition of the complexity of the farming systems in which draught animals are employed. This implies an adaptive 'systems' approach to research. Thus while specific physiological and technical studies may be required to be performed 'on-station', the majority of research needs to be carried out with the farmers themselves. At present the vast majority of research relating to draught animals takes place 'on-station', generally in conditions very different from those of the surrounding farms. The lack of contact with reality of many draught animal research studies is a serious constraint to the improvement of animal power systems. Thus recommendations resulting from 'on-station' studies need to be particularly carefully evaluated in terms of applicability to actual farming systems, and this should be carefully borne in mind when assessing research reports and literature reviews.

It will become evident in the following sections that there is a vast scope for further research and development studies relating to draught animal power. However, there is no need to generate knowledge and experience that already exists. Thus there is an urgent need for the improved reporting of existing knowledge, and for information exchange between workers in this field. FAO (1982) noted that draught animal research had been hindered by the lack of detailed reports of successes and failures, lack of standardized testing procedures, narrow fields of research, insufficient attention to farming background and restricted information flow. It is therefore evident that there is great scope for international cooperation in coordinating research activities

Chapter 8 references, p. 196

and improving information exchange relating to animal traction. If this can be achieved then many of the obvious gaps in knowledge and understanding, as highlighted in the following sections, can be rapidly filled.

2. WORLD UTILIZATION OF DRAUGHT CATTLE

FAO (1982) noted that draught animal power is such a neglected subject that few countries keep statistics on draught animal usage. Thus figures in the following sections should be treated with caution, and should be considered as giving an order of magnitude only. In very broad terms about 250 million draught cattle are used throughout the world, 220 million in Asia, 15 million in Africa and 15 million in Latin America. Although accurate statistics are not available for the Middle East, it is known that in Turkey alone there are about 4 million draught animals. Iraq and Iran have at least this number. Thus about 20% of the world's cattle population is used for draught purposes.

2.1. Draught cattle in developed countries

Animal traction is still employed in the developed countries of North America, Europe and Australasia, although its decline in the past 60 years has been dramatic. Even prior to the competition from tractors, the numbers of draught cattle were decreasing, as horses replaced oxen as sources of power. Thus in the United States between the years 1870 and 1920, the number of draught cattle fell from 1.3 million to 0.3 million, while the number of draught horses increased from 7 million to 17 million (Binswanger, 1984). A major advantage of the horse was its speed, which was sufficient to allow the development of animal powered harvesting equipment. In developed countries the present promotion of draught animal power for forestry and hill-farming, is based mainly on equines (Sasimowski, 1984a; J.P. Morin, personal communication, 1984).

In France, about 1 million draught oxen were employed in agriculture up to the Second World War, and in 1942 there were reported to be 1.9 million

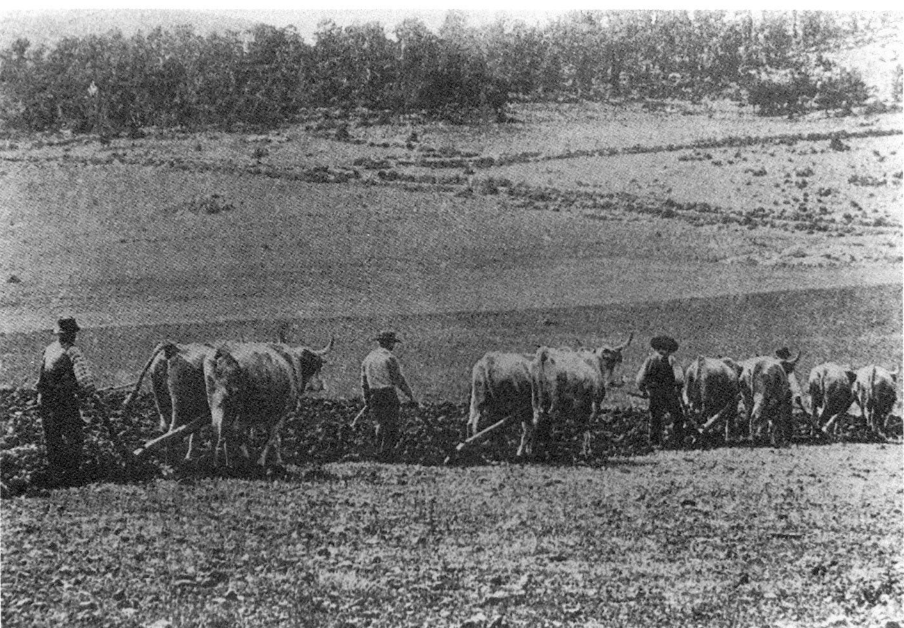

Fig. 8.1. Four pairs of Simmental draught oxen, France, c. 1910.

work cows (Binswanger, 1984). However numbers of draught cattle in France have fallen greatly in recent years, from 118 000 in 1965, to 40 000 in 1970, and to just 9 000 in 1977 (Binswanger, 1984). Nevertheless small numbers of draught cattle are still employed for ploughing and transport in western and eastern Europe, notably in Italy, Yugoslavia and the Balkan States. The traditional large European draught breeds such as the Charolais, Simmental and Chianina were commonly employed on large farms (Fig. 8.1), but now there is a tendency to use local multi-purpose milk/meat/draught animals, such as the Brown Swiss, because draught cattle are now generally restricted to broad-based smallholdings.

2.2. Draught cattle in Africa

The use of draught animals in Africa has been the subject of reviews by CEEMAT/FAO (1972), ILCA (1981), Munzinger (1982), Anderson (1984) and Pingali et al. (1987). A large number of documents exist which describe or evaluate experience from individual countries. Some of these may be traced through the bibliographies of IEMVT (1980), Sargent et al. (1981), Goe and Hailu (1983), Imboden et al. (1983), Bartlett and Gibbon (1984) and Starkey and Goe (1984). Estimates of the total number of draught cattle in Africa range from less than 10 million (ILCA, 1981) to over 16 million (Anderson, 1984).

2.2.1. North Africa

While animal traction has been widely used in North Africa for centuries, cattle are seldom the animals of choice in this zone. In Morocco, Algeria, Tunisia and Libya, donkeys, mules and horses, and to a lesser extent camels, provide most of the animal power used in farming and transport. However, in the Nile valley of Egypt around one million water buffaloes and cattle are employed for ploughing and other agricultural operations, including transport (Ramaswamy, 1981a). While all the North African countries are developing significant large-scale mechanization programmes, animal traction continues to be a major source of power for the small farmers in the region.

2.2.2. West Africa

In West Africa there are three broad zones in which animal traction is used. To the south of the Sahara desert, in the northern part of the Sahel zone where rainfall is less than 600 mm, arable farming is relatively restricted, and where animals are employed for work they are generally donkeys, horses or camels. The south of the Sahel zone and the Sudan zone represents an ecological belt running from Senegal, through part of Mali and Burkina Faso to southern Niger, Chad and northern Nigeria. In this area zebu breeds of cattle can be effectively used in agricultural operations. South of this zone, in the Gambia, southern Senegal, Guinea, Sierra Leone, southwestern Burkina Faso, Ivory Coast, Ghana, Togo, Benin and southern Nigeria, trypanosomiasis and the tsetse fly are major constraints to livestock production. In this area, where work animals are used in agriculture, the small trypanotolerant, humpless taurines, notably the N'Dama are employed. Equines are generally absent from these areas and if zebu cattle are used for work, it is generally in conjunction with trypanocidal drugs.

In most of West Africa animal traction in agriculture was introduced between 1910 and 1935, although before this time draught animals were used for urban transport (Sargent et al., 1981; Starkey, 1981; Payne, 1980). Generally the use of animal traction spread well in areas where it was promoted in conjunction with a distinct cash-crop, such as groundnuts in Senegal or cotton in Guinea and Mali (Sargent et al., 1981). During the period 1945–70 many West African countries invested heavily in mechanization programmes, which

Chapter 8 references, p. 196

generally proved expensive and ephemeral and had little long-term impact on the dominant small-farmer sector of the economies. However, throughout the period there was a slow expansion in the use of animal traction, notably in Senegal where in 1961 a factory was established to produce animal-drawn equipment (Sargent et al., 1981). The period 1973–83 brought both an increase in international aid, after the disastrous drought, and resurgence of government interest in the potential for draught animal power in West African countries. By 1984 the use of draught cattle in agriculture was being actively promoted in all West African countries.

In Senegal up to 20% of farmers use animal power, and about a quarter of a million ploughs are used in the country. Senegal has areas in the three main ecological zones, and in the north equines and zebu breeds are commonly used, while in the southern province of Casamance, N'Dama taurines are used. Attempts to develop a draught cattle breed at Bambey Research Station has yet to have any significant impact on the national situation (Hamon, 1971). The Gambia has had a relatively successful traction programme, with 33% of farmers using oxen and 40% using equines. The use of oxen, mainly N'Dama, has been emphasized (Mettrick, 1978).

In southern Mali a highly successful animal traction programme has been developed mainly for maize and cotton production. In 1984, 170 000 draught oxen were in use, mainly of zebu type (see Fig. 8.2) protected with trypanocidal drugs administered through the veterinary services (Steengaard, 1984). Some use is made of N'Dama and taurine × zebu crossbreeds, and a crossbreeding programme is being initiated using the larger, but trypanosensitive Kouri cattle from Lake Chad region. In Burkina Faso a major animal traction programme from 1973–83 led to a large increase in the use of draught animals, to the present level of about 15% of small farmers. Most of the national herd is of zebu type, and these are used in the north of the country. However in the southwest, where animal traction has been continued with cotton production, the use of trypanocidal drugs is necessary with zebu cattle, and taurine × zebu crosses are often employed (see Fig. 8.3; Imboden et al., 1983).

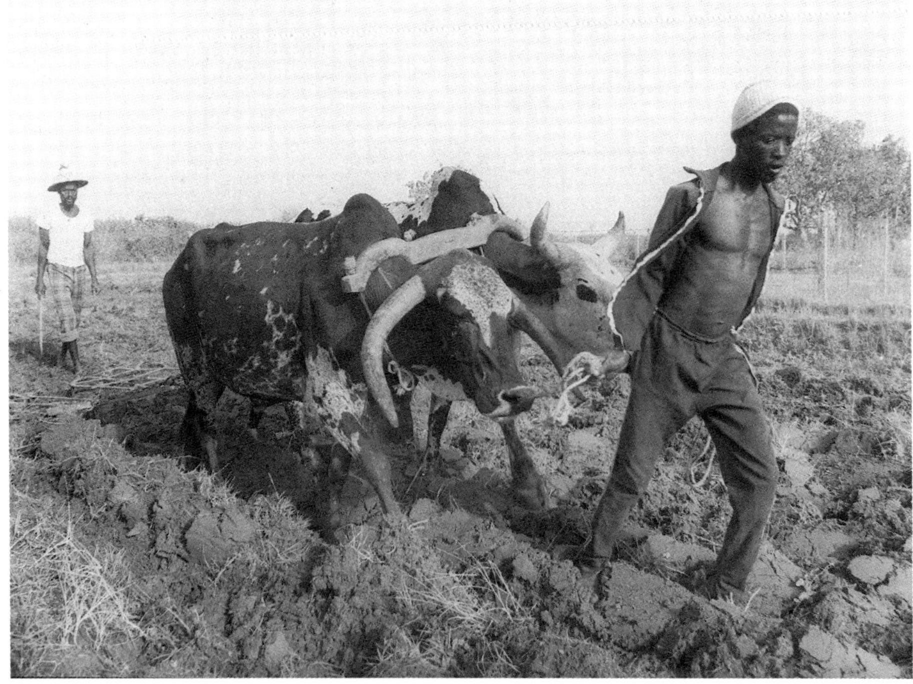

Fig. 8.2. West African zebu oxen with withers yoke harrowing in Mali. (Photo: J. van Acker, FAO.)

In Guinea around 100 000 N'Dama oxen are used for the production of rice, maize, millet and cotton (Bigot, 1983). In neighbouring Sierra Leone interest in the potential for N'Dama cattle for rice production has been stimulated by an active national draught animal research programme (Starkey, 1981, 1982, 1983a). A similar national draught animal programme has also been developed in Togo, which faces problems of very low cattle numbers,

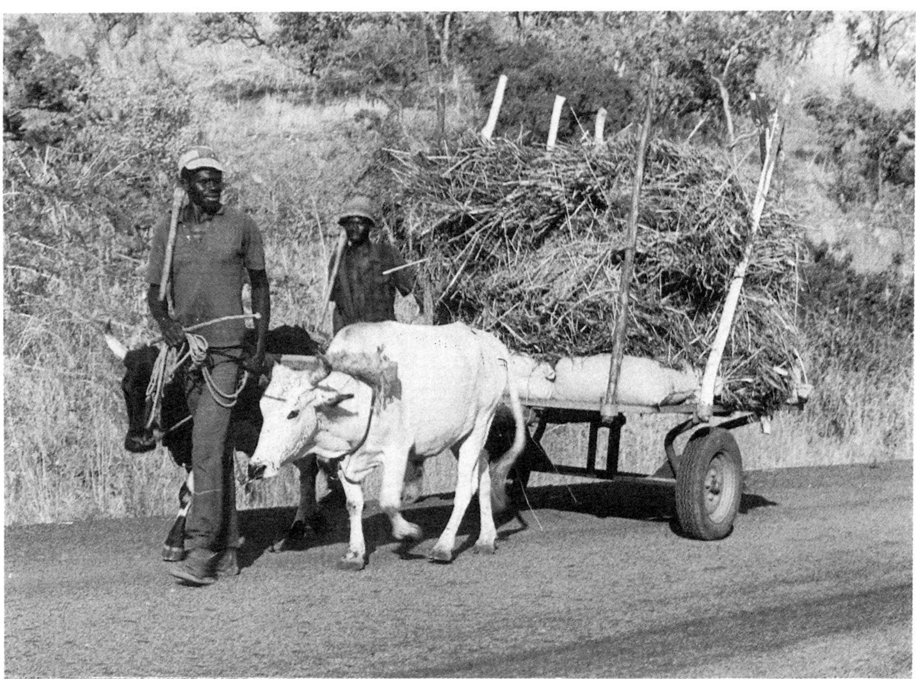

Fig. 8.3. Ox cart in Burkina Faso, pulled by animals of mixed taurine and zebu ancestry. (Photo: P. Starkey.)

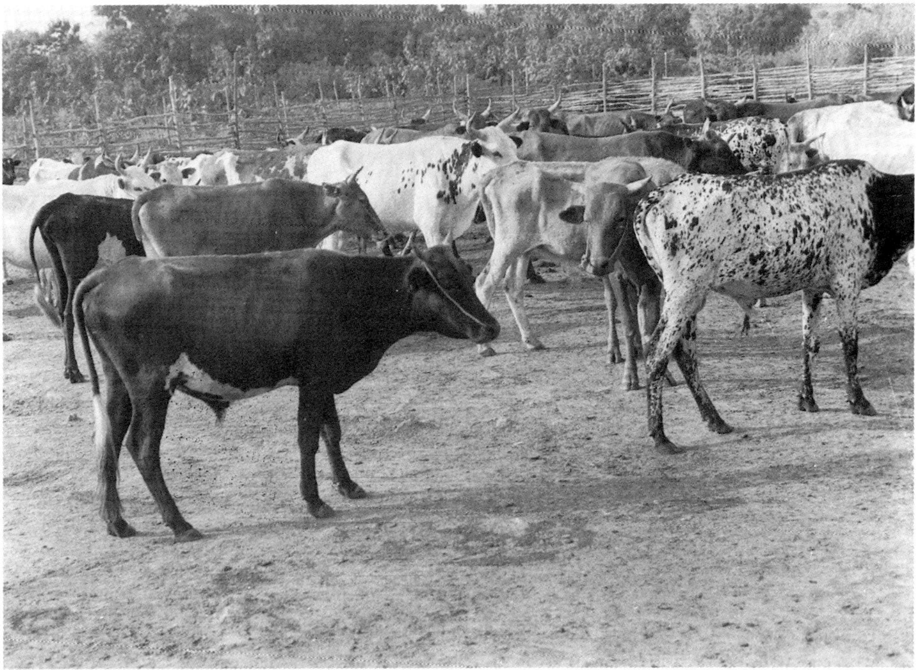

Fig. 8.4. Oxen of taurine and taurine × zebu type at oxen training centre, Togo. (Photo: P. Starkey.)

trypanosomiasis and the unfamiliarity of farmers with cattle husbandry. Between 1976 and 1984, the number of draught animals increased from near zero to 3000. The indigenous taurines of the Somba type are generally used, together with Borgou cattle of Somba × zebu origin, and an up-grading programme using N'Dama cattle has commenced (see Fig. 8.4; Apetofia 1982; Imboden et al., 1983). In northern Ghana another taurine, the small West African Shorthorn has been successfully employed in animal traction extension programmes (Smid, 1982).

2.2.3. Central Africa

Zaire, Central African Republic, Congo, Gabon, Equatorial Guinea and Cameroon have very low cattle populations and are dominated by forest vegetation. However, several small-scale attempts have been made to introduce animal traction into the forest-fringe and savanna ecosystems of this area. In northern Cameroon, Bororo and Aku breeds of *Bos indicus* cattle have been employed successfully, albeit with fairly high initial mortality rates associated with farmer unfamiliarity with cattle husbandry (Wagner and Munzinger, 1982). In Zaire several small draught animal projects have met with varying degrees of success, but have demonstrated that animal traction is technically feasible in this country. N'Dama cattle have been employed in Bas Zaire, indigenous taurines in Kasai Occidental (see Fig. 8.5), Africanders in Kasai Oriental (Fig. 8.6), and zebus in Haut Zaire (Starkey, 1984a).

2.2.4. East Africa

The highlands of Ethiopia are unique in Sub-Saharan Africa in that here animal traction has been used for centuries. Virtually all farmers in the highlands use Ethiopian zebu cattle to plough their land using the traditional ard-type implement (Fig. 8.7). It is estimated that around 6 million draught cattle are used in Ethiopia, a figure that represents about one-half of the total draught animal utilization in the continent.

Animal traction is used in all the countries of East Africa, but there is great variation within and between countries in the extent of its adoption. Dif-

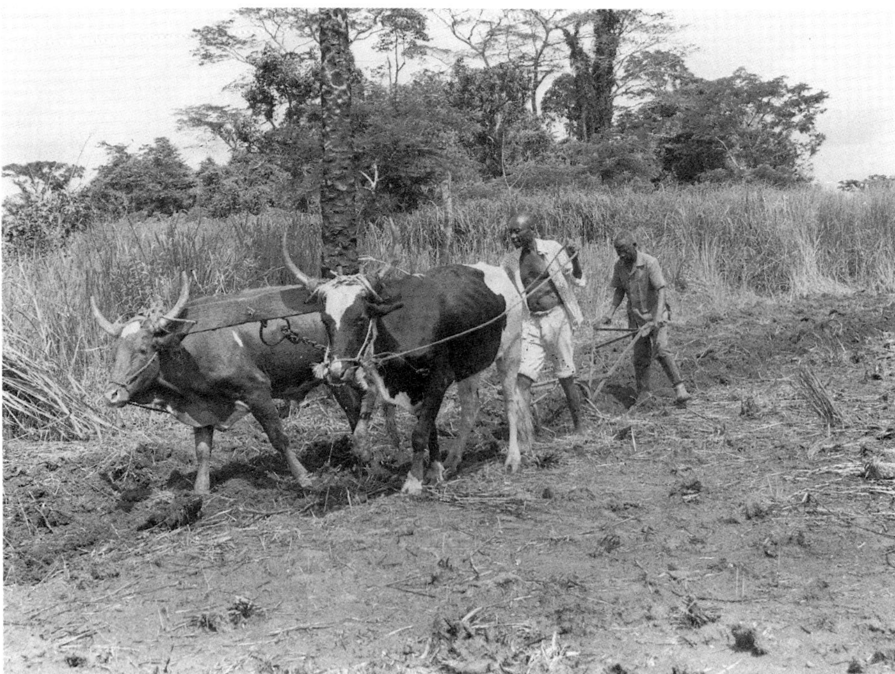

Fig. 8.5. Taurine oxen ploughing on the forest fringe in Zaire. (Photo: P. Starkey.)

ferences in cattle distribution, land use systems, ethnic traditions, and the incidence of trypanosomiasis are associated with the uneven distribution of draught animal utilization. For example in Kenya, the national figure of about 12% of farmer adoption includes areas of Maasai rangeland where no cattle are used for cultivation, and areas, such as Machakos where 80% of the farmers use draught cattle (Starkey and Goe, 1984). In Tanzania, it is estimated that around 300 000 East African zebu cattle are used for work, and they cultivate about 15% of the cropped area (Kjaerby, 1983).

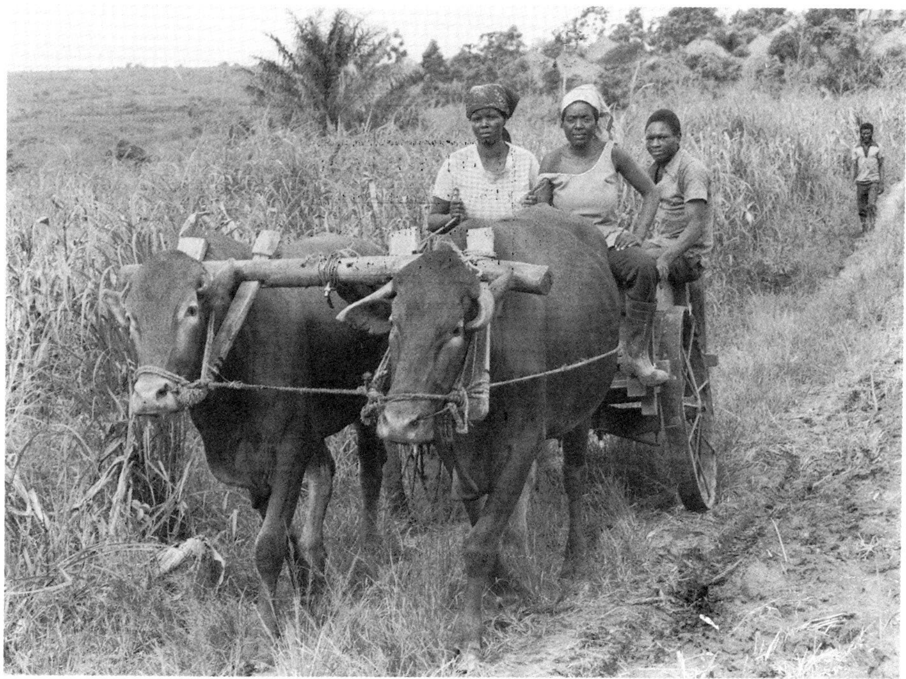

Fig. 8.6. Africander oxen pulling a cart in Zaire. (Photo: P. Starkey.)

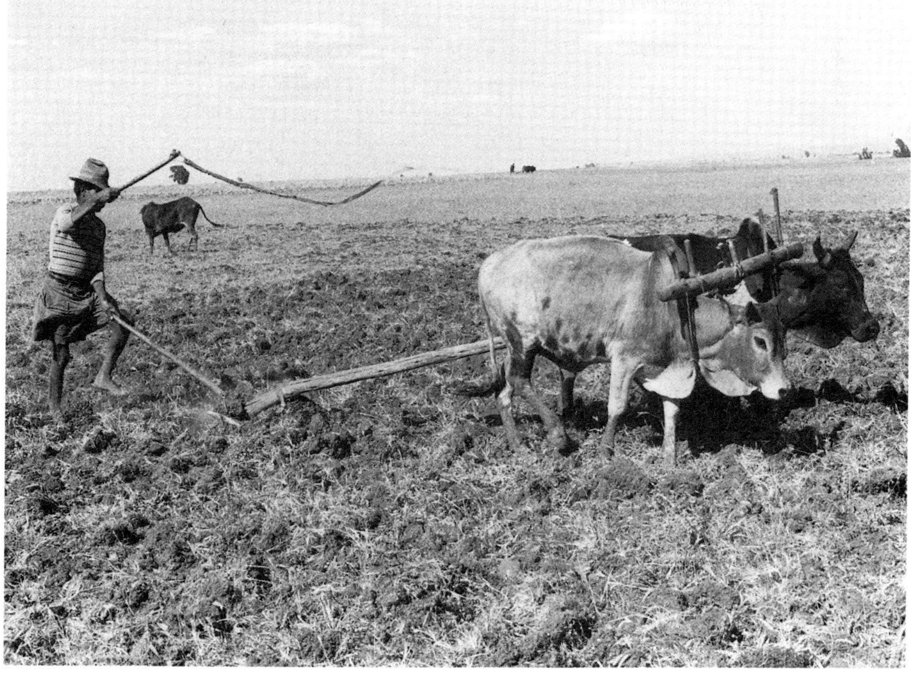

Fig. 8.7. Ethiopian zebu oxen with withers yoke ploughing with maresha ard. (Photo: P. Starkey.)

Chapter 8 references, p. 196

2.2.5. Southern Africa and Madagascar

The use of cattle for transport and cultivation in Southern Africa has a history dating back to the early European settlers. The Africander breed was bred largely as a trek animal. In Zimbabwe, the Tuli, Nkare and Mashona types of sanga cattle are all widely used for draught purposes (Howard, 1979). In Botswana around 360 000 draught cattle are used, mainly of the Tswana breed. Around 80% of farmers use draught animals, and large teams of 6–12 animals are used, often with cows and heifers being included with the oxen and bulls as shown in Fig. 8.8 (Starkey and Goe, 1984). Animal traction was introduced into Madagascar in the last century, and has spread quite extensively, helped by the large population of Madagascar zebu cattle. However, the very small size of holdings (average of 1.2 ha) together with much fragmentation is seen as a constraint to increasing animal traction from current levels of about 330 000 draught cattle (Tran van Nhieu, 1982).

2.3. Draught cattle in Asia

The vast majority, perhaps 90% of all the draught animals of the world are found in Asia. Accurate estimates of usage within most countries are difficult to obtain, and detailed reports on the national status of draught animal power are not available for most Asian countries (Ramaswamy, 1981a). Around 220 million draught cattle are thought to be employed in Asia, in addition to 50 million draught buffaloes (Ramaswamy, 1981a).

India is the major user of draught animal power and estimates of the number of draught cattle in use range from 72 million (Pathak, 1984b) to 110 million (Ramaswamy, 1981a,b). Draught animals are used by about 60% of farmers. The main breeds employed for draught and multi-purpose uses are Nimari, Nagori, Siri, Alambadi, Amritmahal, Kankrej, Hallikar, Kangayam, Tharparkar, Killari, Haryana, Deoni, Ongole and Rathi, although the number of purebred animals is relatively small (Pathak, 1984b).

In Pakistan, while the total cattle population is increasing, the number of

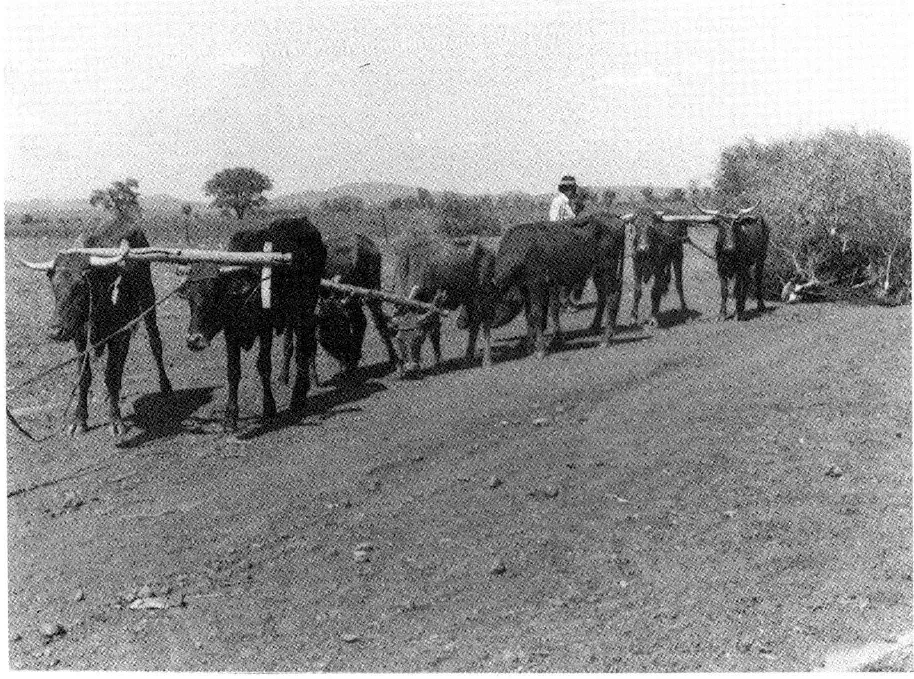

Fig. 8.8. A team of eight oxen, cows and heifers pulling branches as training for ploughing in Botswana. (Photo: P. Starkey.)

draught cattle halved in the period 1965–82, and presently stands at around 4 million (Pathak, 1984b). Most animals are of a nondescript type but with the Tharparkar, Lohani and Dhanni being distinct draught/dual-purpose breeds, and the Sahiwal and Red Sindhi dairy breeds also being employed for work

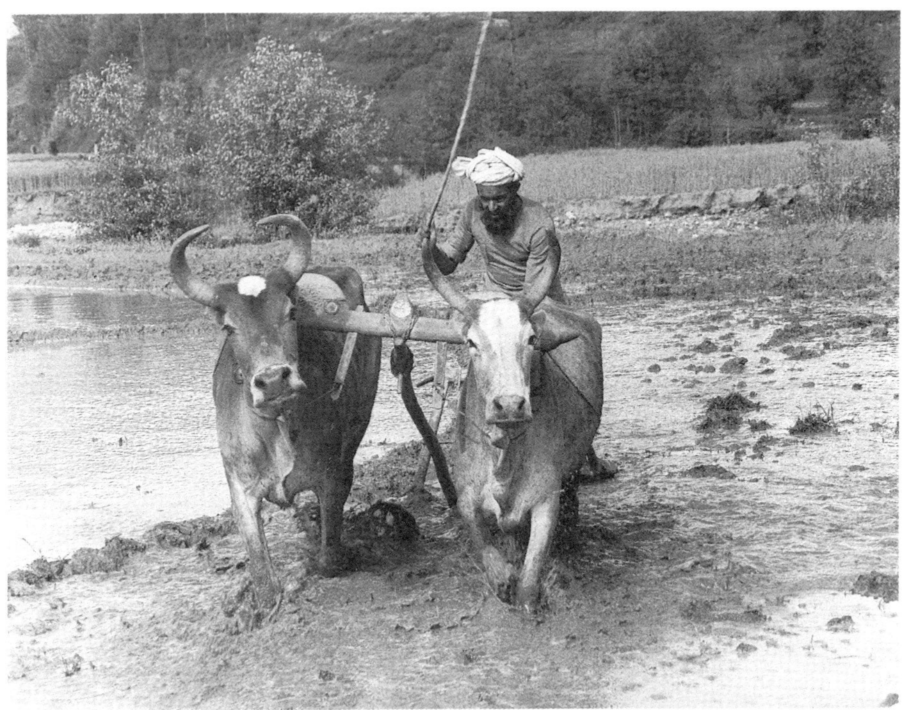

Fig. 8.9. A pair of oxen controlled by one man for puddling in Pakistan. (Photo: F. Mattioli, FAO.)

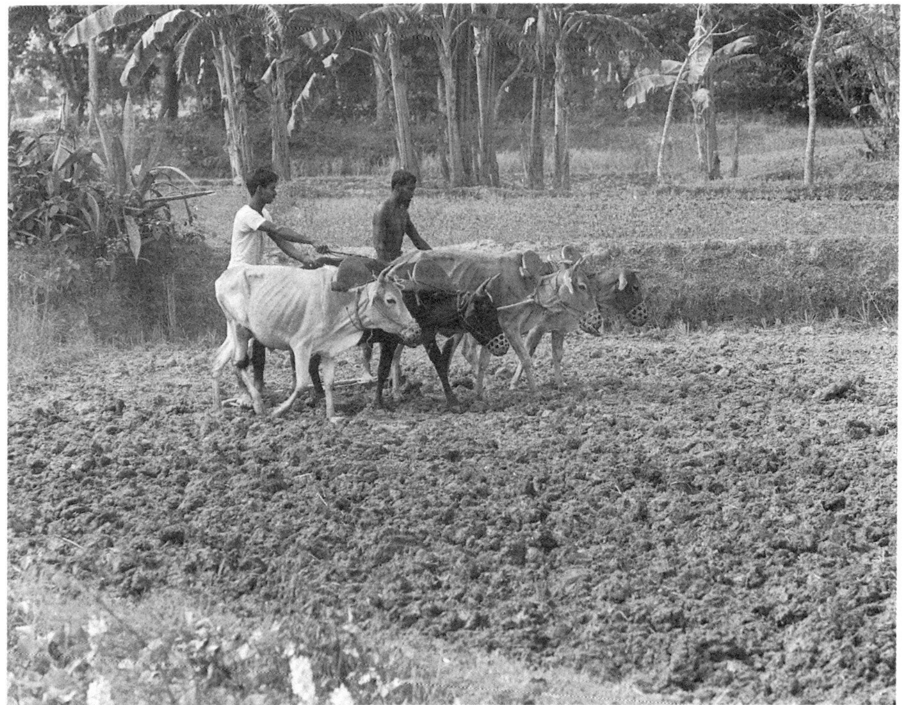

Fig. 8.10. Oxen in poor physical condition used for harrowing in Bangladesh. (Photo: F. Botts, FAO.)

Chapter 8 references, p. 196

purposes (see Fig. 8.9).

In Bangladesh, it is estimated that around 10 million draught animals are employed, mainly of small, nondescript *B. indicus* type (see Fig. 8.10) (Gill, 1981).

The use of draught animals in China has been described by Feng Yang-Lian (1984), who emphasized the importance of the Chinese Yellow cattle as a draught breed. Binswanger (1984) quotes the number of draught oxen as 52 million and draught cows as 600 000. In addition, the number of draught buffaloes is given as 18 million and draught equines as 22 million. Yaks and camels are also used in China.

In southern Asia, notably Sri Lanka, the Philippines, and Thailand, the swamp buffalo is the major draught animal. For example, 2.7 million working buffaloes (carabaos) are used in the Philippines (Binswanger, 1984). In Indonesia about half of the 5 million draught animals are cattle, including the Ongole and Madura draught breeds (Pathak, 1984b). In Sri Lanka estimates on the population of working buffaloes range from 300 000 (Pathak, 1984b) to 850 000 (Farrington and Abeyratne, 1982), although the latter figure is comparable with the total national herd. It has been recommended that with a cattle population of about one million, the use of draught oxen should be actively promoted, in addition to the more popular buffaloes (Farrington and Abeyratne, 1982).

Elsewhere in Asia, 3.5 million draught cattle are employed in Burma, with seven working cattle for every one draught buffalo. The multi-purpose/draught Burmese zebu cattle stand about 1.3 m at the shoulder and have a mean weight at the end of the monsoon of about 440 kg (Fig. 8.11) (M. Hammond, personal communication, 1984). In Nepal around 2 million draught cattle are used, using the system illustrated in Fig. 8.12 (Oli, 1984) and approximately 4 million cattle are employed in Turkey with comparable numbers in Iran and Iraq (C. Hickman, personal communication, 1984). In the Asian states of the Soviet Union, significant numbers of draught cattle are used, but the author

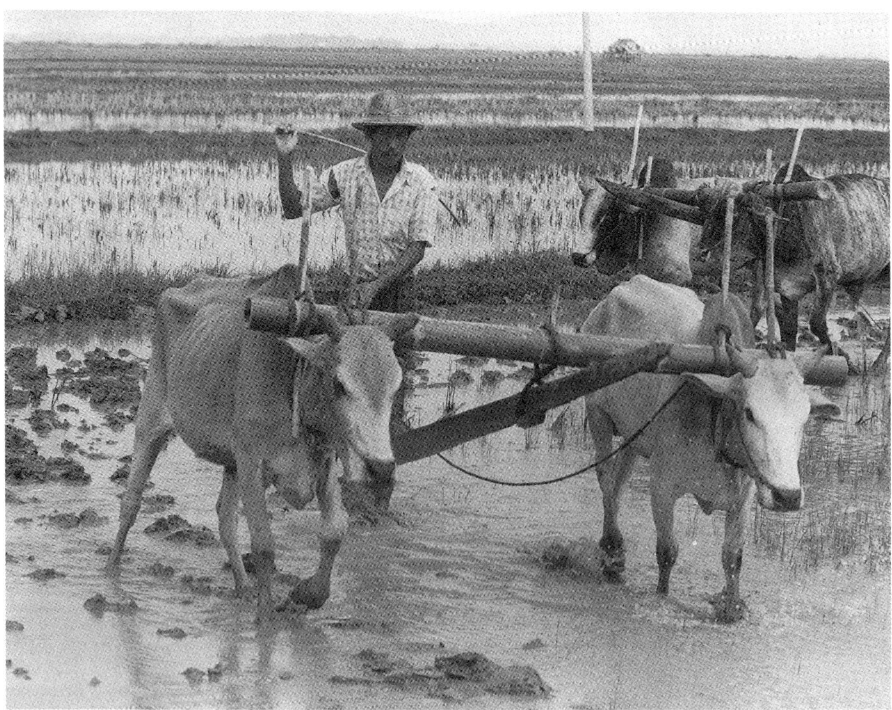

Fig. 8.11. Ploughing in Burma using bamboo withers yoke. (Photo: F. Botts, FAO.)

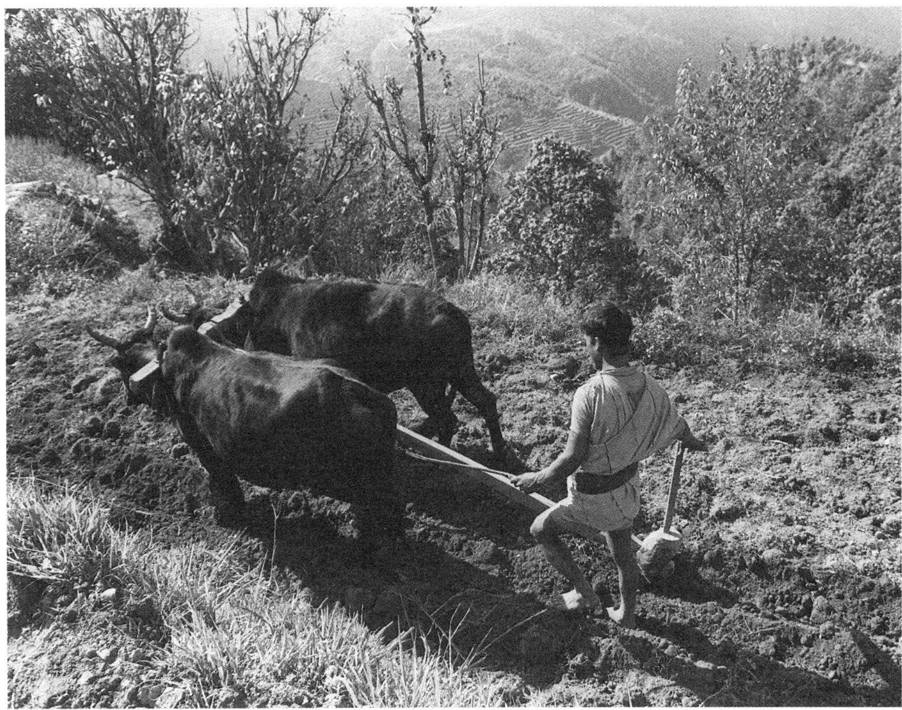

Fig. 8.12. Ox ploughing in Nepal, showing withers yoke and lack of reins. (Photo: F. Botts, FAO.)

is not aware of international publications that quantify this.

2.4. Draught animals in Latin America and the Caribbean

In Latin America and the Caribbean draught animals are used in significant numbers, with perhaps 15 million draught cattle being employed in the region. However, published information concerning draught animals in Central and South America is particularly scarce, and among the main works on animal traction in the English and French languages, the experience of Latin America is almost totally ignored. For example, the reviews on animal traction research by Smith (1981) and Goe (1983), the specialized animal traction bibliographies of Goe and Hailu (1983) and Bartlett and Gibbon (1984), and the general works on draught animals of Watson (1981) neglect the experience of South and Central America, and the Caribbean. The absence of coverage of Latin America by these and other authors is not considered to result from policy decisions, but rather, it is an illustration of both the severe language barrier between Latin America and the francophone and anglophone areas, and also of the acute scarcity of documents in this field. It has already been noted (in the introduction to this chapter) that areas of neglect in the literature tend to remain neglected. However, the development of links between the Centre d'Etudes et d'Expérimentation du Mechinisme Agricole Tropical (CEEMAT), France and Empresa Brasileira de Pesquisa Agropecuaria (EMBRAPA) Brazil (G. Herblot, personal communication, 1984) and between the Centre for Tropical Veterinary Medicine, (CTVM), Scotland and the Escuela Centroamericana de Ganaderia (ECAG), Costa Rica (CTVM, 1984) should ensure that better liaison concerning draught animal research is achieved in coming years.

Some information on the extent of the usage of draught animals in South America has been provided by Ramaswamy (1981a,b). He reports that in Brazil 2.6 million draught cattle are used, mainly in the northeast of the coun-

Chapter 8 references, p. 196

try. In Colombia, 0.5 million draught cattle are used, both in traditional agriculture and forestry. In Peru 100 000 draught cattle are used in the traditional sector (see Fig. 8.13) with more draught power being supplied by equines. Several hundred thousand draught cattle are also used in Argentina and Bolivia. In Chile 40% of agricultural power is provided by draught animals, of which 0.3 million are cattle. Oxen are increasingly being used for

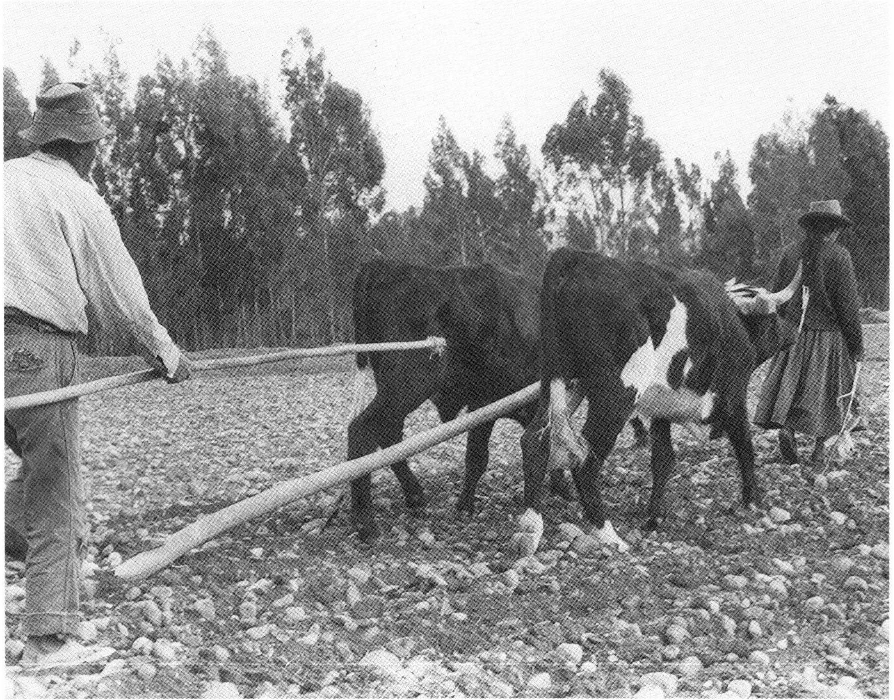

Fig. 8.13. Ox ploughing in Peru, showing simple ard and neck yoke. (Photo: J. van Acker, FAO.)

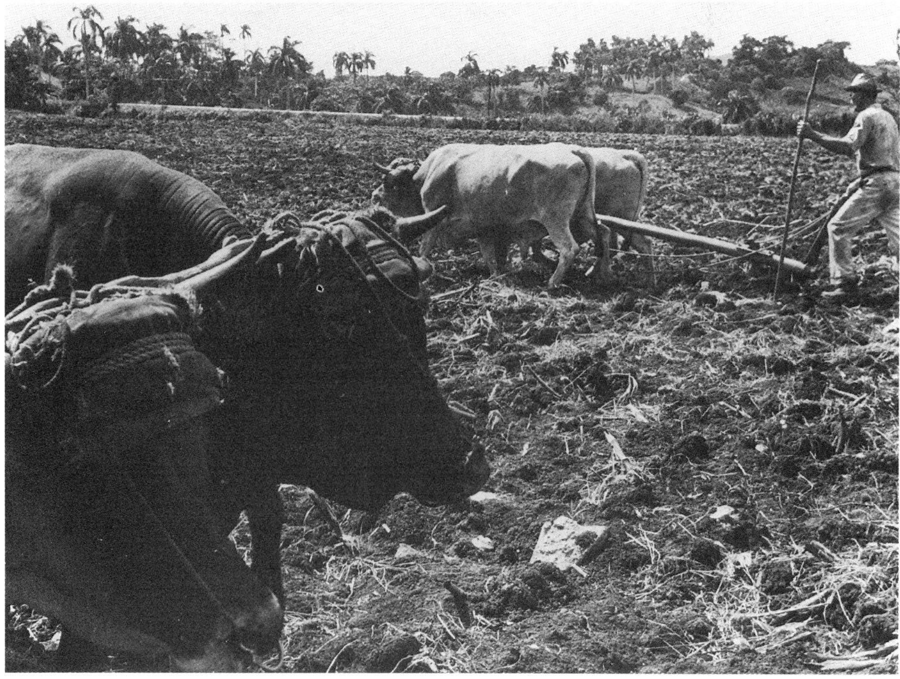

Fig. 8.14. Ox ploughing in Cuba, showing use of neck yokes. (Photo: Prensa Latina, FAO.)

forestry operations in Chile (Rodriguez, 1984).

In Mexico, 4.2 million draught animals are used (Binswanger, 1984), and 2.8 million are said to be draught cattle (Ramaswamy, 1981a,b). Draught cattle are also used in significant numbers in Costa Rica and Cuba (see Fig. 8.14) with a much smaller, but increasing use in Haiti and the Dominican Republic where they are valuably employed for sugar cane harvesting.

3. CHOICE OF TECHNOLOGY AND MANAGEMENT SYSTEMS

3.1. Choice of draught animal technology

Draught animal power is just one option in a spectrum of complementary technology, ranging from the use of hand power and traditional implements to the use of motorized power, particularly two- and four-wheel tractors. Each technology may be appropriate, depending on the social, economic and infrastructural environment in which that technology is to be employed, and these environments will change with time. The present highly mechanized agriculture found in much of North America and western Europe evolved from systems using draught animal technology and this had developed from hand cultivation. This has given rise to the concept of a 'ladder' of mechanization development, with draught animal technology as an intermediate between hand cultivation and fully mechanized agriculture. A useful historical perspective on the development of mechanization has been provided by Binswanger (1984).

In a study on the evolution of farming systems Binswanger and Pingali (1984) argue that animal traction is the natural technology to be employed when population pressures necessitate the development of a grass-fallow system of agriculture. Prior to this, traditional bush-fallow systems, with fire clearance, were used requiring less overall effort than that required for stumping. However, once pressures on land reduce the period of fallow to 1 or 2 years, animal traction becomes almost a necessity. At this stage in agricultural evolution the labour inputs involved in clearing land of weeds for planting is very high, while the costs of maintaining cattle on the grass fallows are low, so that draught animal technology appears an ideal solution.

As agricultural systems further intensify, grazing land becomes less available and the costs of maintaining animals increase. At this point the transition to tractorized mechanization may be practicable, but only in the right conditions. If rural labour remains in plentiful supply, animal traction may be desirable even in very intensively cropped regions (Gill, 1981). Binswanger and Pingali (1984) argue that the direct transition from hand cultivation to tractor cultivation is almost impossible to achieve, and that it is only after land de-stumping and the intensification of agriculture using animal traction, that tractorization becomes economically viable.

The choice of technology of individual farmers will depend on many highly area-specific social and economic factors, and as Binswanger (1984) observed, farmers tend to be the best judges, as outside analysts simply know too little about the farming system. However, the choice of technology is highly dependent on availability of the necessary inputs, and this is greatly influenced by national and regional policies. In developing countries, governments and aid agencies are particularly influential in determining whether or not a technology is practicable, through various controls on importation, local manufacture, distribution, subsidies and credit relating to the necessary inputs. However, Binswanger (1984) points out that despite massive government subsidies, mechanization will not be successful in the long term if the economic criteria needed to justify it are not met. Equally the most successful ex-

Chapter 8 references, p. 196

periences with mechanization in the world, which are those relating to milling, pumping and harvest processing, did not depend on government intervention.

It would appear that the almost universal aspiration of individuals and governments is the introduction of highly mechanized agriculture. However, this is only feasible in the appropriate economic conditions, and for many individuals and districts, these conditions are not likely to be met in the foreseeable future. In such areas draught animal technology may represent the most economically realistic and socially appropriate solution. It is therefore necessary for national governments and develoment programmes to consider animal traction as a potentially valuable system of agricultural development, and the commonly held but mistaken view of draught animal technology as outmoded, as discussed earlier, is to be regretted.

In Sub-Saharan Africa, with the notable exceptions of Ethiopia and Botswana, the vast majority of primary cultivation in farms is still carried out using hand tools. Draught animal technology was generally introduced to African countries during the first half of the 20th century, but in few areas has it been adopted by more than 15% of the farmers. Using the arguments of Binswanger and Pingali (1984), it might be concluded that in most cases, land and population pressures have not reached the levels necessary to justify the adoption of animal traction. However, in many cases it would appear to be associated with the low profitability of food crop production, for areas of high adoption have generally been those with a profitable cash-crop, or easy access to urban markets for the sale of food surpluses (Sargent et al., 1981; Starkey, 1984a). In an assessment of 127 animal traction projects in francophone West Africa, Sargent et al. (1981) concluded that the limiting factors were associated with the heavy cost of investment in animal traction, relative to hand cultivation, and a precondition for the successful adoption of draught animal power was a technological package that ensured higher overall productivity and returns from crop production. Such a conclusion would apply even more to the change to tractorized agriculture.

In Sub-Saharan Africa, many projects of the 1950's, 1960's and 1970's attempted to go straight from hand cultivation to tractorization. The vast majority of these failed, and large sums of money were wasted on large-scale machinery, both by the old colonial governments and new independent African governments. Reasons for failure included the problems of maintenance and spare parts and the inappropriate equipment used, but the most general problem was that the costs involved in operating the tractors were greater than the economic benefits of the cultivation. This problem has been exacerbated by the very serious foreign exchange shortages of most African countries, for the cost of tractor cultivation, involving imported equipment, fuel, lubricants and spare parts, comprises 90% foreign exchange. In comparison, the foreign exchange costs of ox-cultivation have been estimated at 12%, while the foreign exchange cost of hand cultivation is negligible (Starkey, 1981).

Very often in Africa, farmers do not have the financial means to decide to adopt animal traction, and thus a credit provision is necessary (Sargent et al., 1981; Munzinger, 1982). However, another major constraint is the lack of available appropriate equipment (Mettrick, 1978; Starkey, 1981; Kjaerby, 1983). In certain areas the shortage of cattle, and animal health may be a limiting factor (Apetofia, 1982; Imboden et al., 1983; Starkey, 1984a). In certain cases ethnic traditions and ineffective extension services may restrict the adoption of draught animals (Munzinger, 1982) but such constraints can usually be overcome if the economic conditions are highly favourable.

3.2. Choice of species

If draught animal technology is to be adopted, the choice of species will depend primarily on local conditions and the availability of appropriate animals. Sixty per cent of the draught animals in the world are cattle, *Bos taurus, Bos indicus* or crossbreeds, and these are strong but relatively slow moving. The fact that they are generally readily available, well-adapted to their environment and easy to buy and sell, makes them particularly suited to small farms in most parts of the world.

The water buffalo may be preferred to cattle in humid parts of Asia and North Africa, where water is readily available. They are heavier than most cattle breeds, which has the advantage of making individuals stronger, but the disadvantage of higher maintenance feed requirements per individual. Water buffaloes can work for very many years, although the examples of 30–40 year working lives quoted by FAO (1977) would seem to be the exception rather than the rule. Their predilection for water, together with their deliberate movements and large hooves, make them particularly suitable for work in deep rice swamps, and in many southern Asian countries, including Sri Lanka, the Philippines, Indonesia and Thailand, they are preferred to cattle for swamp work. However, buffaloes are generally slower than cattle for upland soils and road transport work, and unless these operations are combined with swamp cultivation and/or suitable wallowing places, cattle are generally preferred for these operations.

Most buffaloes are found in Asia, but significant numbers are also found in Egypt, southern Europe, Australia and certain Latin American countries, where they may be used for work purposes (FAO, 1977).

The introduction of water buffaloes into Sub-Saharan Africa has been attempted, including Madagascar, Mozambique, Nigeria, Senegal, Tanzania, Uganda and Zaire. However, to date no such scheme has flourished away from the close health and husbandry control of a livestock station. The great sensitivity of the Asian buffalo to various diseases including trypanosomiasis, restricts their potential for draught use in Africa, and also in parts of Asia including Vietnam (Finnelle, 1984). The African buffalo, while strongly trypanotolerant, is not domesticated. In general the water buffalo can be recommended as the draught animal of choice where it is to be used mainly in swamps, and where it is readily available. Where buffaloes are not already employed for work, and indigenous adapted cattle are readily available, then it is likely that it would be most appropriate to concentrate resources on the local cattle as draught animals. Any schemes to introduce water buffaloes for work purposes in new areas should proceed with great caution, and then only on a pilot basis until their adaptation to the environmental conditions is proven.

Equines, that is horses, donkeys and mules are the draught animals of choice in many areas. Their ability to move more quickly than cattle makes them particularly suitable for all transport operations, riding, carting and packing. In North America and Europe, horses gained particular preference for harvesting operations, where their speed was a critical advantage (Binswanger, 1984). They are generally considered to be more intelligent and easier to train than draught cattle. They can work for very many years, during which time their users generally develop feelings of attachment associated with their dependability. Unlike cattle, equines are not ruminants and they generally require a higher standard of nutrition than cattle. Equines generally lack the economic and social advantages of multi-purpose use, and also the potential for final disposal at a profit that is associated with draught oxen. Equines seldom thrive in humid climates, and tsetse flies and disease pathogens restrict their distribution in tropical Africa. The harnessing systems used for equines are generally more complicated and more expensive than those used with bovines. Donkeys are particularly adapted to arid and semi-arid ecosystems, and their speed, patience and ability to pull heavy weights, makes them well-suited for transport. Used singly, they can only pull a small plough through light soil, but they can be hitched in teams, and in Botswana up to eight donkeys may be hitched to a single plough. Breeding work on draught equines is still being carried out in Europe, where they are still important in certain areas for both agricultural and forestry operations (Sasimowski, 1984a). In general, in areas where they can thrive, where sufficient feed is available and affordable, where transport is important, and where there is sufficient draught demand to justify single-purpose draught animals, equines are likely to be the draught animals of choice. Elsewhere the almost universal availability of adapted bovines, that are easy to buy and sell and can be maintained for several functions, may make cattle more suitable as draught animals.

Camels may be effectively employed for cultivation, cart transport, pack transport and for riding in arid, sandy areas. The output of a single camel is comparable to a pair of oxen for ploughing sandy soils. Their ability to survive on browse in a harsh environment is legendary. However, camels are not suited to rocky or muddy terrains, or for working heavy soils, and their expense and highly adapted characteristics make them the draught animals of choice only in very distinct and limited ecological zones (Pathak, 1984a).

Yaks are used for draught in China and central Asia, being particularly adapted to high altitudes and low temperatures. Yaks are multi-purpose animals, providing milk and meat, in addition to performing draught and packing operations. They can be successfully bred with Chinese Yellow cattle to produce animals of good draught capability (Feng Yang-Lian, 1984). However, like the camel, the yak is adapted to very specific ecological conditions, and outside its normal range it has few advantages over draught cattle.

In many cases the various types of draught animals are complementary, and can work on the same farm, or in the same area. However, it has been stressed that for the small farmer the criteria of cost, availability and survival will be paramount. In the majority of cases this will mean that cattle are selected, because of their near universal availability, their adaptation to the environment and their ease of purchase, resale and feeding. However, in areas where they are available and have been proven, the specific advantages of horses, donkeys, buffaloes or camels, may make them preferable to cattle. It must be emphasized that the introduction of a novel draught species into an area should proceed with great caution, and on a pilot research basis. Enquiries should be made concerning previous experiences in the region, for there have been many attempts at introduction in the past century, and the absence of an apparently good draught animal is probably for sound ecological or economic reasons. It is particularly risky to introduce draught animal technology at the same time as a novel species, for there is a high risk of an appropriate technology being rejected simply because it is associated with an inappropriate species.

3.3. Choice of breed

While cattle can be classified according to their species, in this discussion the emphasis will be on breed, whether of *B. taurus, B. indicus* or of mixed origin. Inevitably many of the arguments are similar to those used in the determination of the most appropriate species. Thus the breed of choice is likely to be that which is available, affordable and adapted, and which can meet the various social, economic and technical needs of the farmer.

3.3.1. Size of animal

The size of draught cattle ranges from the West African Shorthorn and the Zanzibar Zebu, which stand 1 m at the shoulder and weigh about 200 kg, to the Chianina which stands over 2 m and can weigh over 1500 kg. For absolute strength for draught operations, large animals are desirable, and, for this reason, massive draught breeds were developed in Europe, including Chianina, Charolais and Simmental cattle and Shire horses. As draught power is closely correlated with size, for pure work output and efficiency of draught operations the larger breeds of cattle are to be preferred. Thus for purely commercial operations, such as log-pulling in forestry and sugar cane harvesting in Latin America, the size of the breed will be a key determinant. Large animals are not simply stronger, but also they are able to make more efficient use of poor quality fodder (Lawrence and Mathers, 1985).

However, large animals are not always the most appropriate. Small animals are cheaper, and individually they require smaller quantities of food for maintenance. By using two small animals instead of one larger one, a farmer can reduce the risk of his losing all his draught animal capital in a single incident of disease or accident. Smaller breeds generally have better reproductive performance, and frequently cattle are a source of wealth, with numbers of greater significance than individual size. Thus for a given total herd biomass, small animals are more likely to give higher levels of off-take or replacement rate.

Smaller breeds inevitably have a lower work potential than larger breeds. Thus a farmer using a single small ox can only use a 15 cm plough and in light soil conditions. A larger animal could pull a bigger plough, at a greater depth in heavier soils. The larger the size of the plough, the shorter the total distance a farmer has to walk whilst ploughing a hectare of land, and the greater the overall potential work rate. Thus ploughing with larger animals and larger implements is quicker and, in general, less tiring for the farmer. However, large implements can be pulled by small animals if several are yoked together. While the yoking of many animals may reduce the technical efficiency of the work output (CEEMAT/FAO 1972), it does enable smaller animals to perform heavy draught operations. For example, in Botswana, teams of 6–12 draught cattle or donkeys may be hitched to large ploughs (Starkey and Goe, 1984).

It is concluded that, although large cattle breeds are certainly advantageous for supplying draught power, size is only one of many factors that must be considered in choosing draught animals. A far more critical characteristic of a draught breed is its ability to survive and work in the prevailing environment.

3.3.2. Adaptation

Resistance to disease is perhaps the most important single characteristic of a draught animal for the small farmer. In West Africa, the small N'Dama (see Figs 8.15–8.17) is both trypanotolerant and resistant to streptothricosis (Starkey, 1984b), and where these diseases are prevalent, it is often the preferred breed for work purposes. To the north of the tsetse zone, the larger zebu cattle is preferred for draught. Around the boundary of the tsetse zone in southern Senegal, Mali and Burkina Faso, some farmers use the large zebu animals, and risk the death of their animals through trypanosomiasis. Other farmers use the smaller N'Dama, and accept lower draught power in place of higher security. Some farmers compromise and use zebu × taurine crossbreeds. South of the boundary zone farmers almost invariably use taurines, preferring good disease resistance to body size, even when reasonable veterinary services and trypanocidal drugs are available, as in Togo.

In general, indigenous breeds are likely to be relatively well-adapted to the local tick-borne and infectious diseases, due to years of natural and artificial

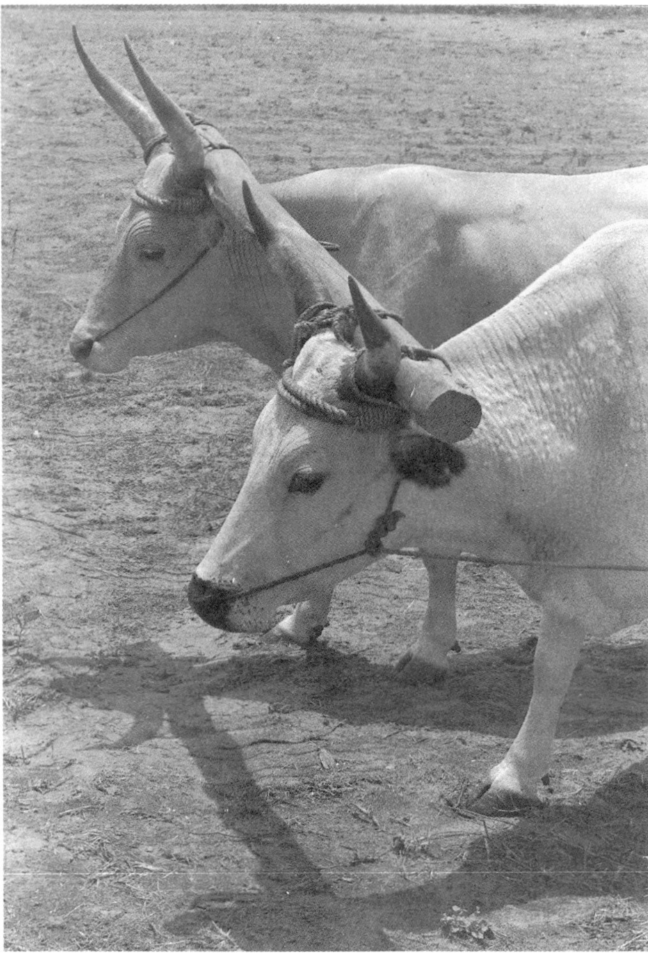

Fig. 8.15. Simple pole neck yoke on N'Dama oxen in the Gambia. (Photo: P. Starkey.)

selection. In addition most indigenous breeds are well-adapted to local climatic conditions. It is not surprising that many research studies have shown that *B. indicus* breeds are better able to withstand high temperatures, water shortages and tick challenges than the classic *B. taurus* breeds of Europe. Such adaptive breed characteristics are clearly desirable in draught cattle in many tropical conditions.

3.3.3. Availability

One of the main advantages of cattle as draught animals is that, generally, they can be easily obtained and easily sold. This allows farmers to profit from the weight gains associated with work oxen, and also allows farmers to quickly replace an animal that is found to be unsatisfactory through temperament, accident or disease. For these benefits to be easily obtained, the draught animals used have to be of the same, or similar breed to other cattle in the area, whether of draught, beef, dairy or multi-purpose type. Any farmer or project adopting a novel breed of cattle for draught purposes must ensure that the benefits of the new draught breed outweigh the significant disadvantage of limited replacement potential.

3.3.4. Research studies on draught cattle breeds

In many countries, government agencies and development projects devote research resources to the testing or identification of alternative draught breeds. One such example is recorded by Tessema and Emojong (1984). Large Friesian × Sahiwal crossbreds were compared with the local East African zebu animals. The larger animals had greater strength, but for the normal ploughing and cultivation operations of the area, a large draught requirement was not critical, and both types were equally effective. However, the larger animals naturally had higher requirements for maintenance feed, and had to be fed expensive feed supplements. It was particularly ironical that the on-station trials were performed in a drought year. Just off the station, up to half of the local zebu population died of starvation, for there was insufficient forage and the local farmers could not afford supplements even when their animals were dying. It was concluded that the larger crossbred animals were not appropriate to the local farming system. However, even if they had been found to be ideal, no realistic multiplication programme could have been initiated that could have made them readily available and affordable on a wide scale within a generation.

In many other countries small numbers of cattle of novel breeds and crossbreeds are being evaluated on research stations for draught performance. The general conclusions of on-station trials are that larger breeds of cattle are stronger. However, frequently such research is not concentrating on the real limiting factors. Very seldom do indigenous cattle reach their genetic potential for size, as nutrition, health and husbandry restrict their growth. The output of the indigenous animals might be significantly improved if more efficient harnessing systems, or alternative equipment were employed. In Africa, many research stations and projects have imported ploughs and then concluded that the local breed is too small for draught work — when a more positive conclusion would be that the imported ploughs were inappropriate, being too large for the available animals. In general it would seem that in very few instances is the genetic make-up of the local cattle the primary limiting factor.

A further example illustrates the danger of overemphasizing the importance of breed. Liberia, which has had no history of using animal traction, wished to initiate a pilot draught animal programme. One aid donor offered to import draught buffaloes while another offered to provide some large *B. taurus* animals from North America. Liberia's indigenous cattle are trypanotolerant taurines, Baoulé and N'Dama, which are well-adapted to the relatively unfavourable environment. Since the aim of the programme was to investigate the feasibility of using work oxen in the villages of Liberia, the available N'Dama cattle would seem ideal, as these are successfully used for work in the neighbouring countries of Sierra Leone, Guinea and Ivory Coast. To have imported exotic breeds would have confounded (in a statistical sense) the technology with the unadapted breed. The almost certain mortality of the animals might have led to the rejection of the technology. To have provided a fair assessment of the disease resistance of the exotic animals, it would have been necessary to use second generation individuals raised in the local environment — which would have delayed the programme by several years. Finally, in the unlikely event of the large exotic animals being able to withstand village conditions in such an unfavourable environment, the resources required to breed large numbers of animals would have been quite disproportionate to the cost of buying the indigenous N'Dama animals. Thus the well-meaning advice of consultants and aid donors, if taken, could have at best delayed, and at worst ruined, the research proposals of Liberia.

3.3.5. Conclusions on choice of cattle breeds

Almost all breeds of cattle, from the dwarf West African Shorthorn to the massive Chianina, Charolais and Simmental, can be successfully used for animal traction. In most cases availability and adaptation to the environment are more critical than size, and so adapted indigenous breeds should be used

Chapter 8 references, p. 196

whenever practicable. If stronger animals are required, it is likely that much can be done to improve the nutrition and husbandry of local stock. Alternative breeds should only be considered when it has been established that larger or more specialized animals are really required and that they can be afforded and adequately managed and fed. In selecting such breeds, adaptation to a similar ecosystem should be an important criterion, as well as any particular multipurpose characteristics that would be desirable in the local socio-economic situation. Experience from nearby areas should be carefully reviewed and evaluated before recommending the introduction of a new breed from a distant area. Similar criteria should be applied when considering upgrading local stock through crossbreeding, which is discussed in later.

3.4. Choice of sex

The word 'ox' refers to a castrated bull of any breed. An ox is considered to be an adult animal, and the term bullock is generally used for a younger castrate. There is sometimes confusion relating to the use of the word 'oxen', and many non-specialists imagine work oxen to be of a special breed or type. Watson (1981) uses the term 'oxen' to refer to working cattle of either sex.

Oxen, that is castrated males, are the draught cattle of choice in most parts of the world. Oxen are more docile than bulls and yet stronger than cows. They are generally readily available as breeding herds of cattle invariably produce a surplus of males. Ideally oxen should be castrated relatively late in life, after 2 years, and perhaps just before training at 3 years. If males are castrated early, they do not develop the strength and conformation associated with a bull.

Bulls ('intact' males) are successfully used for work in certain parts of the world. They are physically stronger than oxen, and they can perform reproductive functions in addition to their work. This is particularly important for the farmer with a small herd of cattle. However, bulls can be more aggressive, unpredictable and less easy to train than oxen, and in general they should be used with caution.

Cows are physically smaller and weaker than bulls and oxen, and if worked without sympathy, their reproductive performance will be significantly reduced. However, with skilled husbandry they can be very profitably used as multipurpose animals.

In Bangladesh about 30% of the 11 million draught animals are females, and Mettrick and James (1981) have developed a relatively complicated mathematical model that takes into account the various costs and benefits of using cows for draught purposes in that country. Using their model, with the available data, it was concluded that despite the drop in calving rate of 15% that was associated with draught utilization, the use of cows was very economically attractive for the small farmers.

Reh and Horst (1982) recorded that in Sine-Saloum in Senegal, N'Dama cows used for draught purposes actually had higher reproductive characteristics than similar cows kept in traditional herds. This was attributed to the fact that the better husbandry associated with draught animals more than compensated for the stresses imposed by the work.

The relative costs and benefits of using bulls, oxen or cows, will vary greatly between areas and between individual farms. For pure draught purposes, the ox is likely to be the best animal, being strong, tractable and without the 2-month interruption in availability that is associated with the calving of draught cows. For pure dairy or reproductive purposes, the cow will probably perform better if it is not made to work. However, with limited capital and feed resources, the small farmer can often compromise, and the combination of work with milk and calf production may be more profitable than either alternative by itself. The costs of multipurpose utilization of cows, will generally be higher than single-purpose use, particularly as a multi-purpose cow will require more feed than a similar individual used for either work or dairy production. Nevertheless the benefits, per cow, will be significantly higher when they are used for more than one function.

Where land, feed resources and thc availability of cattle are not limiting, then the maintenance of separate animals for draught and milk/reproduction purposes is likely to be technically and economically preferable. Thus in much of Sub-Saharan Africa, where the numbers of draught animals employed are low relative to the overall numbers of cattle, and where the availability of grazing land is relatively high, the utilization of cows for work is very low. The use of cows is higher in eastern Botswana, where draught animals are used by almost all farmers. It is even higher in Egypt where land and feed resources for maintaining cattle are very limited. Similarly in much of the Indian subcontinent, cows are used for draught where population pressures are high, and the resources required to maintain cattle, in particular land and feed, are limited.

Where draught work is important, but feed resources are limited, the use of cows can drastically reduce the overall herd size needed to give a given draught output. This is illustrated by the theoretical equations developed by Lawrence (quoted by Smith, 1984 and Lawrence and Mathers, 1985). These show that if young male animals are slaughtered, and all females are used for work, a total of only 63 livestock units are required to maintain 50 working animals. However if only oxen are used, a total of 176 livestock units need to be maintained to ensure the availability of 50 working animals. Further examples are given in Table 8.1, although it should be noted that these are quoted for the illustration of the principle only, as the model contains some assumptions which are, as yet, unproven.

It must be stressed that the use of cows for work necessitates a significantly higher level of feeding and husbandry than is required for work oxen. For this reason it is recommended that programmes introducing the use of draught cattle should start by encouraging farmers to use oxen. Once the necessary animal husbandry skills have become clearly established through the use of work oxen, then the economic advantages of using draught cows may be considered in the light of local needs and resources.

TABLE 8.1

Variations in composition and size of herd that will supply 50 draught animals when changes are made in age of slaughter of males and when females are used for draught purposes

	Strategy				
	(a)	(b)	(c)	(d)	(e)
Age of slaughter of males	6–7	9–10	12–13	6–7	12–13
Working life of oxen in years	3	6	9	3	9
Number of draught oxen per 100 ha	50	50	50	16	30
Number of draught cows per 100 ha	0	0	0	34	20
Calves (0–1 year)	27	14	9	11	7
Young cattle (1–3 years)	54	28	18	22	13
Adult cattle (3+ years)	144	97	82	50	50
Total livestock units[a]	176	113	93	63	58
Carcasses produced per year	27	13	9	11	6

[a] One adult is assumed to be equivalent to five calves or two young cattle.

The following assumptions have been made: (1) females start to breed at 4 years of age; (2) animals start to work at 3 years of age; (3) females are killed at 9 years of age; (4) 40 live calves survive per 100 breeding cows per year; and (5) when oxen are used for work, all male calves are kept but only some females.
Based on model of P. Lawrence quoted by Smith (1980, 1984), Lawrence and Mathers (1985).

Chapter 8 references, p. 196

4. SYSTEMS OF UTILIZING DRAUGHT CATTLE

4.1. Ploughing, harrowing and levelling

The single most important function of draught animals in the world is for ploughing. In much of Africa and Asia ploughing is the only operation performed by draught cattle, although ploughing may be followed by harrowing or levelling to obtain a satisfactory seedbed. Frequently more than one ploughing has to be used, either for weed control or to break up the clods of earth.

The simplest form of ploughing involves the use of a wooden 'ard' with a metal tip for soil penetration. The ard has no mouldboard and so soil is not turned, but it is loosened, often to a depth of 15 cm, and repeated passes at different angles ensure adequate weed control and suitable seedbed preparation. Such a simple ard is used in Peru (Fig. 8.13) and Ethiopia (Fig. 8.7). Using a traditional ard or *maresha,* it takes one man and a pair of Ethiopian zebu oxen between 100 and 200 hours/ha to make up to six passes with the ard for a satisfactory seedbed. Farmers generally use their animals for around 500 working hours a year, with 4–9 hours of ploughing per working day (Gryseels et al., 1984).

Elsewhere in Africa, steel mouldboard ploughs are used, with shares ranging from 15 cm for the smallest ploughs in West Africa to massive 38 cm ploughs used in parts of southern Africa. In Sierra Leone a 23 cm steel mouldboard plough is commonly used, to a working depth of 12 cm, and this is used in rice swamps, riverain grasslands and in 'upland' (non-swampy) soils. On-farm surveys have shown that the pairs of N'Dama oxen average 41 working days a year on ploughing and 3 days a year on harrowing, with other operations being of negligible importance. An average of 6.7 ha is cultivated, representing a rate of 24–30 ox team-hours/ha. Individual sets could plough at rates over 0.5 ha per working day of 4–5 hours, covering 18 ha in a season (Allagnat and Koroma, 1984). These figures involve mainly ploughing for swamp rice cultivation in undeveloped swamps. On-station trials in developed swamps gave figures of 33 ox team-hours/ha for ploughing and 38 ox team-hours/ha for harrowing and levelling (Starkey, 1984c). These figures are similar to the 23–33 team-hours/ha obtained for swamp rice ploughing in the Gambia (Matthews and Pullen, 1975). In Sierra Leone at least two people are used to control the animals, although frequently it is one adult and two or three children (Fig. 8.16). However in neighbouring Guinea, often one person controls the N'Dama oxen for ploughing, which makes the operation far more efficient in terms of human labour (Fig. 8.17).

In Botswana, teams of 6–8 Twsana cattle (often of mixed sexes) are controlled by two persons as they pull large mouldboard ploughs, generally with 30 cm shares. In on-farm trials, this system required 94 animal-hours and 37 man-hours/ha. A further 24 animal-hours and 8 man-hours were required for harrowing, bringing the total to 118 animal-hours/ha and 45 man-hours/ha for overall seedbed preparation (EFSAIP, 1981). Occasionally double-furrow ploughs are used in conjunction with teams of up to 12 oxen. Despite the large teams, actual ploughing rates are generally only 0.3–0.5 ha per working day of up to 6 hours. Animal utilization in Botswana is low. Ridder and Wagenaar (1984) quote figures of 18.5 team-days a year achieving just 4.7 ha of cultivation. Other estimates also suggest limited utilization, with just 12 team-days per year and 6.5 ha of cultivation (Litschauer and Matswe, 1983). The low rates of work are associated with very heavy, baked soils and very few days per year when the soils are considered suitable for ploughing and planting.

In Asia, animals are generally used much more intensively than in Africa. In India, annual utilization rates are generally in the range of 300–1200 team-hours per year, being mainly dependent on the land available to the farmer. Thus farms of 1 ha tend to use their animals for 300 hours per year, while farms of 4 ha would use them for 1200 hours per year (Pathak and Gill, 1984). The 300 ox team-hours/ha generally includes two crops, with ploughing, puddling and levelling being carried out by the animals. The actual time taken for ploughing rice fields in Sri Lanka, derived from an extensive survey, was 149 team-hours/ha for two ploughings and an extra 33 hours for levelling, bringing

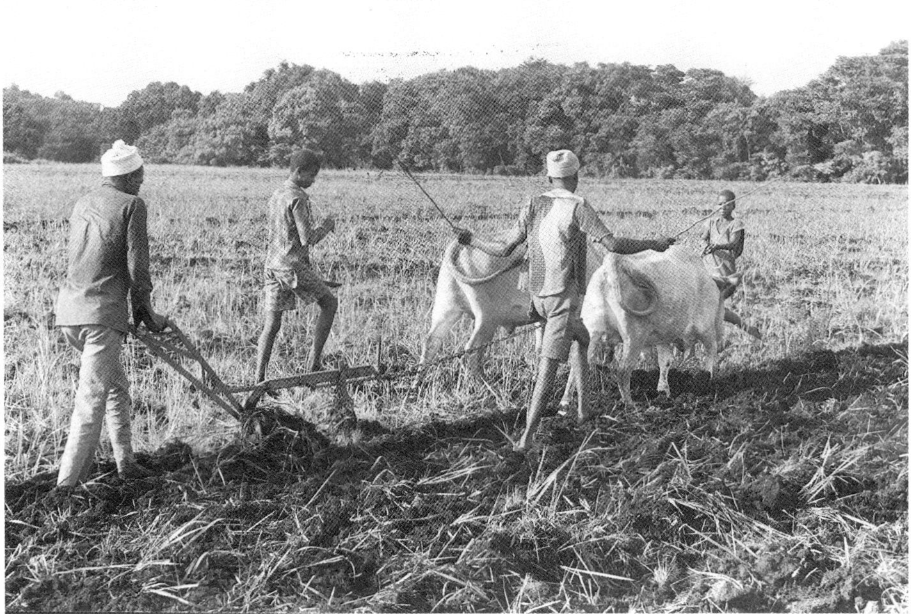

Fig. 8.16. N'Dama oxen being used by four people for ploughing in Sierra Leone. (Photo: P. Starkey.)

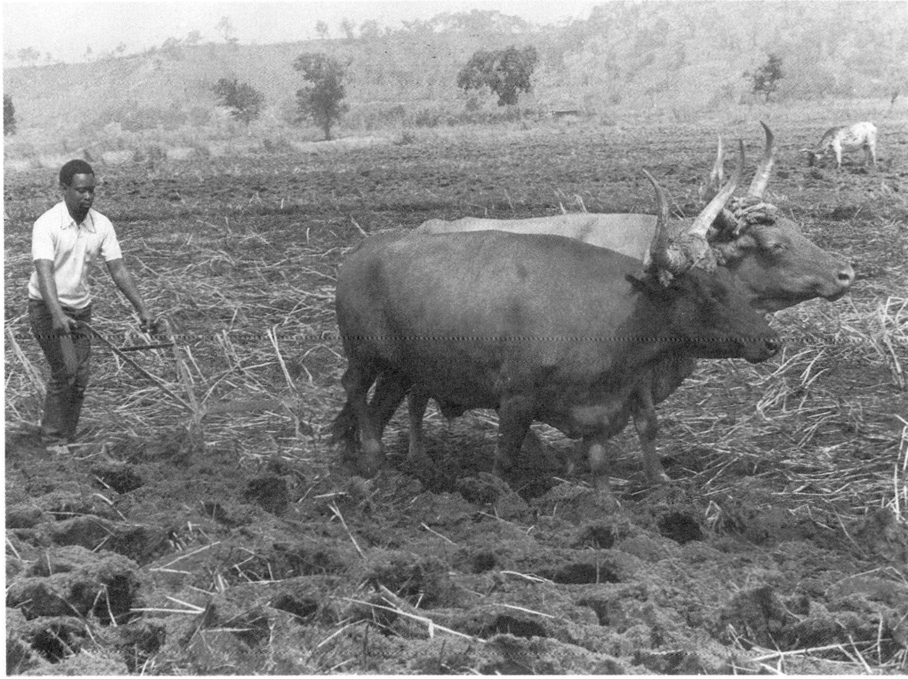

Fig. 8.17. One man controlling N'Dama oxen for ploughing in Guinea. (Photo: P. Starkey.)

the total time for land preparation to 181 team-hours/ha (Farrington and Abeyratne, 1982). These figures are much higher than those quoted for rice production in West Africa where mouldboard ploughs were used (Matthews and Pullen, 1975; Starkey 1984c). In Asia, generally one man controls a pair of animals (Fig. 8.9).

4.2. Ridging, seeding and weeding

Ridging is a specialized form of ploughing, in which soil is turned in both directions to form raised ridges. As it moves through the soil, a ridger forms two half-ridges and on each pass (after the initial run) one ridge is completed and another half-ridge formed. Ridging in untilled soil requires significantly more draught power than comparable mouldboard ploughing, but as the width of work is greater, the number of passes required to cultivate a hectare of land is reduced. Some of the advantages and disadvantages of ridging have been discussed by CEEMAT/FAO (1972) and Viebig (1982). In hard soils, ridging may only be possible after initial ploughing with other implements, but in lighter soils new ridges can be formed by the splitting of old ridges. Ridge cultivation for maize, groundnuts, tobacco and potatoes may be advantageous, particularly if contour ridges are used to conserve storm water and reduce erosion. Ridgers can be used for secondary weeding and re-banking operations. In northern Nigeria, some 40 000 ridgers are used as the main, and often the only, cultivation implement (CEEMAT/FAO, 1972), and ridging land by splitting old ridges takes 15 ox team-hours/ha (Phillips, 1977). However, generally ridging is much less common than other forms of ploughing, and figures of Le Moigne (1980) indicate that only 2% of the cultivation implements in francophone West Africa are ridgers. In the Gambia, ridging used to be very common, but it is declining as there appear to be no significant yield benefits of ridge cultivation, and conventional seed planters cannot be used on ridges (Mettrick, 1978).

Draught oxen can be used to pull seed planters, and this has been heavily promoted in Senegambia, where in 1977 there were reported to be 233 000 seeders in use, a number comparable with the total number of ploughs and toolbars (Sargent et al., 1981). This very high usage of seeders is exceptional, and associated with a short planting season, easily grown cash-crops and the large-scale local production of appropriate seeding implements. In other West African countries the ratio of seeders to ploughs is generally less than 1:10 (Sargent et al., 1981), and in many countries seeders are hardly used at all. Generally seeders are expensive, complicated, and sensitive to both variations in seed size and soil conditions, and in some circumstances can give very uneven results (Starkey and Goe, 1984). The economic case for seeders is weakened by the fact that generally human seeding can be achieved relatively quickly and accurately. In Sierra Leone, seeders were evaluated for maize, rice, groundnut and cowpea production, but they were found to give very erratic results unless soil conditions were ideal. It was concluded that seeders could not be justified on economic grounds by themselves, but if they led to the use of inter-row weeding, the total package was highly profitable (Starkey, 1981). Inter-row weeding using oxen is generally very effective, with enormous savings in human labour. For example, in trials in Sierra Leone, it was found that hand weeding of groundnuts required 403 man-hours/ha, while the use of oxen reduced this to just 76 man-hours/ha (Starkey, 1981). Elsewhere in West Africa time savings of 50–60% have been reported, when draught cattle are used for weeding (Sargent et al., 1981). The very high efficiency of inter-row weeding has prompted the development and promotion of multi-purpose toolbars, to which ducks-foot weeding tines can be connected (Mettrick, 1978; Sargent et al., 1981; Starkey, 1981).

Despite potentially very great savings in labour, inter-row weeders are seldom employed on a very large scale, and there are several important reasons for this. First, inter-row weeding requires straight line planting, which requires either an expensive and relatively complicated seeder, or a labour-intensive method of marking lines with strings or large rake-like markers. Secondly, line planting generally is associated with mono-cropping, and many farmers prefer to inter-crop. Thirdly, inter-row weeding requires very good control of animals, for crops can be badly trampled by the animals or uprooted by the weeder if the operation is not well-controlled. Fourthly, weeding is frequently the work of women, while the use of oxen is often the responsibility of men, so that the labour savings of one sex may necessitate an increase in the responsibilities of the other sex. Finally inter-row weeding is particularly suited to crops of relatively wide spacing (maize, groundnuts and cotton), for it is more difficult for animals to walk down the much narrower rows associated with high-density cereals like rice and wheat.

In Burkina Faso, it was found that while farmers were encouraged to buy a weeder when they bought their ploughs, they very seldom used this until they had become accustomed to using draught animals for 4 or 5 years. Until this time, they did not have the confidence that their animals would not ruin their crops (Barrett et al., 1982). Such fear is understandable, but can be overcome by ensuring high standards of training. Thus in one extension scheme in Zaire, farmers accepted immediately the use of line planting with strings, and inter-row weeding of maize (Fig. 8.18). In this case they considered the use of inter-row weeding to be one of the major benefits of adopting animal traction and the great labour saving of weeding more than compensated for the labour-intensive method of row-planting (Starkey, 1984a).

It has been argued that when animal traction leads to increases in planted areas, it can place a severe additional strain on the women, who may be expected to weed and harvest the increased areas. For this reason, the promotion of ox weeding techniques may be particularly important in areas where there are strong traditional labour divisions for the various farming operations (Bar-

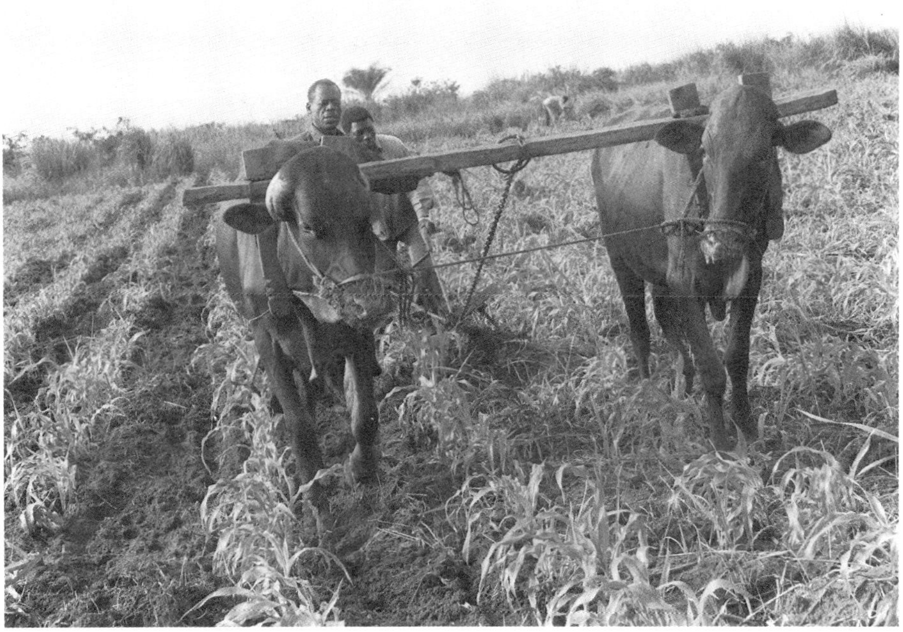

Fig. 8.18. Africander oxen weeding maize in Zaire. (Photo: P. Starkey.)

Chapter 8 references, p. 196

rett et al., 1982). With the notable exception of Senegambia, draught animal weeding is relatively limited, although its potential benefits seem to have been clearly demonstrated. The slow rate of adoption of ox weeding has been ascribed both to lack of research (Chambers, 1980) and to a lack of emphasis on such techniques by extension services (Sargent et al., 1981).

4.3. Harvesting, processing, irrigation, earthworks and forestry

In Senegambia about 90 000 lifting implements are employed for raising groundnut crops for harvesting. This represents a high use of animal power for a harvesting operation, and this is associated with both availability of suitable equipment, and the profitability of the crop (Le Moigne, 1980). Elsewhere there is relatively little use of draught animal power for harvesting. While certain publications give impressive illustrations of draught animal reapers, mowers, binders and equipment for harvesting roots and tubers, they acknowledge that their use is extremely limited, with most examples being either experimental prototypes or technology developed for temperate farming systems prior to the shift to tractor power (CEEMAT/FAO, 1972; Viebig, 1982; Pathak, 1984c). As Binswanger (1984) noted, in the United States and Europe crop harvesting equipment was generally pulled by horses and as such equipment spread the ratio of draught cattle to draught horses declined. In general, the high draught requirement and speed required for harvesting equipment means that draught cattle are seldom used for such operations.

Draught cattle are frequently used for threshing operations, particularly in Asia and in Ethiopia. The most simple method is the trampling of cut stalks by unharnessed animals (Fig. 8.19), although sledges or other drawn implements may increase the efficiency of the operations. Animal gears for crop processing including threshing, grinding and chopping have been used for many years in Europe and parts of Asia, but their distribution is limited. However, this is an area of recent research, development and promotion

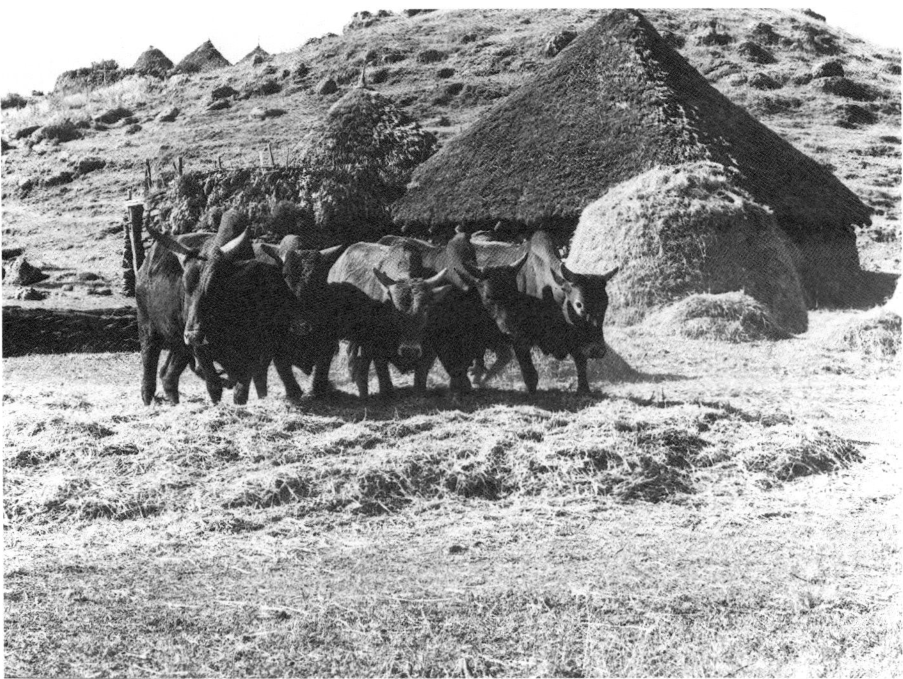

Fig. 8.19. Ethiopian zebu cattle being used for threshing. Note stock of conserved teff straw in background. (Photo: P. Starkey.)

(United Nations, 1975; Löwe, 1982; P. Löwe/GTZ, personal communication, 1984).

For centuries, draught cattle have been used for raising water for irrigation in North Africa, the Middle East and Asia. In general, the animals are attached to horizontal poles, and as they walk round in circles a pumping system raises the water. While in many places such operations are being replaced by mechanical pumps, efficient animal-powered systems of water raising are still being developed, although frequently emphasis is on the use of donkeys (Starkey and Goe, 1984). Such rotational systems are much more efficient than the laborious 'bucket haulage systems', where pairs of draught cattle simply repeatedly walk away from a deep well pulling a long rope and so raising a container of water (Fig. 8.20).

In the rice-growing areas of Asia and Africa, draught cattle are often used for bund formation, and equipment for this has been described by CEEMAT/FAO (1972), Viebig (1982) and Pathak (1984c). Draught cattle may also be used for other earthworks including terrace formation and the excavation of ponds. The use of an earth scoop developed at ILCA in Ethiopia is illustrated in Fig. 8.21. While land development work represents only a very small proportion of the total utilization of draught animal power, it is an area of research interest, particularly in view of its potential importance in soil and water conservation (Anderson, 1983).

The use of draught cattle in various forestry operations, notably log extraction, is increasing in many countries including Chile (Rodriguez, 1984), Malawi (E. May, personal communication,1983) and Tanzania (Humar, 1984).

4.4. Transport

The use of draught animals for transport has frequently preceded their employment for cultivation (Imboden et al., 1983; Binswanger, 1984). However, once a new mobile power source (either animal power or mechanical power) is introduced for crop cultivation, it rapidly becomes used for transportation, as it meets an important rural need (Binswanger, 1984). In rural areas,

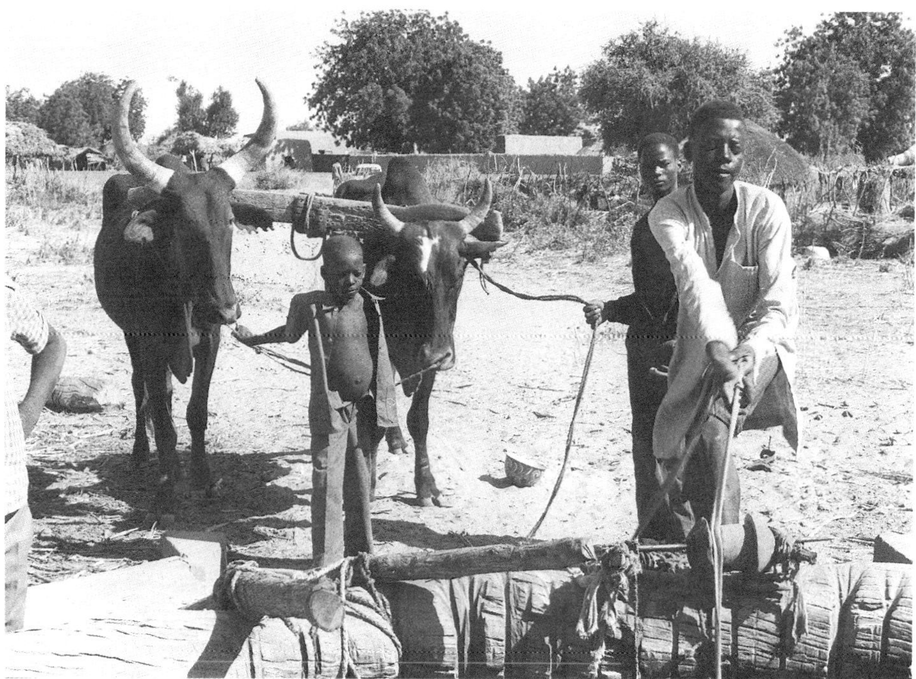

Fig. 8.20. Oxen in Niger used to pull water from a very deep well. (Photo: P. Starkey.)

Chapter 8 references, p. 196

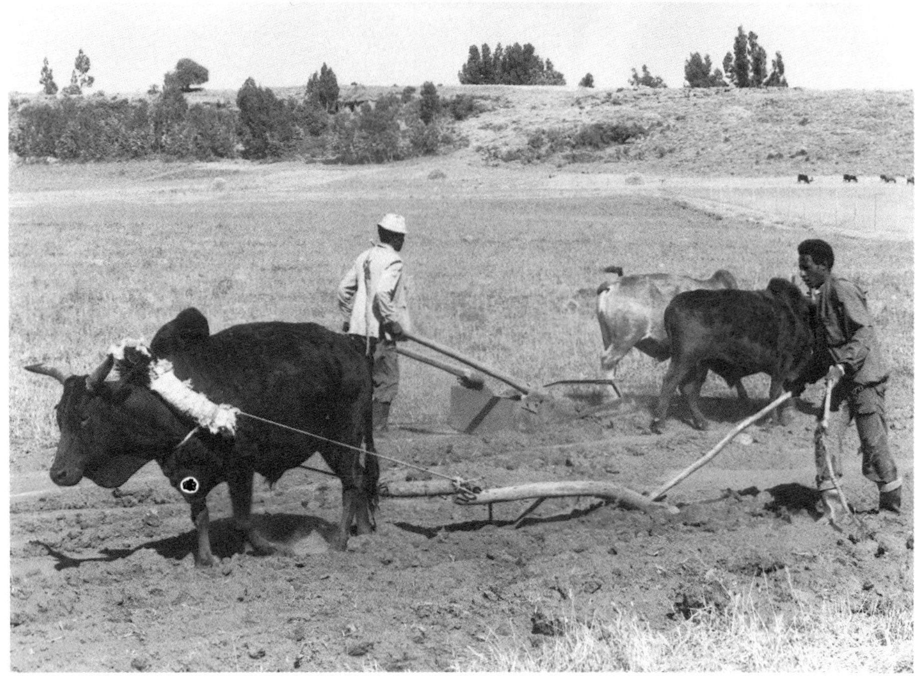

Fig. 8.21. Use of single Ethiopian zebu ox using withers yoke. Note also use of earth-moving scoop. (Photo: P. Starkey.)

where draught cattle are kept mainly for ploughing, the use of ox carts allows animals to be efficiently employed throughout the year, so keeping the animals in training. The relative costs of ox carts and other forms of transportation (human or motorized) are frequently such that an ox cart can be economically justified in rural areas if used just 50 times a year (Ramaswamy, 1981a; Starkey, 1981).

The relatively low capital cost of ox carts and their relatively slow speed makes them particularly suited to work with short distances and long loading times. For example both in Indian cities (Ramaswamy, 1981a) and on large-scale farms in Zambia (Dixon, 1985), ox carts have been found to be economically preferable to capital-intensive motorized transport.

The world utilization of animal-drawn vehicles has been reviewed by Ramaswamy (1981a). Ox carts are particularly important sources of transport in India and China, where 15 million and 10 million animal drawn vehicles are used respectively. While the majority of these carts are used in rural areas, some 3 million bullock carts are used in the cities of India, often being employed for 300 days a year for urban transport (Ramaswamy, 1981a).

The work achieved by draught cattle in transport operations is very variable, depending on animal size and condition, cart design and the nature of the terrain. Williamson and Payne (1959) quoted various authors giving examples of daily distances and loads. For example, sustainable distances of 34–38 km daily have been recorded for military ox carts in Africa and India, and Indian draught breeds can pull 1½ ton loads for up to 60 km on rough roads in a single day. While such performances are clearly possible for animals in good condition, ox carts are more commonly employed for shorter journeys, often between villages or between fields or water sources and the villages. In Africa, carts for two oxen are generally designed to carry about 1 ton (CEEMAT/FAO, 1972).

Cart design is an area with very great scope for improvement (Ramaswamy, 1981a). Families in Costa Rica take a special interest in building ornate carts.

In Asia, the traditional large wooden wheels are rapidly being replaced by technically more efficient pneumatic tyres and roller bearings (Ramaswamy, 1981a; Pathak, 1984c). In Africa, wheel and axle designs remain a major constraint. Traditional skills for making wooden wheels do not generally exist (Starkey, 1984a). Metal wheels with wooden bearings have been developed (Fig. 8.6), but they are frequently found to be unsatisfactory (Starkey and Goe, 1984). Pneumatic tyres on carts (Fig. 8.3), are considered very efficient, but repairing punctures in isolated villages is often found to be a major problem, and the foreign exchange costs of tyres may be considerable. In Kenya, the use of old tyres filled with sawdust has been advocated by research workers, but the practice has remained at the prototype stage for several years (Starkey and Goe, 1984). In some countries, research workers and farmers have found that sledges overcome many of the problems associated with wheels and axles (Kjaerby, 1983; Starkey, 1984a). Throughout Africa, workers in institutions, universities, agricultural development projects and village associations are actively working to improve the designs of ox carts. However, there is almost no coordination and liaison, and consequently there is a great deal of duplication of effort and considerable wastage of resources (Imboden et al., 1983; Starkey and Goe, 1984). As a result, the potential to improve the utilization of draught cattle for transport in Africa is particularly great.

While most other draught animals (horses, donkeys, mules, camels, yaks and llamas) are used as pack animals, cattle have never been commonly used in this way. While a need exists for field to village transport in areas where tracks cannot be easily developed or maintained, packing is considered much less efficient than haulage, and the use of sledges might be more appropriate than pack-harnessing (Ramaswamy, 1981a). Nevertheless the use of cattle as potential pack animals is an area of research interest (Smith, 1981; Lawrence and Mathers, 1985).

5. THE BREEDING OF DRAUGHT CATTLE

5.1. The problems of breeding for draught

The genetic improvement of draught cattle has received very little attention in recent years, and current scientific knowledge on this topic is extremely limited. The scientific literature on the genetics of draught cattle is minimal, as can be noted by the small number of references on breeding in animal traction bibliographies, such as those of Goe and Hailu (1983) and Bartlett and Gibbon (1984). The reasons for this are various. One could rightly observe that the whole subject of draught animal power has been neglected, and with it most subcomponents including breeding. However, the very complexity of breeding for draught power in different social, economic and ecological systems, makes the formulation of breeding policies particularly difficult. Seldom are cattle maintained exclusively for draught, and so selection and breeding programmes must establish complex criteria to balance the various requirements for multi-purpose utilization. In particular the most obvious draught characteristics are strength and power which are very closely correlated with size. While increased size would be relatively easy to select for, it would not always be appropriate to do so, for increasing size means increasing the feed requirements per animal, and increasing the cost or value of each animal, something which may not be desirable in traditional farming systems. The fact that draught characteristics relate to adult animals, and are not easily identifiable prior to maturity, makes both the selection of breeding stock, and genetic improvement slow processes. The very common practice of castra-

Chapter 8 references, p. 196

tion of draught cattle effectively prevents the possibility of using proven individuals as sires. Farmers generally obtain their animals for draught training from small, relatively isolated herds, very often the farmer's own, and in such circumstances the logistical problems of initiating any smallholder-based selection and breeding programme would be formidable. The financial incentives to encourage private sector genetic improvement programmes for draught animals are minimal, for the timescale for realization of benefits would be very long and much greater than for other animal production enterprises (such as pigs, poultry and beef), and the small-farmer sector has limited resources to invest in more costly improved genotypes. Finally, with so many draught characteristics being greatly influenced by environmental exposure and the history of the individual, the practicalities of identifying the better genotypes represented in phenotypes is daunting.

5.2. Selection criteria

In order to select individuals for breeding future generations, it is necessary to define the characteristics of an outstanding draught animal.

The most important characteristic, which is actually easy to overlook, is the ability simply to *survive* in the particular environment in which it is to live and work. This must include the ability to live in the prevailing climate, facing the local pathogenic challenges, using locally available feed resources and requiring only such services that are readily available and economically affordable by the farmer. These survival characteristics are precisely those universally selected by most farmers and by nature, and have resulted in the present use of highly adapted draught animals in most countries in the world.

Sadly, the primary importance of survival as a selection criteria has been frequently neglected by draught animal programmes. Research workers and agricultural development projects tend to look first at more obvious characteristics such as size and strength, and this had led to wastage of research and aid funds. The proposed importation of water buffaloes and North American cattle breeds into remote, tsetse-infested villages in West Africa (Sierra Leone and Liberia) illustrates this point well. The buffaloes have proven draught characteristics superior to the local N'Dama, and the cattle from the United States would also be significantly stronger than the small N'Dama. The aid donors concerned sincerely wished to improve draught capability in these countries, but veterinary services were virtually unavailable in the remote villages, and had the schemes been accepted, the chances of survival of the imported animals would have been minimal.

It should be noted that the criterion of survival is related to the prevailing social, economic and physical environment, and as the environment improves, so the selection criteria may be modified. Thus where good veterinary services are readily available and affordable, animals less resistant to disease may be considered. For example, in Togo, the provision of trypanocidal drugs by the veterinary services has allowed the use of larger zebus and zebu × taurine crossbreds, even though it is acknowledged that the smaller taurines have a greater ability to survive (Apetofia, 1984).

The second major characteristic is the ability of the animals to work effectively within the prevailing environment. This second generalization also represents many complex and interacting criteria, for it is not simply strength that is required, but the ability to give satisfactory work performance in the available time, under the local climatic and farming conditions.

Body size and strength are of particular importance in determining maximum working power, and the two characteristics are closely related. In a review of work in francophone Africa (CEEMAT/FAO, 1972), it was concluded that power output depends on a whole range of factors characterizing the animals and their environment, but in broad terms, sustained average traction is directly related to the weight of the animal, being in the order of 10–15% body weight. When draught cattle walk fast, maximum instantaneous effort is approximately equal to body weight, but it is nearer 50–70% of body weight if animals are moving at their normal speed (CEEMAT/FAO, 1972). In horses, clear correlations have been established between body mass and strength (Dyrendahl and Bengtsson, 1984). However, while in animals generally, the relationship between size and strength is clearly established, it has been noted that the correlation is not a simple one. The larger the animal, the greater its strength; but relative draught capacity actually decreases with body size, so that smaller animals are stronger relative to their weight than large animals (Lawrence and Mathers, 1985).

Conformation is clearly important for draught purposes, and desirable physical attributes have been described by various authors including Williamson and Payne (1959), CEEMAT/FAO (1972), Howard (1979), Watson (1981) and Reh (1982). It is generally agreed that a draught bovine should look powerful, compact and sturdy, with well-developed muscles, particularly those of the hindquarter/back (CEEMAT/FAO, 1972) and the forequarter/shoulder (Howard, 1979). For animals selected mainly for ploughing, short legs are desirable, but longer legs may be preferable for inter-row cultivation and transport (Williamson and Payne, 1959; Howard, 1979). The chest should be broad and deep, and the neck strong. Reh (1982) recommends that the presence of a hump is a desirable characteristic where withers yokes are used, but Goe (1983) argues that a hump is certainly not necessary, and by implication it can be undesirable as it encourages the use of inefficient withers yoking systems. Where head and neck yokes are used, the horns are particularly important as they provide the attachments for the ropes securing the yoke. In these cases the horns must be strong and relatively long — at least 15 cm — although Reh (1982) accepts a lower minimum of 10 cm. Horns that are directed forwards and upwards are desirable (Starkey, 1981). It is universally agreed that draught animals need to be selected to have strong, hard hooves, although the literature does not elaborate on precisely how such selections should be made.

Having established criteria for a desirable conformation, it is possible to give weights to the importance of each characteristic, and so develop a selection index (Bowman, 1974). Indeed Sasimowski (1984b) has proposed such a scoring system, based on ten general conformation characteristics. However, considerable caution should be exercised in any selection based primarily on conformation, for during a quarter of a century of detailed and systematic measurements and assessments of different anatomical features in draught horses, the only conformation characteristic that statistically correlated with draught capacity was the live weight of the animal (Dyrendahl and Bengtsson, 1984).

Temperament is an extremely important characteristic, and certain desirable behavioural qualities have been given by Pathak (1984a,b,c). In general, wild or excitable, lethargic or lazy animals are rejected in the early stages of training, as soon as these characteristics become apparent. However, Williamson and Payne (1959) counsel against the early rejection of animals showing fierceness or nervousness, as these characteristics may simply indicate a useful degree of spirit and courage. In horses, special 'temperament' tests have been developed (Sasimowski, 1984a), but similar routines are rare, or absent from draught cattle selection programmes. While temperament is clearly important, it may be very largely a phenotype characteristic, related to the upbringing, for it is widely recognized that animals brought up in close contact with men are generally more tractable than those raised in ranches or in big herds.

Chapter 8 references, p. 196

5.3. Evaluation of performance

Once desirable characteristics have been selected, there still remains a means of ascertaining which are the best draught animals with these characteristics, whose genes should be maximized in future generations. This necessitates an objective method of evaluating the performance of individuals.

In recent years, draught horses have undergone performance testing in several European countries. In some cases the tests have been voluntary, but in others they have been compulsory (FAO, 1982). The tests fall into two major categories evaluating *maximum efficiency* and *draught aptitude*. In a maximum efficiency test, ergometers measure maximum draught power, and in Wangen, Sweden a large circular capstan ergometer has been used, with horses walking round with increasing, quantified loads. Elsewhere a loaded cart and dynamometer have been used to measure maximum performance. In a draught aptitude test in Sweden, a weighted cart is pulled round a varied course in a forest, which is taken at normal speed and includes an obedience test. Associated measurements during the test include heart rate, respiration and degree of sweating. Such testing procedures have generated much interest and enthusiasm among draught horse users (Dyrendahl and Bengtsson, 1984).

However, similar large-scale evaluation tests have not been undertaken with draught cattle. On a small-scale research basis, evaluation of the performance of draught cattle has included the use of loaded carts (Howard, 1979) and a treadmill (Lawrence and Mathers, 1985). On a large scale, subjective estimates of draught cattle performance have been made within the context of ploughing competitions, for example in Sierra Leone (Starkey, 1983a,b), but none of these system of evaluation has been linked to a breeding programme.

At an Expert Consultation on Draught Animals (FAO, 1982) it was noted that there was a distinct need to develop standardized performance testing procedures for draught animals in Africa and Asia. However, it was considered that sophisticated performance-testing stations, such as those developed for European horses, would be inappropriate, as draught cattle selection programmes in developing countries would probably be based on relatively small and widely dispersed herds.

5.4. Heritability

The phenotypic characteristics of good draught animals are a result of an interaction between the genotype of the individual and its environment. The heritability is a measure of the proportion of the variation between the individuals of a population that can be ascribed to the genotype. In more precise terms it is the ratio of additive genetic variance to phenotypic variance. A heritability approaching 1.0 would indicate that a trait is highly heritable, and selection procedures should yield very rapid genetic progress. A heritability near to zero would suggest that the variation in a trait is primarily a result of environmental effects, and the selection of particular phenotypes (measurable characteristics) is unlikely to result in significant changes in the genetic make-up of the population. It is therefore of great interest to obtain estimates of the heritabilities of different draught characteristics, for there is little point in allocating scarce resources to selection programmes, if the phenotype is not a reliable guide to the genotype.

The actual size of an animal is determined by its genetic composition and its environment, and in particular its past environmental history of nutrition and disease. In general the heritability for final weight in cattle is high, being estimated at between 0.6 and 0.7 (Preston and Willis, 1974). This implies that in general selection for increased size should lead to genetic progress in this trait. However, it should be stressed that if the estimates of heritability come from different individual herds, and within each herd the animals have similar environmental histories then such heritability estimates cannot be applied to, say, market animals coming from different herds, for in such circumstances the phenotypic variation attributable to the environment is likely to be much greater.

A useful historical example of genetic selection for large size for draught power can be seen in the different European beef breeds. During the 19th and early 20th century pure beef breeds, such as the Aberdeen Angus, were being selected for meat quality, and in particular a high proportion of tasty fat. At the same time the Charolais and Chianina were selected for draught power, and this led to the development of a large frame, a high proportion of muscle and very little fat. Changing consumer tastes and the need for improved efficiency of beef production have made these 'draught' characteristics desirable in the meat trade, so that the genetic progress in draught power is being widely exploited with the use of the large 'draught' breeds for beef production.

Apart from relatively high heritability of physical size, there seems very little objective evidence on the heritability of other draught characteristics in cattle. Preston and Willis (1974) note that any correlation between conformation scores of cattle and production traits, including final body weight are low or even negative. The lack of correlations between anatomical conformation and draught ability has already been noted, albeit in reference to horses (Section 5.2).

In the conclusions of the FAO Expert Consultation on Draught Animals it was stated that the 'heritability of draught traits seem to be fairly high' (FAO, 1982). At this consultation, Sasimowski (1984b) stated that 'another proof is the well known fact that bad-pulling parents of a draught breed have progeny with poor pulling ability'. Sasimowski was referring mainly to work with horses, and whether or not such terms as 'proof' and 'fact' are scientifically appropriate with relation to equines, a much greater degree of caution would seem applicable when considering draught cattle, on which much less work has been carried out. However, it is of interest to note that commercial horse breeders consider racing attributes to be highly heritable, and for this reason successful racehorses attract extremely high stud fees. While the characteristics of racehorses are clearly very different from those of draught cattle, there may be certain similarities in the general principles of selecting for a combination of anatomical, physiological and behavioural characteristics.

Of the various adaptive characteristics desirable in draught animals, many appear to be breed-related. For example many studies have been carried out comparing the disease resistance, tick resistance, and heat-stress resistance of different cattle breeds. However, even in such a well-researched area as trypanotolerance, the genetic basis and heritability is not well-understood (Schote, 1982; Starkey, 1984d). Nevertheless in areas where particular adaptive characteristics are desirable, efforts should be made to obtain such estimates of heritabilities as are available, with a view to including those adaptive attributes of high heritability in any selection programme.

5.5. Systems of breeding and selection for draught

The FAO Expert Consultation on Draught Animals, recognizing the apparent high heritability of draught traits, recommended to FAO and member countries that mass selection for desirable draught characteristics be initiated, in association with nucleus-herd schemes. It also noted that selection should be made within the environment in which the animals work, and that sophisticated performance stations were not required in developing countries (FAO, 1982). Mass selection, which is also known as individual selection, in-

Chapter 8 references, p. 196

volves the performance testing of individuals and the selection for breeding of those animals which excel.

The organizational problems associated with the recommendation for mass selection programmes are formidable. First, objective testing systems for draught cattle have yet to be adequately developed. Thus performance testing systems will need to be developed, preferably ones that can be easily used in isolated areas. Secondly, as cattle are seldom maintained exclusively for draught purposes, the selection procedures will probably have to be multifactorial. Thirdly, the nearly universal practice of castrating draught bulls will make mass selection among the majority of working animals an impossibility. Finally systems will have to be developed to enable the numerous small farmers, each owning very few draught animals, to benefit from the resultant genetic progress. Clearly mass selection as a means of assisting the small farmer, is likely to be a slow and difficult process.

Mass selection is just one option, and with the large number of castrates used, is clearly not ideal. However, other breeding systems also have their disadvantages. Pedigree selection involves choosing preferred breeding stock on the basis of the performance of parents or grandparents. However, pedigree selection necessitates not just performance testing, but record keeping of the performance of different generations, which may be difficult in the rural areas of developing countries. It is also impracticable when the majority of draught animals are castrates. In some farming systems family selection is employed, particularly when heritability is low. Family selection involves breeding with the siblings of selected individuals and so can be used when the selected individual is castrated. Thus the brothers and sisters of a particularly good draught animal could be retained for breeding. However, as cattle have such small family sizes, and generation times are so long, such a selection procedure is far from ideal. Nevertheless it is one option open to cattle-raising farmers using draught oxen, although rapid genetic progress cannot be assured. Progeny testing involves selected breeding on the basis of the performance of offspring. Thus if the offspring of one bull are found to be above average draught animals, the bull can be selected to serve more cows to produce more offspring. The main problem is that draught characteristics are normally assessed relatively late in life, perhaps 5 years after the initial siring, so that by the time a bull has been shown to have outstanding progeny, many years will have passed and future reproductive performance is consequently limited. Schemes using artificial insemination are best able to use progeny testing, for with artificial insemination, reproduction can continue after the natural life of the original bull. However, artificial insemination in developing countries represents a very high cost form of reproduction that, to date, has been restricted almost exclusively to dairy and beef production.

No breeding system can work effectively without the reliable evaluation of performance, the detailed recording of such performance, and the controlled and selected reproduction of the chosen individuals. Finally for genetic progress to be effective, a large population of animals needs to be involved. This requires a very high degree of organization, and, by implication, of funding also.

This is not to suggest genetic progress is impossible. On the contrary, despite all the constraints associated with small herds, castrated draught animals, multi-purpose requirements, and lack of performance testing and systematic recording, many breeds have been developed in the world that are extremely well-adapted to their work and their environment. For example, the Ethiopian zebu has been proven as an adapted, multi-purpose/draught animal for generations. Similarly many Indian breeds have specific draught/multi-purpose/adapted characteristics that have been developed over many centuries. This proves that genetic progress is certainly attainable, and modern techniques will make much faster rates of improvement possible. Nevertheless the obstacles have been emphasized to make it clear that within-breed selection is a very long-term activity, and dramatic improvements in draught animal power are more likely to come from changes in management and systems of utilization, than from selection within breeds.

5.6. Crossbreeding

Crossbreeding has much greater potential for achieving rapid genetic changes than within-breed selection, for, from the very first cross, the favoured characteristics may be displayed in the offspring. Crossbreeding is generally undertaken to combine the better attributes of two (or more) breeds, and also to benefit from the advantages of heterosis ('hybrid vigour'). Very often the objective of crossbreeding is to combine the adapted characteristics of an indigenous breed with more productive characteristics of an exotic breed. However, it must be emphasized that crossbreeding by itself does not necessarily result in the ideal combination of characteristics. Very often, the crossbreeding combines the disease susceptibility of the exotic animals with the relatively low performance of the indigenous breed, so that animals are produced that are insufficiently adapted for village conditions, yet insufficiently productive to justify the resources required to maintain them.

Natural crossbreeding occurs at the interface of the distribution zones of different breeds, and this is particularly noticeable in West Africa. Here, around the margin of the zones of zebu dominance and the more tsetse-infested areas of the taurine breeds, exist natural crossbreds. All grades exist between pure zebu and pure taurine, but the crossbreds are common in relatively limited ranges, and they experience particularly heavy selection. To the north of the zones they are selected against mainly by the farmers, who prefer the larger zebu animals. To the south they face the natural selection of trypanosomiasis, and are less able to withstand this than the trypanotolerant taurines. In only a few areas do relatively stable populations of zebu × taurine crossbreds thrive.

This natural example illustrates one of the major problems of crossbreeding, that of ensuring long-term continuity. In the few cases where the exotic purebred is well-adapted, the up-grading programme can continue using purebred bulls to produce higher and higher grades of crosses until the indigenous population becomes almost pure exotic breed. However, in most cases the higher grades are insufficiently adapted, and if left to breed among themselves, the crossbreds will produce some animals that are high grades (and relatively unadapted) and some that are low grades (and relatively unproductive), with high selective forces operating. In some cases, this has led to the creation of new breeds (such as the Australian Milking Zebu and the Australian Friesian Sahiwal), but in other cases, on large stations, rotational crossbreeding is employed so that the higher grades and lower grades are never produced. This is impracticable under village conditions, and so introducing crossbreds often results in either the loss of genetic progress through back-crossing with the indigenous breed, or the undesirable production of some non-adapted high grades through *inter-se* matings. The difficulties experienced with crossbreeding may be illustrated by the fact that while most developing countries have one, or more, crossbreeding programmes, relatively few have progressed satisfactorily beyond the confines of experimental stations and large farms.

Nevertheless, the use of crossbred exotic × indigenous cattle has been cited as a major means to improve the efficiency of animal traction (ILCA, 1981). The argument is that the larger and heavier crossbreds are better suited to animal traction, and that they have demonstrated adequate performance in

---

Chapter 8 references, p. 196

trials in tropical countries (Goe and McDowell, 1980; ILCA, 1981). However, it has already been noted here that crossbreds are not always sufficiently well-adapted to their environments, and that in African countries, crossbreds have yet to be introduced on any large scale. As there are very few crossbreeding programmes specifically for animal traction, it is necessary to look at the 'by-products' of crossbreeding programmes for dairy and beef production.

Most countries in which dairy production is practicable have crossbreeding programmes involving one of the major world dairy breeds such as Friesian-Holstein, Jersey and Sahiwal. In tropical countries the crosses of these breeds are generally larger than the pure indigenous animals, and therefore it is thought that the surplus males produced by a dairy programme could be suitable for use in animal traction programmes. For this reason crossbred dairy × indigenous animals are often evaluated on research stations, and the author has observed draught operations performed by Friesian × zebu crossbreds at research stations in Ethiopia, Kenya and Tanzania. In all cases was it concluded that the larger crossbred animals were technically proficient at draught work on the stations, but also that they required greater quantities of food for maintenance. In all cases reservations were expressed at the problems smallholders might have in maintaining the crossbred animals in good condition in the villages, and it was also noted that the availability of the crossbreds was very limited. ILCA has also investigated the use of zebu × Friesian cows for milk and draught (Fig. 8.22); initial results suggest that it is technically possible with a high standard of management (Anderson, 1983).

In Ivory Coast, a long-term crossbreeding programme was carried out between the highly adapted and disease-resistant N'Dama and the high producing Jersey dairy breed (Letenneur, 1978). It was initially intended as an upgrading programme, but very high mortality was observed in animals which had over 50% Jersey genes. It was concluded that the optimum combination was three-eighths Jersey and five-eighths N'Dama. At this grade, the females were reasonable milk producers, and the males made good draught animals, and their disease resistance was such that they could thrive with reasonable

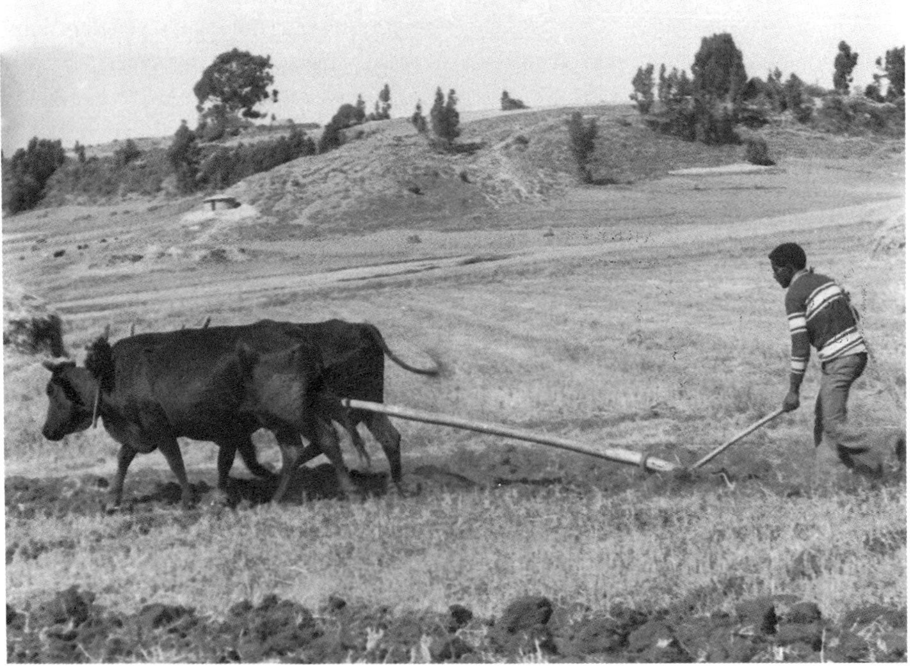

Fig. 8.22. Crossbred Ethiopian zebu × Holstein-Friesian cows being used for ploughing at ILCA, Ethiopia. (Photo: P. Starkey.)

stockmanship. However, the main problem was in developing a breeding system that could succeed off the research station. To ensure that the optimum inclusion of Jersey genes was not exceeded, it was necessary to devise a relatively complicated breeding programme, for example using three-eighths or five-eighths bulls on F_1 females. A more practicable solution was to simply back-cross the three-eighths bred animals with pure N'Dama in the villages, to ensure continued adaptation to local conditions, and combine this with the sustained supply of crossbred animals from the research station.

In India, which has numerous multi-purpose/draught breeds, and several specialized dairy breeds, crossbreeding dairy programmes have become very well-established. However, only 10% of the animals in India are crossbred, and the proportion is not likely to increase above 15% in the next 20 years (ESCAP/FAO, 1983). In other countries the proportions of crossbred cattle are generally well below these levels, and in the foreseeable future, the vast majority of the world's draught animal power will continue to be provided by indigenous breeds.

While crossbreeding for dairy production generally involves the smallholder sector (large-scale commercial dairy farmers generally use purebred animals), crossbreeding for beef production is often restricted to the large-scale farmers. This may explain the very limited number of reports of crossbred beef animals being evaluated for animal traction. For example, in Botswana, where 80% of all farmers use draught animals, but where cattle ownership is highly skewed, a major, long-term evaluation of crossbreeding involving Tuli, Tswana, Brahman, Simmental, South Devon, Africander and Bonsmara breeds, concentrated entirely on beef production rather than draught characteristics (APRU, 1978; Lipton, 1978).

One of the few crossbreeding programmes initiated specifically to produce draught animals is being developed in Togo. At different ranches indigenous Borgou taurines and zebus are being crossed with N'Dama, to produce a disease-resistant draught animal (personal observation; Apetofia, 1982, 1984). The optimum combination of N'Dama, zebu and Borgou genes will be decided following the evaluation of the different grades.

One problem associated with crossbreeding, or any genetic improvements, is that the improved animals are inevitably more expensive due to shortages of supply, larger size, or costs of production and distribution. For example, the expense of the draught/multi-purpose Renitelo breed developed on Madagascar has been cited as a major constraint to its widespread adoption (Tran van Nhieu, 1982).

5.7. Disease resistance

The ability of his draught cattle to survive is of paramount importance to the small farmer. For this reason disease resistance must be a major criterion in any breeding or selection programme designed to improve smallholder animal traction.

In West and Central Africa, trypanosomiasis, transmitted by the tsetse fly is a major problem to livestock, and it is a particularly serious threat to working animals for the additional stresses of work or related undernutrition may reduce resistance to the disease challenge. In this area many draught animal programmes have experienced high mortality, particularly in cases where zebu cattle have been used in areas of trypanosomiasis risk, as in southern Senegal, Togo and southern Burkina Faso (personal observation; Reh, 1982). In these areas trypanocidal drugs are now being routinely administered to working animals to prevent the repetition of earlier high rates of death. However, the use of the natural resistance of the N'Dama is now being recommended, and in addition to use in its normal range, it is being multiplied for

Chapter 8 references, p. 196

draught use in Togo and Zaire (Starkey, 1984a). The N'Dama is small (adults 230–370 kg), but it is strong and it has been widely proven as a draught animal in Guinea, Guinea Bissau, Senegal, the Gambia, Mali, Sierra Leone and Ivory Coast where a total of about 250 000 N'Dama draught animals are employed (Figs 8.15–8.17); (Starkey, 1984b). The N'Dama is most famous for its trypanotolerance, but it is also resistant to streptothricosis and is generally highly adapted to survive under difficult West African conditions (Starkey, 1984b).

When the N'Dama is crossed with larger breeds such as the Jersey, zebu and Sahiwal, its disease resistance decreases (Letenneur, 1978; Djabakou et al., 1982; Starkey, 1984b). However, if crossed with other small trypanotolerant breeds such as the Baoulé it retains its trypanotolerance (Roelants and Pinder, 1982).

Although the N'Dama is particularly noted for its disease resistance, most other indigenous cattle breeds in tropical countries are also relatively well-adapted to their environments as a result of generations of natural and artificial selection. Disease resistance is seldom absolute, and thus it is difficult to detect within an indigenous population. It becomes most obvious when exotic breeds are introduced, and it is found that even second and third generation crossbred animals show themselves to be significantly more susceptible to local diseases than the indigenous population. For example, in Sierra Leone the disease streptothricosis was not considered a major problem. It was only after Sahiwals had been introduced for crossbreeding, and suffered severely from this disease, that it was realized the disease existed as a permanent challenge, but one that seldom produced clinical symptoms due to the resistance of the indigenous animals. Similar types of disease resistance probably exist in many indigenous cattle breeds, and it is important that such characteristics are not inadvertently lost through crossbreeding or selection for a single characteristic such as large body size.

It should be noted that for genetic disease resistance to express itself in the phenotype, an environmental challenge by the appropriate pathogen may be required. Such challenges may be absent from strictly controlled animal breeding stations and ranches, and they may also be absent from different parts of a country. Thus there is a significant danger when draught animal programmes rely on cattle from stations or on transported stock, for they may not be able to withstand the disease challenge of the new environment. For example, draught animal programmes in Burkina Faso, Sierra Leone and Togo all experienced high mortalities when indigenous stock were taken from ranches or nearby areas to new local environments. In such cases it may be assumed that the animals had not had the necessary early pathogenic challenges to enable them to express any genotypic disease resistance.

5.8. Multi-purpose requirements

In certain circumstances, cattle are required specifically for draught purposes. For example in forestry industries cattle may be technically and economically more efficient than machinery, and the draught cattle are maintained commercially for their draught work (Rodriguez, 1984; E.D. May, personal communication, 1983). In such cases breeding programmes can concentrate on developing good draught characteristics, combined with environmental adaptation, and it is likely that such programmes will lead to physically larger animals.

In a few other specific cases, emphasis may be placed exclusively on draught characteristics, combined with appropriate adaptation. These include areas with low cattle populations, such as Togo and Zaire, that are specifically multiplying cattle for use in draught animal programmes. Another example is India where for many years the emphasis on breeding and crossbreeding has been for milk production, and this has led to the feeling that the draught breeds have been neglected. Thus the Haryana, the Ongole and Hallikar breeds are to be selected specifically for draught purposes in five state livestock farms (Pathak, 1984b).

However, in the vast majority of farming systems in developing countries, cattle perform several functions, and highly specialized animals are not preferred. Thus there is a tendency for many breeding stations in Asia to breed for multi-purpose use, including milk and work functions (ESCAP/FAO, 1983; Pathak, 1984b). The author is unaware of any specific selection indices utilized in multi-purpose breeding, and in the light of difficulties in performance testing for draught, it is assumed that these programmes select primarily for milk yield and body size, with screening for adequate body conformation and adaptive characteristics, prior to final utilization in the breeding programme.

There may be good socio-economic reasons why large, specialized draught animals are not required. In many social and economic systems in the world, cattle play an important role as an indicator of wealth or status, and cattle are a prerequisite for certain traditional ceremonies and transactions. In such cases, absolute numbers of animals are generally more important than their quality, and there is little advantage of having large animals. Two small animals may well be preferable to a single one twice the size, particularly as the risk of losing all the wealth represented by the live weight of cattle is reduced if it is spread between more than one animal. In addition, a larger number of smaller animals is likely to have a higher reproductive potential than a comparable weight of larger animals. Thus there are often significant social and economic pressures acting against the breeding of larger or more specialized draught animals. For example in Madagascar the relatively large Renitelo breed has been developed from Limousin, Africander and zebu, and it is acknowledged to be particularly good as a draught animal. However, the Renitelo is larger and relatively more expensive, and smallholders continue to use mainly the smaller and cheaper Madagascar zebu for their draught operations (Tran van Nhieu, 1982).

6. PROSPECTS AND PRIORITIES

6.1. Prospects for draught animal utilization

After many years of relative neglect, the importance of draught animal power is being increasingly recognized by national governments, agricultural institutions and development agencies. Ramaswamy (1981a), classified countries and regions on the basis of the prospects for draught animal utilization. The major categories represented adoptive, complementary, declining and reviving models.

Most of Sub-Saharan Africa, with the exception of Ethiopia, would be classified as adoptive, as in these countries farmers are often in the process of making the transition from hand cultivation to draught animal power, as discussed by Binswanger and Pingali (1984). In Sub-Saharan Africa the overall level of draught animal utilization is low, but is steadily increasing, and the doubling of the numbers of draught cattle in many countries in the region by the year 2000 would not seem unrealistic.

Using Ramaswamy's categorization, Ethiopia and many Asian countries, including India, China and Bangladesh, would fall within the model of complementarity. In these countries, draught animal power has been traditionally used for centuries, and it is likely to remain extremely important in the coming years. While other forms of mechanical power including tractors, trucks

Chapter 8 references, p. 196

and power tillers have been introduced in specific social and economic circumstances, this has been alongside the continued widespread use of animal traction, and the different power sources are generally considered to be complementary, within these countries. The *proportion* of overall power supplied by animals may well decrease by the year 2000, but this is likely to be due to the overall increase in the total farm power requirement, which will be associated with increased use of motorized power, as well as increased efficiency of draught animal utilization. However, the actual numbers of draught animals are not likely to decrease significantly, and indeed their overall power contribution may well increase due to improved efficiency of their use. Various studies (Binswanger et al., 1980; Gill, 1981; Mettrick and James, 1981; Ramaswamy 1981a,b; Farrington and Abeyratne, 1982) have shown that in many cases in these countries, for both the small farmer and for national, social and economic development, increased and improved utilization of draught animals is more attractive than the increased use of motorized power sources. Thus, in the period up to the year 2000, increases in motorized power will be complementary to increases in the efficiency of the use of animal traction, and the overall numbers of draught cattle employed will remain relatively constant.

In certain countries, including the Philippines, Thailand, Indonesia and Pakistan, draught animal power has been the major traditional source of farm power, but in recent years it has been declining, as draught animal populations have decreased and the numbers of motorized implements have increased. Such declines have been associated with many complex social and economic conditions, including population pressures, government fiscal policies and the relative prices of animals, crop harvests, power tillers and human labour. However, in some of these countries, specific measures are being taken to reverse the decline in the use of animal power, and various programmes in these countries are actively promoting the use of animal traction. Thus it is likely that the rate of decline will be reduced, and in certain areas the use of draught animals may actually rise again.

Most of the Latin American countries are classified by Ramaswamy (1981a) as revival areas. In these countries, draught animals have been traditionally used, but while they are still used by many small farmers, total numbers have declined as national policies have encouraged the more wealthy and innovative farmers to adopt motorized power sources. However, Ramaswamy argues that there is now a greater awareness of the social and economic advantages of the use of animal traction, and there is consequently a revival in the overall utilization of draught animal power in these countries. On this basis, overall numbers of draught cattle may be expected to increase slowly in the Latin American region.

6.2. Prospects for breeding programmes and breed utilization

It has been stressed that the efficiency of draught animal utilization is constrained more by the environment than by the genetic make-up of the animals. Thus greater efficiency in the use of animal power is likely to be achieved more quickly through improvements in general management, nutrition and health, than by breeding programmes. In most situations where draught animals are used, environmental adaptation, low cost and ease of purchase and sale are of particular value, and so locally adapted indigenous breeds will continue to be numerically most important for draught purposes. To date, such breeds have tended to be neglected by animal scientists and draught animal programmes, but as their importance becomes increasingly realized, it is likely that greater attention and resources will be given to the improvement of local breeds.

As few draught cattle are maintained exclusively for work, most breeding programmes for draught will have to involve complex multi-purpose selection criteria. However, at present there appear to be no proven, objective and quantifiable parameters that correlate with draught qualities, other than physical size and in many farming systems large body size is not a particularly desirable characteristic. Mass selection programmes for draught characteristics will be hampered by the common practice of castrating draught cattle. Thus the combination of multi-purpose use, castration and lack of reliable selection criteria suggests that genetic progress through within-breed selection for draught will be slow. The main exception is in circumstances where large size and strength are clearly required (as in forestry operations and harvesting sugar cane) and in such cases, within-breed selection should yield rapid results, as body size is both easily measured and of high heritability.

Crossbreeding and up-grading programmes for draught using larger exotic animals and adapted indigenous breeds are only likely to be successful in the few cases where the higher exotic grades can be adequately managed, fed and worked at village level. An example of producing draught animals by crossbreeding has existed in Bhutan for several centuries (Hickman, 1982; Hickman and Tenzing, 1982). Here the Mithan is traditionally crossed with the local Siri zebu breed to supply superior F_1 milk animals and draught F_1 males. Back-crossing to selected Siri males with compulsory Siri purebreeding in certain regions of the country, assures continuation of the system. If the higher grades are *not* well-adapted, then their production through *inter-se* matings within village herds is undesirable. Given the difficulties of managing crossbreeding programmes at village level, a long-term system of ensuring the supply of appropriate grades from breeding stations may be necessary, but the expense of this may create economic disadvantages that outweigh the genetic benefits. Crossbred ‘by-products’ from dairy improvements schemes can be used for draught, in appropriate management conditions, but the relatively small numbers involved in such schemes means that such programmes are unlikely to make significant changes in draught animal populations in the foreseeable future.

Thus it would seem that in the year 2000, the vast majority of the world’s draught cattle will still be of adapted indigenous types, and that consequently these will be taken increasingly seriously by draught animal specialists in the coming years. While national selection and crossbreeding programmes should certainly take account of national draught requirements, it is unlikely that in the short term, the overall efficiency of utilization of draught animals will be greatly affected by efforts in genetic improvement programmes.

6.3. Research priorities and information exchange

Insufficient adaptive research has been carried out relating to producing more efficient draught animals. The relatively limited resources devoted to draught animal research, whether on breeds, equipment or management and feeding systems have often been wasted on on-station trials of little relevance to the realities of the surrounding farming systems. Numerous examples could be cited of technical specialists (agricultural engineers, animal nutritionists, breeders) who have produced technically excellent results in machinery, feeding systems or breed utilization which have been completely inappropriate in the context of the local farming systems. The major constraints on the development of draught animal power generally have significant social and economic components, and are seldom simple technical problems. Thus research in the key areas of draught animal equipment, harnessing, breed utilization, nutrition and management systems should normally be carried out in cooperation with the farmers themselves. It is therefore recommended that all new draught animal research programmes should start with farmer con-

Chapter 8 references, p. 196

sultation, and should be pursued, preferably on a multi-disciplinary farming systems basis, in very close cooperation with the farmers, and wherever practicable using primarily the resources (animals, equipment, farmland) of representative potential beneficiaries of the research.

Inevitably such adaptive on-farm research will be highly area-specific, since the unique combinations of social, economic, environmental and agricultural constraints to draught animal utilization will differ with each location. Nevertheless valuable general lessons and conclusions will be produced from each location, and these should be shared, whether they be based on successes or failures. At present, information exchange relating to draught animals is minimal, with consequential duplication of effort and repetition of mistakes. With the growing interest of national governments, agricultural institutions and donor agencies in the development of draught animal power, there are likely to be an increasing number of research, development and extension programmes concerned with animal traction. At present, such programmes are generally carried out in relative isolation, without liaison with similar development activities in the region. Faster overall progress would be made in both extension and research, and fewer mistakes would be made, if there were closer liaison and information exchange from the outset of such programmes. It is therefore recommended that a small percentage of any budget for draught animal power development be specifically allocated for the promotion of information exchange, through publications, visits and liaison meetings.

The continued need for draught animal power in the coming years is clearly evident. Research and development programmes should aim to increase the efficiency of draught animal utilization, through appropriate improvements in management, nutrition, harnessing, breed utilization, equipment design and equipment use that optimize the use of local resources. However, before new programmes are initiated, close attention should be paid to what information and lessons have already been acquired in the region. It may well be that searching for existing experience, the subsequent dissemination of such knowledge and the continued active liaison between draught animal programmes, is the most cost-effective means of improving the overall efficiency of draught animal utilization.

7. REFERENCES

Allagnat, P. and Koroma, B., 1984. Socio-economic survey of the use of ox traction in the Mabole Valley, Bombali District. Sierra Leone Work Oxen Project, Freetown, Sierra Leone (unpubl.), 119 pp.

Anderson, F.M., 1983. An overview of ILCA's animal traction research in Ethiopia. Reprint of paper presented at Third Annual Farming Systems Research Symposium, Kansas State University 31 Oct.–2 Nov. 1983. International Livestock Centre for Africa, Addis Ababa, Ethiopia, 8 pp.

Anderson, F.M., 1984. Draught animal power in Africa: an overview. In: Animal Energy in Agriculture in Africa and Asia. Animal Production and Health Paper 42, Food and Agriculture Organization, Rome, pp. 132–137.

Apetofia, K., 1982. Aperçu sur la traction animale au Togo. In: E. Karbe and E.K. Freitas (Editors), Trypanotolerance: Research and Implementation. GTZ, Eschborn, F.R.G., pp. 231–237.

Apetofia, K., 1984. Les animaux de trait dans les régions à trypanosomiase. In: Animal Energy in Agriculture in Africa and Asia. Animal Production and Health Paper 42, Food and Agriculture Organization, Rome, pp. 124–127.

APRU, 1978. An Integrated Programme of Beef Cattle and Range Research in Botswana, 1970–1977. Animal Production Research Unit, Gaborone, Botswana, 141 pp.

ARC, 1980. The Nutrient Requirements for Ruminant Livestock. Commonwealth Agricultural Bureaux, Farnham Royal, U.K.

Barrett, V., Lassiter, G., Wilcock, D., Baker, D. and Crawford, E., 1982. Animal traction in Eastern Upper Volta: A technical, economic and institutional analysis. International Development Paper 4, Michigan State University, U.S.A., 118 pp.

Bartlett, J. and Gibbon, D., 1984. Animal draught technology: An annotated bibliography. University of East Anglia School of Development Studies, Norwich, U.K., 76 pp.
Barton, D., Jeanrenaud, J.P. and Gibbon, D., 1982. An animal drawn tool carrier for small farm systems. Discussion Paper 110, School of Development Studies, University of East Anglia, Norwich, U.K., 20 pp.
Bigot, Y., 1983. Project de recherche sur la mecanisation agricole en Afrique sub-Saharienne. Rapport de Mission Effectuée en Guinée du 20–30 novembre 1983. World Bank, Washington, DC (unpubl.), 39 pp.
Binswanger, H.P., 1984. Agricultural mechanization: a comparative historical perspective. Staff Working Paper 673, World Bank, Washington, DC, 80 pp.
Binswanger, H.P., Ghodake, R.D. and Thierstein, G.E., 1980. Observations on the economics of tractors, bullocks and wheeled tool carriers in the semi-arid tropics of India. In: Proc. International Workshop on Socio-economic Constraint to Development of Semi-Arid Tropical Agriculture, 19–23 February 1979, Hyderabad, India. ICRISAT, Hyderabad, India, pp. 199–212.
Binswanger, H.P. and Pingali, P.L., 1984. The evolution of farming systems and agricultural technology in Sub-Saharan Africa. Discussion Paper. Report ARU 23, World Bank, Washington, DC, 44 pp.
Bowman, J.C., 1974. An Introduction to Animal Breeding. Edward Arnold, London, 76 pp.
CEEMAT/FAO, 1972. The employment of draught animals in agriculture. Food and Agriculture Organization, Rome, 249 pp.
CTVM, 1984. Draught Animal News No. 2. Centre for Tropical Veterinary Medicine, Edinburgh, 14 pp.
Chambers, R.J.H., 1980. Socio-economics of improved animal-drawn implements and mechanization: Chairman's summary. In: Proc. International Workshop on Socio-economic Constraints to Development of Semi-Arid Tropical Agriculture, 19–23 February 1979, Hyderabad, India. ICRISAT, Hyderabad, India, p. 237.
Dixon, D., 1985. The Farming World. Transcript of programme broadcast 15 January 1985. British Broadcasting Corporation, London.
Dyrendahl, S. and Bengtsson, G., 1984. Performance testing of draught horses: initiatives and experience of the North Swedish Horse Association. In: Animal Energy in Agriculture in Africa and Asia. Animal Production and Health Paper 42, Food and Agriculture Organization, Rome, pp. 37–43.
Djabakou, K., Fimmen, H.O. and Karbe, E., 1982. Comparative trypanotolerance of West African taurine and zebu cattle. In: E. Karbe and E.K. Freitas (Editors), Trypanotolerance; Research and Implementation. GTZ, Eschborn, F.R.G., pp. 23–28.
EFSAIP, 1981. Report No. 5 1980–1981. Evaluation of Farming Systems and Agricultural Implements Project, Sebele, Botswana, 149 pp.
ESCAP/FAO, 1983. Draught Animal Power, Vol. V, Renewable Sources of Energy. ST/ESCAP/270, Economic and Social Commission for Asia and the Pacific, Bangkok, Thailand, 116 pp.
FAO, 1977. The Water Buffalo. Animal Production and Health Paper 4. Food and Agriculture Organization, Rome, 283 pp.
FAO, 1982. Report of the FAO Expert Consultation on Appropriate Use of Animal Energy in Agriculture in Africa and Asia, 15–19 November 1984, Rome. Food and Agriculture Organization, Rome, 44 pp.
Farrington, J. and Abeyratne, F., 1982. Farm power in Sri Lanka. Development Study 22. Department of Agricultural Economics and Management, University of Reading, U.K., 272 pp.
Feng Yang-Lian, 1984. The use of draught cattle in China. In: Animal Energy in Agriculture in Africa and Asia. Animal Health and Production Paper 42, Food and Agriculture Organization, Rome, pp. 21–27.
Finnelle, P., 1984. Surra (Trypanosomiasis) in buffaloes in Vietnam. In: Animal Energy in Agriculture in Africa and Asia. Animal Production and Health Paper 42. Food and Agriculture Organization, Rome, pp. 129–131.
Gill, G.J., 1981. Farm Power in Bangladesh, Vol. 1. Development Study 19, University of Reading, Department of Agricultural Economics and Management, Reading, U.K., 248 pp.
Goe, M.R., 1983. Current status of research on animal traction. World Anim. Rev., 45: 2–17.
Goe, M.R. and Hailu, M., 1983. Animal Traction: A Selected Bibliography. International Livestock Centre for Africa, Addis Ababa, Ethiopia, 42 pp.
Goe, M.R. and McDowell, R.E., 1980. Animal traction: Guidelines for utilization. International Agricultural Development Mimeograph 81, Cornell University, Ithaca, NY, 84 pp.
Gryseels, G., Astatke, A., Anderson, F.M. and Assemenew, G., 1984. The use of single oxen for crop cultivation in Ethiopia. ILCA Bulletin 18, International Livestock Centre for Africa, Addis Ababa, Ethiopia, pp. 20–25.
Hammond, M., 1984. (personal communication). Team Leader, International Rice Research Institute, P.O. Box 1369, Rangoon, Burma.
Hamon, R., 1971. Création, amelioration et performances d'une race de bovins de trait au CNRA de Bambey. In: Colloque sur l'Elevage, Ndjamena, Chad, 8–13 December 1961. Institut d'Ele-

vage et de Médicine Vétérinaire des Pays Tropicaux, Maisons-Alfort, France, pp. 503–514.

Herblot, G., 1984. (personal communication). Directeur Information, Documentation, Centre d'Etudes et d'Experimentation du Machinisme Agricole Tropical, 92160, Antony, France.

Hickman, C.G., 1982. Cattle breeding in Bhutan. Ceres (FAO), March–April.

Hickman, C.G. and Tenzing, D., 1982.The classical breeding system in Bhutan, J. Am. Husbandry Bhutan, 3–17.

Howard, C.R., 1979. The draft ox: management and uses. Zimbabwe Rhodesia Agric. J., 77: 19–34.

Humar, I.F., 1984. Oxen logging potential in Tanzania. Report of Animal Logging Mission to Tanzania, 7–22 July 1984. Food and Agriculture Organization, Rome (unpubl.), 52 pp.

IEMVT, 1980. Bibliographies: Traction animale et culture attelée en Afrique. Institut d'Elevage et de Médecine Vétérinaire des Pays Tropicaux, Maisons-Alfort, France (mimeo), 9 pp.

ILCA, 1981. Animal traction in Sub-Saharan Africa. Bulletin 14, International Livestock Centre for Africa, Addis Ababa, Ethiopia, 17 pp.

Imboden, R., Starkey, P. and Goe, M., 1983. Rapport de la mission de consultation preliminaire a l'établissement d'un réseau de cooperation technique dans les pays en voie de développement (TCDC) en matière de développment, recherche et formation pour l'utilisation de l'energie animale. Food and Agriculture Organization, Rome, 92 pp.

Kjaerby, F., 1983. Problems and contradictions in the development of ox cultivation in Tanzania. Research Report 66, Centre for Development Research, Copenhagen, Denmark, 163 pp.

Lawrence, P.R. and Mathers, J.J., 1985. The Work Output and Nutritional Requirements of Draught Animals. Centre for Tropical Veterinary Medicine, Edinburgh, 100 pp.

Le Moigne, M., 1980. Animal-draft cultivation in Francophone Africa. In: Proc. International Workshop on Socio-economic Constraits to Development of Semi-Arid Tropical Agriculture, 19–23 February 1979, Hyderabad, India. ICRISAT, Hyderabad, India, pp. 213–220.

Letenneur, L., 1978. Crossbreeding N'Dama and Jersey cattle in Ivory Coast. World Anim. Rev., 27: 36–42.

Lipton, M., 1978. Employment and Labour Use in Botswana. Ministry of Finance and Development Planning/EDF, Gaborone, Botswana, 495 pp.

Litschauer, J.G. and Matswe, S., 1983. 1982 ALDEP Program: Baseline data and evaluation. Ministry of Agriculture, Gaborone, Botswana, 90 pp.

Löwe, P., 1982. Animal powers as a complementary use of draught animal power. Paper presented at FAO Expert Consultation on Appropriate Use of Animal Energy in Africa and Asia, November 1984, Rome (unpublished).

Löwe, P./GTZ., 1984. (personal communication). German Appropriate Technology Exchange, GTZ, D-6236 Eschborn 1, Post frach 5180, F.R.G.

Mathers, J.C., 1984. Nutrition of draught animals. In: Animal Energy in Agriculture in Africa and Asia. Animal Production and Health Paper 42, Food and Agriculture Organization, Rome, pp. 60–65.

Matthews, M.D.P. and Pullen, D.W.M., 1975. Cultivation trials with ox-drawn implements using N'Dama cattle in the Gambia. National Institute of Agricultural Engineering, Silsoe, U.K., 62 pp.

May, E.D., 1983. (personal communication) from Chief Forestry Officer, Department of Forestry, P.O. Box 30048. Lilongwe, Malawi.

Mettrick, H., 1978. Oxenization in the Gambia. Overseas Development Administration, London, 67 pp.

Mettrick, H.M. and James, D.P., 1981. Farm Power in Bangladesh, Vol. 2. University of Reading, Department of Agricultural Economics and Management, Reading, U.K., 145 pp.

Morin, J.P., 1984. Comite d'Études et de Propositions pour le Développement des Activities Paysannes, Savioe, France.

Munzinger, P. (Editor), 1982. Animal Traction in Africa. GTZ, Eschborn, F.R.G., 490 pp.

NAS, 1977. Leucaena. Promising forage and tree crop for the tropics. National Academy of Sciences, Washington, DC, 115 pp.

NRC. 1970. Nutrient requirements of beef cattle. National Research Council, National Academy of Sciences, Washington, DC.

Oli, K.P., 1984. Utilisation of draught animal power in the hill agriculture systems of Nepal. Paper presented Livestock Workshop, Lumle, Nepal, 17–19 January 1984. Pakhribas Agricultural Centre (unpubl.), 5 pp.

Pathak, B.S., 1984a. Management and utilisation of camels for work. In: Animal Energy in Agriculture in Africa and Asia. Animal Production and Health Paper 42, Food and Agriculture Organization, Rome, pp. 46–51.

Pathak, B.S., 1984b. Report of the Preparatory FAO Mission for the Establishment of a TCDC Network for Research, Training and Development of Draught Animal Power in Asia. Food and Agriculture Organization, Rome (unpubl.).

Pathak, B.S. 1984c. Selection and application of draught animal equipment. In: Animal Energy in Agriculture in Africa and Asia. Animal Production and Health Paper 42, Food and Agriculture Organization, Rome, pp. 67–79.

Pathak, B.S. and Gill, B.S., 1984. Management and utilization of cattle for work. In: Animal Energy in Agriculture in Africa and Asia. Animal Production and Health Paper 42, Food and

Agriculture Organization, Rome, pp. 8–20.
Payne, I., 1980. Trees and disease. New Scientist, 3 January 1980.
Phillips, T.A., 1977. An Agricultural Notebook, with Special Reference to Nigeria. Longman, Harlow, U.K., 312 pp.
Pingali, P., Bigot, Y. and Binswanger, H., 1987. Agricultural Mechanization and the Evolution of Farming Systems in Sub-Saharan Africa. World Bank, Washington, DC, in association with Johns Hopkins Press, Baltimore, 217 pp.
Preston, T.R. and Willis, M.B., 1974. Intensive Beef Production (2nd Edition). Pergamon, Oxford, 566 pp.
Ramaswamy, N.S., 1981a. Report on draught animal power as a source of renewable energy. Food and Agriculture Organization, Rome (unpubl.), 150 pp.
Ramaswamy, N.S., 1981b. Draught animal power in the Third World. URJA, July 1981, pp. 26–37.
Ramaswamy, N.S., 1984. Draught animal power in developing countries with special reference to India. In: Animal Energy in Agriculture in Africa and Asia. Animal Production and Health Paper 42, Food and Agriculture Organization, Rome, pp. 140–143.
Reh, I., 1982. Basic aspects of the use of draught animals: animal husbandry and animal health. In: Peter Munzinger (Editor), Animal Traction in Africa. GTZ, Eschborn, F.R.G., pp. 65–132.
Reh, I. and Horst, P., 1982. Possibilities and limits of the use of trypanotolerant cattle for draught purposes. In: E. Karbe and E.K. Freitas (Editors), Trypanotolerance: Research and Implementation. GTZ, Eschborn, F.R.G., pp. 217–222.
Ridder, N. de and Wagenaar, K.T., 1984. A comparison between the productivity of traditional livestock systems and ranching in Eastern Botswana. ILCA Newsletter 3, International Livestock Centre for Africa, Addis Ababa, Ethiopia, pp. 5–7.
Rodriguez, E.O., 1984. Extracción de trozas mediante bueyes y tractores agrícolas. Estudio FAO, Montes 49, Food and Agriculture Organization, Rome.
Roelants, G.E. and Pinder, M., 1982. Susceptibility to trypanosomiasis among a range of cattle breeds. In: E. Karbe and E.K. Freitas (Editors), Trypanotolerance: Research and Implementation. GTZ, Eschborn, F.R.G., pp. 29–32.
Sargent, M.W., Lichte, J.A., Matlon, P.J. and Bloom, R., 1981. An assessment of animal traction in francophone West Africa. Working Paper 34, Department of Agricultural Economics, Michigan State University, 101 pp.
Sasimowski, E., 1984a. Management and utilisation of equine animals for work. In: Animal Energy in Agriculture in Africa and Asia. Animal Production and Health Paper 42, Food and Agriculture Organization, Rome, pp. 30–35.
Sasimowski, E., 1984b. Breed improvements in draught animals. In: Animal Energy in Agriculture in Africa and Asia. Animal Production and Health Paper 42, FAO, Rome, pp. 52–59.
Schote, W., 1982. Trypanotolerance and heredity. In: E. Karbe and E.K. Freitas (Editors), Trypanotolerance, Research and Implementation. GTZ, Eschborn, F.R.G., pp. 188–192.
Smid, J., 1982. The use of draught oxen in northern Ghana. In: P. Munzinger (Editor), Animal Traction in Africa. GTZ, Eschborn, F.R.G., pp. 453–476.
Smith, A.J., 1980. The role of draught animals in agricultural systems in developing countries. In: C.R.W. Spedding (Editor), Vegetable Productivity. Institute of Biology, London, pp. 247–262.
Smith, A.J., 1981. Draught animal research: a neglected subject. World Amin. Rev., 40: 43–48.
Smith, A.J., 1984. The integration of draught animals into agricultural systems. In: Animal Energy in Agriculture in Africa and Asia. Animal Production and Health Paper 42, Food and Agriculture Organization, Rome, pp. 1–7.
Starkey, P.H., 1981. Farming with Work Oxen in Sierra Leone. Ministry of Agriculture and Forestry, Freetown, Sierra Leone, 88 pp.
Starkey, P.H., 1982. N'Dama cattle as draught animals in Sierra Leone. World Anim. Rev., 42: 19–26.
Starkey, P.H., 1983a. Introducing the ox. Ceres, 96: 36–40.
Starkey, P.H., 1983b. The training of draught cattle. Appropriate Technology, 10 (1): 28–29.
Starkey, P.H., 1984a. The use of draught animal power in the Kasai Occidental and Kasai Oriental regions of Zaire. Work Oxen Project, Freetown, Sierra Leone (unpubl.), 40 pp.
Starkey, P.H., 1984b. N'Dama cattle — A productive trypanotolerant breed. World Anim. Rev., 50: 2–15.
Starkey, P.H., 1984c. The use of draught animals for swamp rice cultivation in Sierra Leone. International Rice Commission Newsletter 33: 2.
Starkey, P.H., 1984d. The care and feeding of draught cattle. Appropriate Technology, 11 (2): 25–26.
Starkey, P. and Goe, M., 1984. Report of the Preparatory FAO/ILCA Mission for the Establishment of a TCDC Network of Research, Training and Development of Draught Animal Power in Africa. Food and Agriculture Organization, Rome, 54 pp.
Steengaard, S., 1984. Second Mali Sud Agricultural Development Project: Implementation of livestock component and aide memoire. World Bank, Washington, DC (unpubl.), 9 pp.

Tessema, S. and Emojong, E.E., 1984. Feeding of draught oxen for improved and more efficient power. In: Dryland Farming Research, The Kenya Experience. E. Africa J. Agric. For., 44: 400–407.

Tran van Nhieu, J., 1982. Animal traction in Madagascar. In: P. Munzinger (Editor), Animal Traction in Africa. GTZ, Eschborn, F.R.G., pp. 427–449.

United Nations, 1975. Animal-Driven Power Gear. United Nations Division of Narcotic Drugs, Geneva.

Van Niekerk, B.D.H., 1975. Supplementation of grazing cattle. In: Potential to Increase Beef Production in Tropical America. CIAT, Cali, Colombia, pp. 83–97.

Viebig, U., 1982. Basic aspects of harnessing and the use of implements. In: Peter Munzinger (Editor), Animal Traction in Africa. GTZ, Eschborn, F.R.G., 135–221.

Wagner, C.M. and Munzinger, P., 1982. Introduction of draught animals in North-West Cameroon by the Wum Area Development Authority. In: P. Munzinger (Editor), Animal Traction in Africa. GTZ, Eschborn, F.R.G., pp. 377–402.

Watson, P.R., 1981. Animal Traction. Peace Corps, Washington, DC, 242 pp.

Williamson, G. and Payne, W.J.A., 1959. An Introduction to Animal Husbandry in the Tropics. Longman, Harlow, U.K., 447 pp.

Chapter 9

Breed Identification and Development

J. DOUGLAS MacKECHNIE and KLAUS MEYN

1. BREED DEFINITION AND HISTORY

1.1. Introduction

> Who would grow spirited stallions for the olympic prizes or strong bulls for the plow, let him choose carefully the females who will be their dams.
> (Virgil, 70–19 BC)

The two subtypes of domestic cattle, *Bos indicus* and *Bos taurus,* are fully fertile with each other, both male and female. They are composed of many different breeds which have been formed through natural or artificial selection since the first domestication of cattle in Anatolia/Turkey, some 10 000 years ago (Epstein, 1972). The breeds, in turn, are subdivided into populations, strains or lines.

The term 'breed' is not uniformly applied in the classification of cattle populations. The term either

(1) describes the cattle population of a certain area with varying degrees of uniformity;
(2) expresses uniformity in a few traits effected by simple gene action such as colour, colour pattern, head form, horn form, polledness, pretending uniformity also with regard to the production traits; or
(3) means the result of a systematic breeding programme based on set goals with emphasis on production traits. Cattle breeds of this category are selected with varying degrees of homozygosity (inbreeding, line-breeding, outbreeding, selection from crossbred foundations); there is no standard definition for differentiating between a gene pool from a crossbred foundation and the uniformity required using the term 'breed'.

1.2. Indigenous breeds

The first category comprises the indigenous breeds of the 'Old World' — Asia, Europe and Africa — which were developed before genetic principles were sufficiently understood by cattle producers (Mason, 1951; Joshi and Phillips, 1953; Joshi et al., 1957; Faulkner and Epstein, 1957; Mason and Maule, 1960; Hammond et al., 1961; Payne, 1964; Mahadevan, 1966; Wilkins, 1984). Little is known about their history. Natural selection in their production environment and the needs of cattle producers over time have formed these breeds. The emphasis in selection was laid on adaptability and the requirements of the people, usually draughtpower, meat and milk.

The existence of many indigenous breeds is endangered through current

Chapter 9 references, p. 219

changes in the production environment, the improved transfer of knowledge and the easier transfer of genetic material. For example, a recent FAO publication about the livestock breeds in the USSR (Dmitriev and Ernst, 1989) states that from 1945 to 1985 five breeds have disappeared completely, with a further nine classified as vanishing breeds, and nine as declining breeds. These breeds have given way to the more productive, specialized breeds of the developed countries which require high levels of feeding and management, and which are less adaptable to areas of limited feed resources and extremes of climate.

Programmes have been designed to conserve cattle genetic resources (cf. Vol. 1, 1 Vol 11, Chapter 1); however, due to inadequate analytical methods little is known about the real loss in genetic variability that has occurred and that must be expected in view of current development trends.

1.3. Breeds with uniformity in physical traits of simple gene action

Cattle breeds in the second category were formed on the basis of physical traits expressed by simple gene action, mainly colour, colour pattern and horn forms. The first such 'breeds' were identified during the Sumerian, Assyrian, Babylonian and Egyptian cultures about 3000–2000 BC (Kräußlich, 1981, p. 32). Cattle breeds were also formed during the Roman Empire some 2000 years ago. For example, one of the roots of the Chianina breed, the largest sized cattle breed on Earth, goes back to ancient Roman cattle.

Although utility to the cattle owners has always been the main objective for breeding, some breeds have passed through selection for a certain 'stamp', such as uniform colour in Red Danish cattle and the dominant white in the Charolais; white head in Hereford and Simmental; white back and belly line in the Hereford, Pinzgauer and Telemark; and polledness in Aberdeen Angus and Galloway. These genes exist in small frequencies in native cattle populations elsewhere, and have been stabilized by means of close line- or inbreeding. For the Hereford, it is on record that the Hewer brothers stabilized the colour pattern of the breed, while Hugh Watson did this for the Aberdeen Angus (Winnigstedt et al., 1961, p. 310).

1.4. Systematic breeding programmes

Cattle breeds of the third category, which were developed through systematic breeding programmes, are the main subject of this chapter. The production traits of cattle are not affected by simple gene action but are influenced by many genes. The task of breed improvement is to increase the frequency of yield-increasing genes, and this requires biometric approaches. This phase originated in the British Isles, when individual breeders in the 18th century started to improve their cattle through close inbreeding and subsequent rigid selection (Winnigstedt et al., 1961). Robert Bakewell (1725–95) pioneered this development with his Longhorns. His selection principles included: (1) a clear definition of the breeding goal, (2) selection and mating of animals which corresponded best with the breeding goal, (3) systematic progeny testing of the best sires (leasing of bulls under the condition that their offspring would be tested), and (4) fixation of the breeding goal through inbreeding.

During the 19th century the Colling brothers and subsequently Bates for the Dairy Shorthorn, and Booth and son as well as Cruikshank for the Beef Shorthorn, applied these principles. As a result, the Shorthorn had a major influence on the cattle industries of the U.K., France, Belgium, Holland, the German North Sea Coast, Denmark and the overseas territories. Another pioneer of modern cattle breeding was Benjamin Tomkins (1769–1815), the breeder of the Hereford.

Four other British cattle breeds emerged from rigid selection for specialized production goals and some physical uniformity in the late 18th and early 19th centuries:

(1) The *Jersey* was already known for its high-fat milk during the 17th century. Because importations of cattle into Jersey were stopped from France in 1763 and from the U.K. in 1789, in order to prevent disease, the breed was selected within a small population (10 000 cattle) and for the specific use of high butterfat and milk production. Breeding work was so successful that exportations to the U.K. and the U.S. started at the beginning of the 19th century.
(2) The *Guernsey*, originating from the neighbouring Channel Island, like the Jersey was separated from importations in 1789. Close inbreeding in the herd of Alfred La Patourel mainly contributed to the standardization of colour, type and production in this breed. Exports to the U.S. started as early as 1830.
(3) The *Ayrshire,* a dairy breed originating from the southwest corner of Scotland, surfaced in 1814 as a breed with standardized type and specialized production. Exports to the U.S. commenced as early as 1822.
(4) The *Galloway* is regarded as the oldest stabilized beef breed in the U.K. with no infusion of foreign blood during known times.

2. PRESENT IMPORTANCE OF CATTLE BREEDS

2.1. Overview

The worldwide emphasis on the productivity and further specialization of cattle breeds, the easier movement of genetic material (live animals, semen, embryos) and the improved flow of information have facilitated an enormous transfer of breeds between countries, continents and climatic zones. Breeds which show a high productivity under favourable management conditions and which also comply with the demand for specialization are being favoured. They are mainly the European dairy, dual-purpose and beef breeds that are supported by strong breed societies, recording programmes, AI organizations and traders of live animals, semen and embryos (Table 9.1). These breeds are rapidly penetrating the commercial dairy units in the temperate zones, the arid tropics and subtropics, and the temperate tropical highlands.

Cattle producers in areas with climatic and nutritional stress and socio-economic problems have tended to stay with the locally adapted multi-purpose breeds. There are gaps in the breed spectrum with regard to highly productive dairy and dual-purpose cattle in the hot and humid tropics: further breed formation from crossbred foundations is necessary, because local tropical cattle breeds lack productivity, particularly in milk, and the high-yielding breeds of the temperate zone lack sufficient adaptability to these environments.

2.2. Temperate zone

In the temperate zone the factors that favour further breed identification are:

(1) changing input and product prices;
(2) policy decisions such as the milk quota system in Canada, the EEC and other European countries;
(3) better information regarding the availability and utility of different genotypes; and
(4) ecological considerations and recreational factors entering cattle farming.

Chapter 9 references, p. 219

TABLE 9.1

Important cattle breeds in the world

Dairy	Dual-purpose	Beef
1. *Bos taurus*		
Holstein-Friesian	Simmental	Charolais
Red Cattle	Red and White	Limousin
Jersey	Montbéliard	Hereford
Ayrshire	Brown Swiss	Blonde d'Aquitaine
Guernsey	Normandy	Aberdeen Angus
	Pinzgauer	Shorthorn
	Criollo	Galloway
		Highland
		Belgian Blue
		Piemontese
		Chianina
		Marchigiana
		Red Steppe
		N'Dama
		West African Shorthorn
2. *Bos indicus*	Sahiwal	Hariana (draught)
	Red Sindhi	Kankrej (draught)
	Tharparkar	Boran
	M'Bororo	Brahman
		Gir
		Indubrazil
3. Taurindicus crosses		Africander (sanga)
Jamaica Hope Auhole		Tuli (sanga)
Australian Milking Zebu		Santa Gertrudis
		Beefmaster
		Droughtmaster
		Brangus
		Braford
		Simbrah

Technical progress in plant, feed and animal production has led to:

(1) lower costs of concentrate feeds in relation to forages;
(2) faster progress in productivity for dairy than for beef cattle;
(3) a trend towards larger units and more specialized production; and
(4) higher intensity in the production systems.

2.2.1. Dairy breeds

As a consequence, dairy cattle have gained ground against the dual-purpose breeds. Large-framed dairy cows with well-suspended udders and a good milkability such as the Holstein-Friesian have conquered most of the world's modern dairy operations, and this trend continues. Their population is estimated at over 100 million head. More than nine dairy cows out of ten in North America and more than five dairy cows out of ten in the EEC are Holstein-Friesian. The popularity of the breed (Holstein-Friesian, Holstein, Friesian, Black and White, etc.) is assisted by strong breed promotion through breed organizations and traders.

Among the other dairy breeds of the world, the Red Holstein of Canada and the U.S.A. is closely related to the black Holstein-Friesian, but it is penetrating into the Red and White populations of western Europe, which are originally of a dual-purpose type. The Scandinavian populations of Red Cattle appear to have a high frequency of dairy genes; they are making rapid progress in selection, and should, therefore, have a good chance in developing separately from the Holstein-Friesian. The other important dairy breeds of the world, such as the Jersey, Ayrshire and Guernsey, are mostly on the decline — the Jersey in Denmark and New Zealand, and the Ayrshire in Finland being the major exceptions (Table 9.2).

2.2.2. Commercial crossbreeding for beef

Because of the emphasis on dairying the beef qualities of dairy breeds are being neglected. Therefore, commercial crossbreeding of dairy cows with large-sized beef breeds has gained importance. Following a period of crossbreeding with the Hereford and Aberdeen Angus, e.g. in the U.K., the more popular breeds are now those that can produce large, but lean carcases without causing undue calving difficulties. The Charolais, Simmental, Blonde d'Aquitaine, Gelbvieh, Piemontese, Chianina, Marchigiana and Belgian Blue are the most popular breeds in this line.

2.2.3. Beef breeds

The trend among the beef breeds is threefold:

(1) for crossbreeding with dairy cattle and intensive stall fattening, the large-sized continental breeds are in the lead;
(2) for pasture fattening, the traditional British beef breeds such as the Hereford, Aberdeen Angus and Shorthorn appear to be quite appropriate, both as purebred cattle and as crossbreds with the dairy breeds; and
(3) for extensive grazing situations the hardy British and French breeds have become specifically popular.

2.2.4. Dual-purpose breeds

The need to consider the use of different cattle populations or breeding systems or to introduce outside genes may also arise from policy changes. The EEC dairy policy may serve as an example: For many years, EEC price decisions favoured dairying over beef so that the dairy breeds gained over the dual-

TABLE 9.2

Breed distribution in the EEC (1985–6)

	Registered pedigree[a] 1985 ('000 head)	Artificial insemination[a] 1985 ('000 first inseminations)	Milk recorded[b] 1986 ('000 cows)
Holstein – Friesian	4 397	10 381	6 760
Red and White	902	1 799	972
Simmental	658	2 767	931
Brown Swiss	388	570	375
Normandy + Montbéliard	159	924	310
Jersey	72	188	131
Red Cattle	63	224	117
Ayrshire		14	43
Other breeds	—	—	—
Dairy and dual-purpose breeds	7 425	17 539	9 927
Beef breeds	620	4 172	—
	8 101	21 711	9 927

[a] From COPA/COGECA (1985)[b] from ICRPMA (1988a,b).

Chapter 9 references, p. 219

purpose breeds. The situation has changed since milk quotas were introduced. Suddenly, milk producers may only sell limited quantities of milk, but they are free to sell as much beef as they want. In areas with smaller farm sizes and good beef prices, e.g., in southern Germany, milk producers reacted by turning towards the dual-purpose breed, the Simmental, which helps them to maximize income. It is expected that increasing milk yields per cow will reduce the number of cows kept in the EEC, and, in turn, the number of calves suitable for beef production. Beef prices may, therefore, be expected to be more stable than milk prices, and will favour dual-purpose rather than dairy breeds.

Among the dual-purpose breeds, the Simmental, its close relative the French Montbéliard, and the more dairy-oriented Brown Swiss have kept remarkably stable, while other breeds such as the Normandy, Red Poll and Pinzgauer have declined. Other dual-purpose breeds, such as the Belgian Blue and Gelbvieh on the one hand and the Red and White (MRY) on the other, are being re-oriented towards single-purpose beef or milk.

2.2.5. Hardy breeds

As rapid productivity increases on the fertile soils leave more and more marginal land idle, the trend towards recreational and ecological animal husbandry offers new opportunities for the use and development of hardy beef breeds, such as the Galloway, Highland, Salers and others.

2.3. Tropics and subtropics

The tropics and subtropics have had less breed identification and development than the temperate zone, although about two-thirds of the world's cattle are kept there. Due to lack of organization and interest, too little work has gone into identifying the productivity of indigenous cattle populations and organizing breeding programmes. Furthermore, gaps of knowledge exist with regard to productivity and the economic competitiveness of taurindicus crosses. Because of the powerful breeding organizations for temperate breeds and the availability of their breeding stock, semen and embryos, there is little incentive to carry out cumbersome but necessary evaluations of the local breeds and/or their crosses with temperate zone cattle. Frequently, the opinion prevails that environmental conditions have to be fitted to the requirements of high-yielding animals, rather than that the genotype best suited for the existing economic and ecologic conditions should be found. In environments where high-energy, protein-rich feed rations are economically feasible, there is less need for breed identification than in the more extensive production systems based on pastures and forages.

Studies on the productivity of indigenous tropical and subtropical cattle have shown a low gene frequency for milk yield (Mahadevan, 1966); conversion ratios in intensive fattening are also inferior to the temperate zone breeds. But although temperate zone cattle appear to be productive in hot and dry environments at high levels of feeding and management, their performance is not satisfactory in the humid tropics and under conditions of suboptimum feeding and management.

2.3.1. Zebu cattle

In their countries of origin in Asia and Africa, the zebu breeds have had little or no benefit from breed organizations, while government breeding efforts lacked continuity. Breed identification in earlier years did, however, lead to the exportation of the Sahiwal, Tharparkar and Red Sindhi breeds for dairy breeding purposes to Africa, the U.S. and Australia; the Kankrej, Krishna Valley and Gir breeds for the formation of the Brahman to the U.S.; the Kankrej and Gir as genetic bases of the Indubrazil breed; the Ongole as the ancestor of the Nellore breed in Brazil; and also maintained the purity of the Gir in Brazil and Australia.

The African zebu has produced a few local breeds which are subject to systematic selection, the Boran (beef) breed of eastern Africa being the leading one.

2.3.2. Sanga and other indigenous cattle

The Africander — draught/beef breed belonging to the sanga group of cattle (taurindicus) — has had some influence on tropical cattle breeding in the U.S. and in Australia. A second sanga breed, the Tuli, is known for its high fertility under marginal conditions and meets some interest in other tropical ranching areas.

The N'Dama, a humpless, trypanotolerant *B.taurus* breed, was identified in the 1920's as suitable for beef production in tsetse-infested areas. The van Lancker family from Zaire has carried out systematic selection since 1928, and the breed is used in many development projects in areas where tsetse flies occur.

The potential of the Criollo cattle, which became adapted to their new environment following importation to the tropics and subtropics by the Spanish starting in the 16th century, seems to have been neglected up to recent years because of inadequate selection work and promotion (Wilkins, 1984).

2.3.3. Synthetic breeds

There have been many efforts to select taurindicus beef breeds from crossbred foundations. The best-known is the Santa Gertrudis, a synthetic breed of the Brahman and the Shorthorn, developed by William Kleeberg Jr. on King Ranch, Texas. Other breed formations of importance are the Bonsmara (3/16 Hereford, 3/16 Shorthorn and 5/8 Africander) in South Africa and the Droughtmaster (Hereford, Shorthorn, Santa Gertrudis, Bonsmara, Brahman) in Australia.

The list of taurindicus beef breeds also includes (Cunha et al., 1963) Beefmaster, Brangus, Braford and Charbray in the U.S.A. and Simbrah in Australia.

There is still a lack of taurindicus dairy and dual-purpose breeds suitable for tropical environments. So far, the focus has been on systematic crossbreeding in order to exploit hybrid vigour combined with the right taurindicus gene combination (Mason, 1977). Most results are available from India. Attempts to develop and stabilize breeds such as the Jamaica Hope have failed to reach enough critical mass and are affected by competition with the Holstein-Friesian at an improved management level (Wellington and Mahadevan, 1977). The Australian Milking Zebu (Hayman, 1977), a synthetic breed derived from the Jersey and the Sahiwal, may be one exception.

3. TOOLS OF SELECTION

3.1. Background

Starting with the development of modern cattle breeding in Britain, the following selection tools were introduced and have accelerated genetic progress and its distribution over time:

livestock shows,
stud book registrations,
the formation of breed societies and the development of cooperative breeding schemes,
productivity recording,

Chapter 9 references, p. 219

artificial insemination,
progress in biotechnology,
advances in population genetics,
computerization, and
government assistance.

3.2. Shows

During the 19th century, show competitions at the local, regional, national and international levels provided the driving force of the growth of organized cattle breeding and the opening of markets. In particular, the British Royal Agricultural Show, which was inaugurated in 1839 and held annually since, helped to set the breed standards (Winnigstedt et al., 1961). Cattle shows also gained importance in continental Europe, the U.S., Canada, Latin America, South Africa, Australia and New Zealand. Even today, show ring results are important criteria for selection in regions such as Latin America and Japan.

Along with the shows, cattle breeding became international. It is reported that Angler cattle from northern Germany were shown at the World Exhibition in Paris in 1856 (Hofmann, 1980), and Aberdeen Angus cattle from Scotland at the World Exhibition — also in Paris — in 1878. Furthermore, Aberdeen Angus and Hereford cattle from Scotland dominated the show ring at the Chicago Fatstock Show in the same year. This initiated the decline in popularity of the Shorthorn breed in the United States (Winnigstedt et al., 1961). Shows nowadays have a lesser influence on selection plans in the leading cattle breeding countries. Their main function is breed and herd promotion. However, the growing trend of demonstrating progeny groups of AI bulls to the cattle producers contributes to current selection work.

3.3. Stud books

Stud books or herd books were founded in the 19th century by private individuals, farmers' organizations or parastatals ahead of breed societies. The first stud book was started in 1822 by George Coates in the U.K. for the Shorthorn breed — some 52 years before the formation of the breed society. Similarly, stud book registration for the other British breeds started earlier than the formation of breed societies (Table 9.3). Stud book registration independent of the breed society was typical for countries in the British Empire, but in other countries it was and still is carried out by the respective breed society. In the centrally planned economies of Eastern Europe, pedigree registration is done by parastatal companies charged with implementing the breeding programmes, while in countries with developing cattle breeding industries, they are frequently handled by governments.

The purpose of stud books is to maintain accurate records on the animals that meet the rules of entry requirements. A registration certificate is also

TABLE 9.3

Beginning of stud book registration in the U.K.

Shorthorn	1822
Jersey	1833
Hereford	1848
Aberdeen Angus	1862
Ayrshire	1877
Guernsey	1878

From Hammond et al. (1961).

issued. Each animal requires some form of identification so that each certificate can be associated with a particular animal. The most common methods of animal identification are tattoos, colour diagrams, brands, ear notches, ear tags, neck tags and leg bands. The challenge is a numbering system that (a) provides space for internationally unique numbers, (b) can be read at a distance, (c) lasts for an animal's lifetime, (d) cannot be removed or changed, (e) is adaptable to computers, and (f) is economical. Experimental work is being done with transponders both in ear tags and as a subcutaneous device. Transponders are electronic devices that can retain information such as a unique animal number. This information can be retrieved by another electronic device which may be portable and powered by a battery. National numbering systems for stud book and other recorded cattle should be harmonized, in order to simplify sire evaluation programmes.

Pedigree recording organizations are dependent upon the accuracy of breeding and birth records supplied by the breeders for authentic pedigrees. There are some easy checking procedures including the verification of gestation dates and blood-typing. Most blood-typing laboratories can verify the parentage in at least 85% of the cases. A frequent practice is to verify the accuracy of a pedigree system by blood-typing every 1000th application for registration as a spot checking procedure. Even more accurate verification methods for pedigrees may be expected from genetic fingerprinting methods currently being researched.

In the early days, herd books which contained all officially registered animals were published regularly. Today, very few are published in printed form due to the large cost and limited use. An official herd book is maintained by all pedigree-recording organizations. This may be a few typed copies, a computer generated copy, records on microfiche or computer tapes. In each case the records must be complete, accurate and easily retrievable. The requirement to maintain a complete pedigree history of all animals ever registered and recorded varies from country to country.

3.4. Breed societies

Following the formation of the Jersey Society in 1866, breed societies gained momentum in the 1870's and 1880's in Britain, North America and con-

TABLE 9.4

Formation of breed societies in Europe and the U.S.A.

	Europe		U.S.A.
Breed	Year	Country	
Jersey	1866	Jersey	1868
Holstein-Friesian	1874	NRS – Holland	1873
Shorthorn	1874	Great Britain and Ireland	1882 Shorthorn Association 1889 Polled Shorthorn Association 1910 Milking Shorthorn Association
Red and White	1874	MRY–Holland	
Ayrshire	1877	U.K.	1876
Hereford	1878	U.K.	1881
Aberdeen Angus	1879	U.K.	1893
Normandy	1883	France	
Danish Red	1885	Denmark	
Guernsey	1888	Guernsey	1877
Red Poll	1889	U.K.	1883
SRB	1891	Sweden	

From Hammond et al (1961).

Chapter 9 references, p. 219

tinental Europe (Table 9.4). In the case of the Holstein, Ayrshire, Guernsey and Red Poll, the breed societies in the United States were founded earlier than those in their countries of origin. During the 20th century the formation of breed societies occurred in Latin America, New Zealand, Australia, Japan, Italy, Spain, the African continent and elsewhere. In 1985, the population of pedigree cattle in the European Economic Community had reached 8.1 million head, of which 92% were dairy and dual-purpose and 8% beef cattle.

Breed societies have helped to promote the worldwide expansion of the British dairy and beef breeds, the continental Friesian and the Brown Swiss in the first half of the 20th century. Meanwhile, the Simmental was able to penetrate into southeastern Europe and Russia, and became established in South-West Africa. The international expansion of the large-sized continental beef and dual-purpose breeds occurred during the 1960's and 1970's. Those breeds originating from France (Charolais, Limousin, Blonde d'Aquitaine), Germany, Austria and Switzerland (Simmental, Gelbvieh), Italy (Chianina, Marchigiana and Piemontese) and Belgium (Belgian Blue) became popular in North and South America, Australia, New Zealand and Africa because they produced leaner carcases on feedlot rations than the traditional beef breeds and had more milk to feed to the calves. Breeds with strong organizations behind them, such as the Holstein-Friesian, Charolais and Simmental, were more successful in the export market than breeds with lesser organizational strength.

For want of effective breed organizations, few zebu and taurindicus breeds have ever gained a global role in the tropics and subtropics. Only the Brahman (zebu) and Santa Gertrudis (taurindicus), both originating from Texas, have made an impact in more than one continent.

The traditional tasks of breed societies are to establish a breed description and ideal breed type; formulate a breeding goal; carry out stud book registrations based on breed type classification; and organize show competitions and generally promote the breed. Some breed societies in continental Europe are also involved in marketing breeding stock and, more recently, in performance recording, AI breeding plans and embryo transfer operations.

The role of breed societies in the present-day breeding industry varies considerably. On the one hand, breed societies follow traditional patterns catering for a small breeders' élite, for instance by applying stringent up-grading rules for the operation of closed herd books and in order to reserve the bull market to a few stud breeders. The dangers of this approach are too great an emphasis on traditional show ring points and too little relevance to actual production conditions; limited genetic progress; and little impact on the whole industry. On the other hand, breed societies are part of integrated AI breeding/extension organizations. Normally these organizations reach out to a large proportion of the cattle industry and utilize modern tools of animal breeding. Such cooperative AI breeding organizations exist in Scandinavia, and conditional Europe. In the German-speaking countries one of the most important activities of the breed societies is the marketing of their breeders' surplus stock.

The breed improvement policies and programmes determine the changes a breed can undergo during successive generations. Changes that improve performance or sales appeal of a breed affect the profits of the breeders. The first step is to identify the traits that are important, rank them in order of priority, identify where the breed is now and what the objective is for the next 10 or 20 years. Limitations are the collection of data over space and time and its cost. Furthermore, the larger the number of traits, the slower will be the progress in each of them. To maximize progress the important traits are normally combined in an index taking the heritabilities and economic weighting of the traits into consideration.

The success or failure of breed improvement programmes depends very much on the acceptance by the breeders involved. Breeders must be involved in establishing the goals and there must be an effective information/publicity programme. This needs to be followed up by regular reports on the progress being made.

3.5. Livestock recording

It soon became obvious to cattle breeders that pedigree recording and type classification alone does not produce satisfactory genetic gains. The need to quantify productivity became evident. In addition, production records were required for farm management purposes.

3.5.1. Milk recording

The first milk-recording association in the world was started in 1892 in Kildebrönde, Denmark (Kräußlich, 1981). From there, organized milk recording rapidly spread in continental Europe, Britain, the United States, Canada, New Zealand, Australia, Japan, Israel and a number of developing countries. The International Committee for Recording the Productivity of Milking Animals (ICRPMA) was founded in 1950, originally grouping the western European milk-recording organizations. During the 1980's, ICRPMA has become a true world organization with the main dairy cattle breeding countries joining as members. In 1989 Interbull, the organization responsible for the conversion of breeding values between countries, was added to ICRPMA.

Despite its considerable cost, the importance of milk recording increases all over the world. In 1986, the total number of milk-recorded cows in ICRPMA member countries was about 13.6 million (at that time still excluding the U.S.A.). High densities of milk recording are reported from Jersey (89%), Norway (80%), the Netherlands (74%), Israel (73%), Denmark (72%) and Sweden (72%). The largest number of milk-recorded cows are kept in the U.S.A. (about 4.8 million) and in the EEC (about 9.9 million) (Table 9.2).

Milk-recording programmes are labour-intensive, involve the use of computers and must be well-planned and managed in order to balance the expectations of the cattle producers with costs. The ICRPMA accepts two methods of recording: method A with sampling and measuring being carried out by a recorder, and method B with the farmer himself taking the samples. Method B is mainly practised in Scandinavian countries. Because of the growing use of farm computers and automatic measuring devices, the forms of milk recording are in a process of change.

A typical milk-recording programme requires monthly data collection. It is also necessary to collect and analyse a milk sample monthly. At very little extra costs, additional data can be collected to provide reports that are valuable for the management of a dairy herd. These reports are of special value to large herds when cows can no longer be readily identified and individually treated by the herdsmen involved with their day-to-day care.

Table 9.5 lists a number of traits that are included in a milk-recording programme in Canada. The collection of a representative milk sample permits an analysis for butterfat, protein and somatic cells. Somatic cell counts are used to detect mastitis at an early stage, and are very popular among dairy producers in countries for markets with stringent hygienic standards.

Milking speed of a cow is important for the dairyman, especially in large commercial operations. A number of countries operate testing programmes for the milking flow of cows with subsequent genetic evaluation for selection purposes. Many milk-recording programmes also provide feeding recommendations based on a feed analysis of the forages and concentrates fed. The weight of the cow, her milk yield, milk composition, age and stage of gestation are required for a more accurate recommendation.

Generally, it is not practical to weigh cows with a scale. However, heartgirth measurements are sometimes used to estimate the body weight and height measurements are sometimes taken as an expression of size. Height can best be measured at the withers. One method is to measure height at a specific time such as first test after first calving or better still at first test after 36 months of age. Most breeds of dairy cattle reach 95% of their wither height by 24 months of age, which should also be a preferred time for taking the measurement. Table 9.6 lists normal weights and heights at different ages of well-grown animals for four dairy breeds in Canada.

TABLE 9.5

Some suggested traits for a recording programme

Trait	Information needed	Frequency of collection
Any heritable trait	Cow unique identification: cow ancestry, birth date, and supplementary ID	Once per lifetime
Milk yield	Cow supplementary ID,	Monthly
	24 Hour milk yield	Monthly
	Calving dates	Once per lactation
	Dry dates	Once per lactation
Butterfat test	Milk sample analysis	Monthly
Protein test	Milk sample analysis	Monthly
Somatic cell counts	Milk sample analysis	Monthly
Ease of calving	Subjective score + sex and sire of calf	Once per calving
Milking speed	Milk yield + time to milk	Once per lactation
Weight	Actual weight or heartgirth measurement	Once per lactation
Height	Height at withers	±30 days from specified age, e.g., 36 months
Days open	Breeding dates and service sires	Monthly
Retained placenta	Yes or no	Once per calving
Milk fever	Yes or no	Once per calving
Ketosis	Yes or no	Once per calving

TABLE 9.6

Normal growth in weight and height of female dairy cattle (Canada)

	Ayrshire		Guersey		Holstein		Jersey	
Age	Weight (kg)	Height (cm)	Weight (kg)	Height (cm)	Weight (kg)	Height (cm)	Weight (kg)	Height (cm)
1 month	40	73	35	72	51	78	30	69
2 months	54	77	46	76	67	82	41	73
4 months	90	86	78	85	110	92	72	83
6 months	133	94	118	94	161	101	110	92
8 months	176	101	159	101	210	107	147	99
10 months	213	106	194	106	250	113	178	104
12 months	244	110	222	110	287	117	204	107
18 months	329	118	301	118	383	125	273	115
24 months	409	123	371	122	485	131	332	119
3 years	439	124	409	127	528	134	388	122
4 years	469	127	449	128	559	135	407	123
5 years	490	128	479	129	603	136	425	124

Performance records are designed for breed improvement, but they are also important for marketing breeding stock. If the records are authentic they have an impact on the value of the animals and their offspring. This is a real incentive for breeders who sell breeding stock to enroll in production-recording programmes. Milk-recording organizations carry a special responsibility to make sure that the data recorded are accurate. Verifications by the recording organizations should, therefore, be a routine procedure.

3.5.2. Beef recording

Beef recording in cattle is by no means as popular as milk recording. Sizeable programmes exist only in France, Canada, the United States, Australia, Italy, Britain, New Zealand and South Africa (ICRPMA, 1988a,b). For dual-purpose cattle, beef recording is part of the selection programmes in southern Germany, Switzerland, Austria and the Scandinavian countries. ICRPMA set up a beef-recording committee in 1984 with the objective of harmonizing international beef recording.

Beef-recording programmes on farms normally include the traits of reproduction (calving ease, stillbirths, multiple births, first calving age, calving interval), weaning weights, bulling heifer weights, and weights at different ages of young bulls and fattening stock. Other traits of interest are conformation scores at the point of selection for breeding and at slaughter. Furthermore, field recording in Bavaria, Germany, extends to carcass gradings and weights in contracted slaughterhouses and liveweights and kilo prices of calves sold for fattening.

3.5.3. Fertility recording

Several countries with established AI services have developed fertility-recording programmes covering the following traits:

(1) male fertility measured by the non-return-rate (for example 56 days) of the females inseminated with the semen by a certain bull;
(2) female fertility measured by the non-return-rate of the daughters (for example 56 days) of a certain bull;
(3) calving ease;
(4) stillbirths; and
(5) multiple births.

These records are used to analyse the efficiency of AI services, herd management problems and genetic differences between AI bulls.

Calving ease is important in the management of a herd and the mortality rate of newborn calves. If there has been a lot of emphasis on growth, size and certain rump formations, difficult calvings may be frequent enough to warrant the identification of sires who do not sire calves that contribute to this problem at birth.

3.5.4. Health recording

Because of the joint data banks between AI and health records, a genetic analysis of health records is possible in some Scandinavian countries (Bratt, 1988, Solbu, 1988), particularly with regard to mastitis and ketosis.

Recent research studies on the financial impact of disease on a typical dairy herd list mastitis with about ten times the impact of any other disease and more than the total of all other diseases combined. An analysis of the culling reasons for dairy cows reveals that fertility is the main culling reason in dairy herds.

3.5.5. Conformation trait recording

The collection of data for conformation traits is both difficult and expensive.

Chapter 9 references, p. 219

Measurements can be taken for a few traits such as height at withers, weight, size of udder, etc., but most other traits require a subjective rating. It is much more difficult to maintain uniform standards with a subjective rating both between different evaluators and during an extended time period.

A number of conformation traits have a direct effect on the longevity of animals and are therefore important for breed improvement. Other conformation traits are keenly sought after by some breeders and therefore become very important economically. Because of these conformation fanciers the buying and selling of breeding stock is one of the true examples of supply and demand determining the market price in agriculture.

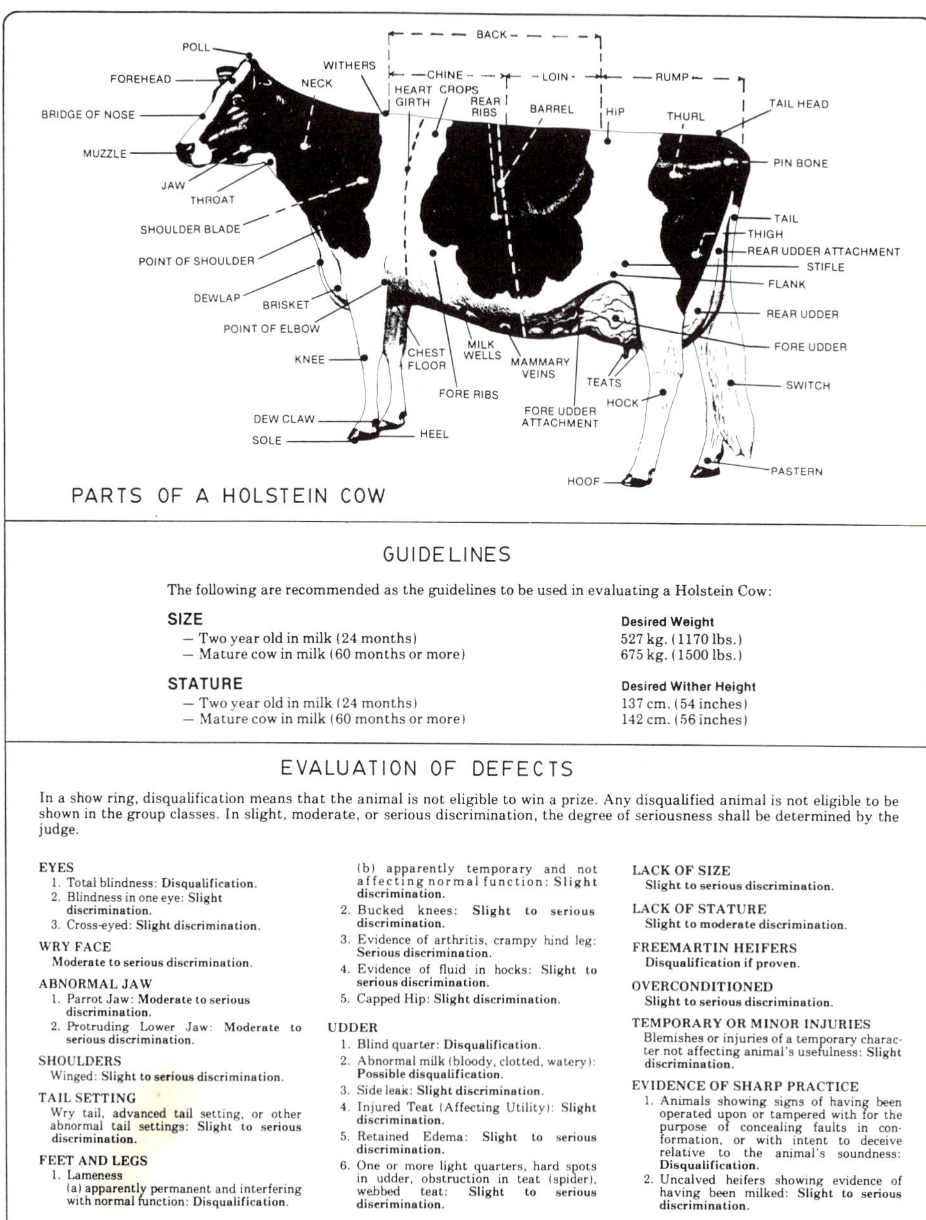

GUIDELINES

The following are recommended as the guidelines to be used in evaluating a Holstein Cow:

SIZE	**Desired Weight**
– Two year old in milk (24 months)	527 kg. (1170 lbs.)
– Mature cow in milk (60 months or more)	675 kg. (1500 lbs.)
STATURE	**Desired Wither Height**
– Two year old in milk (24 months)	137 cm. (54 inches)
– Mature cow in milk (60 months or more)	142 cm. (56 inches)

EVALUATION OF DEFECTS

In a show ring, disqualification means that the animal is not eligible to win a prize. Any disqualified animal is not eligible to be shown in the group classes. In slight, moderate, or serious discrimination, the degree of seriousness shall be determined by the judge.

EYES
1. Total blindness: **Disqualification.**
2. Blindness in one eye: Slight **discrimination.**
3. Cross-eyed: **Slight discrimination.**

WRY FACE
Moderate to serious discrimination.

ABNORMAL JAW
1. Parrot Jaw: **Moderate to serious discrimination.**
2. Protruding Lower Jaw: **Moderate to serious discrimination.**

SHOULDERS
Winged: **Slight to serious discrimination.**

TAIL SETTING
Wry tail, advanced tail setting, or other abnormal tail settings: **Slight to serious discrimination.**

FEET AND LEGS
1. Lameness
   (a) apparently permanent and interfering with normal function: **Disqualification.**
   (b) apparently temporary and not affecting normal function: **Slight discrimination.**
2. Bucked knees: **Slight to serious discrimination.**
3. Evidence of arthritis, crampy hind leg: **Serious discrimination.**
4. Evidence of fluid in hocks: **Slight to serious discrimination.**
5. Capped Hip: **Slight discrimination.**

UDDER
1. Blind quarter: **Disqualification.**
2. Abnormal milk (bloody, clotted, watery): **Possible disqualification.**
3. Side leak: **Slight discrimination.**
4. Injured Teat (Affecting Utility): **Slight discrimination.**
5. Retained Edema: **Slight to serious discrimination.**
6. One or more light quarters, hard spots in udder, obstruction in teat (spider), webbed teat: **Slight to serious discrimination.**

LACK OF SIZE
Slight to serious discrimination.

LACK OF STATURE
Slight to moderate discrimination.

FREEMARTIN HEIFERS
Disqualification if proven.

OVERCONDITIONED
Slight to serious discrimination.

TEMPORARY OR MINOR INJURIES
Blemishes or injuries of a temporary character not affecting animal's usefulness: **Slight discrimination.**

EVIDENCE OF SHARP PRACTICE
1. Animals showing signs of having been operated upon or tampered with for the purpose of concealing faults in conformation, or with intent to deceive relative to the animal's soundness: **Disqualification.**
2. Uncalved heifers showing evidence of having been milked: **Slight to serious discrimination.**

THE HOLSTEIN-FRIESIAN ASSOCIATION OF CANADA

Fig. 9.1. Guidelines and evaluation of defects card.

Type classification programmes were introduced in North America by the dairy cattle breeds in the 1930's and 1940's. These programmes became very popular and played a useful role in both the changing of certain traits and in marketing cattle. In the 1950's evaluations were restricted to milking age cows, and reports were summarized according to sires utilizing computers. Undoubtedly, these programmes have made a significant contribution in breeding cows with more tightly attached udders, reduced the incidence of sickle hocks and changed other traits such as height and size.

The success or failure of a type classification programme depends largely

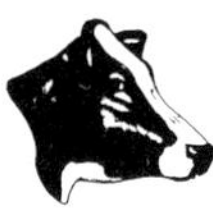

CANADIAN HOLSTEIN COW SCORE CARD

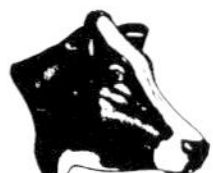

	Perfect Score
1. GENERAL APPEARANCE **(Attractive individuality indicating femininity, vigor, strength, stretch, size, and stature, with harmonious blending and proportional balance of all parts, and impressive carriage. Consider all parts of a cow in evaluating general appearance.)**	20
2 DAIRY CHARACTER **(Evidence of milking ability, angularity, and general openness, without weakness; freedom from coarseness, giving due regard to stage of lactation)** HEAD — clean cut; eyes large and bright; ears carried alertly; resulting in a head with Holstein Breed Character NECK — long and lean, blending smoothly into shoulder; clean cut about the throat, dewlap, and brisket WITHERS — well defined and wedge-shaped, with the dorsal processes of the vertebrae rising slightly above the shoulder blades RIBS — wide apart; rib bones wide, flat, and long FLANKS — deep and refined THIGHS — incurving to flat from side view; from the rear view, wide apart, providing ample room for the udder and its rear attachment SKIN — loose and pliable. Hair fine UDDER — soft and pliable; free from excess tissue or edema BONE — flat, strong, and clean cut	14
3 CAPACITY **(Head with adequate strength and size; Mid-section relatively large in proportion to size of animal, providing ample capacity, strength and vigor.)** HEAD — broad muzzle with large, open nostrils; jaws meeting properly; strong lower jaw; broad forehead SHOULDER BLADES — set smoothly against chest wall and withers, forming neat junction with the body CHEST — wide floor, resulting in ample width between legs HEART GIRTH — large and deep; full at elbows with well sprung fore ribs blending smoothly into the shoulders CROPS — well filled BACK — strong and straight, with vertebrae well defined LOIN — broad and slightly arched; vertebrae well defined; attachment to hip bones high and wide MID-SECTION — long ribs highly and widely sprung, with depth and width tending to increase toward rear	14
4 FEET AND LEGS **(Clean and strong boned, with shape and movement of feet and legs resulting in proper carriage of the animal)** FEET — short and well rounded, with deep heel; toes slightly spaced LEGS — Pasterns strong, of medium length, and flexible — Fore Legs straight and wide apart, with feet squarely placed — Hind Legs nearly perpendicular from hock to pastern from the side view, straight and wide apart from the rear view; hocks cleanly moulded — Bone flat, strong, and flinty, with tendons well defined	12
5 RUMP **(Long, wide, and clean cut, blending desirably with the loin)** HIPS — wide but not prominent, slightly higher than pins PINS — wide apart and free from patchiness THURLS — high and wide apart, giving consideration to stage of lactation TAIL-HEAD — refined, carrying out level with backline and set slightly higher than pins TAIL — long and slender	10
6 MAMMARY SYSTEM **(A strongly attached, well balanced, level udder of fine texture indicating heavy production and a long period of usefulness.)** UDDER — symmetrical, of moderate length, width, and depth; slight quartering on sides MEDIAN SUSPENSORY LIGAMENT — strong, showing definite cleavage between halves UDDER TEXTURE — soft, pliable, elastic, and well collapsed after milking FORE UDDER — firm and smooth attachment to body wall; of moderate length; quarters evenly balanced REAR UDDER — attached high, wide, and strong; slightly rounded; uniform width from top to floor; quarters evenly balanced TEATS — uniform size, of medium length and diameter, cylindrical, and plumb; from side view teats placed in centre of each quarter, and from rear view teats slightly closer to inside than outside of each quarter MAMMARY VEINS — long, tortuous, and branching. Udder veining is desirable	30
Scores for parts are not assigned in type classification TOTAL	100

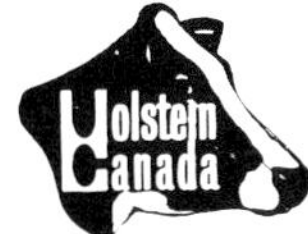

Approved by

THE HOLSTEIN-FRIESIAN ASSOCIATION OF CANADA

Fig. 9.2. Example of a score card.

Chapter 9 references, p. 219

upon the people evaluating the cows on the farms. When more than one person is required to perform these duties, the difficulties in applying uniform standards occur. The North American type classification programmes have been very successful in overcoming these difficulties.

Several breed societies have identified the traits of importance to them, the ideal for each trait and the weight to be applied to each. Some societies have drawn up an ideal model mature cow and a score card for each trait. This exer-

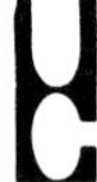

HOLSTEIN ASSOCIATION OF CANADA
120982

TYPE CLASSIFICATION REPORT

STABLE NAME OR NO.	OWNER	POST OFFICE
STELLA	D. SMITH	BRANTFORD

REGISTRATION OR NIP NO.	SIRE	DAM	BIRTH DATE (DAY / MONTH / YEAR)	LACTATION NO.	PREV. CLASS
3195921	333688	2920310	16 / 07 / 77	3	GP

GENERAL CHARACTERISTICS

STATURE UPSTDG. 9 8 (7) 6 5 4 3 2 1 LOWEST — STYLE STYLISH 9 8 7 (6) 5 4 3 2 1 LACKS STYLE

SIZE LARGE 9 8 (7) 6 5 4 3 2 1 SMALL — DAIRYNESS DESIRED 9 8 (7) 6 5 4 3 2 1 NOT DESIRED

DESCRIPTION OF PARTS-CIRCLE (0)-AS APPROPRIATE — DEFECTS - TICK AS SLIGHT (✓) OR PRONOUNCED (✓✓)

FRONT END
HEAD DESIRED 9 8 (7) 6 5 4 3 2 1 UNDESIRED

HEAD: 01 NARROW; 02 COARSE; 03 SHORT; 04 WRY FACE; 05 WEAK JAW; 06 LACKS CHARACTER
NECK: 07 SHORT; 08 THROATY

MID-SECTION
CHEST WIDE 9 8 (7) 6 5 4 3 2 1 NARROW
LOIN STRONG 9 8 7 (6) 5 4 3 2 1 WEAK

SHOULDER: 09 WINGED; 10 HEAVY
BODY: 11 WEAK CROPS; 12 WEAK BACK; 13 NARROW HEART; 14 SHALLOW; 15 NOT WELL SPRUNG; 16 CLOSE RIB
LOIN: 17 NARROW; 18 LOW

RUMP
THURL WIDTH WIDE 9 8 (7) 6 5 4 3 2 1 NARROW
PIN SETTING 9 8 7 6 5 (4) 3 2 1 (LOW — DESIRED — HIGH)

RUMP: 19 SHORT; 20 COARSE PELVIS; 21 HIGH PELVIS; 22 NARROW PINS; 23 WRY TAIL ✓; 24 LOW THURLS
TAIL-HEAD: 25 HIGH ✓; 26 COARSE; 27 ADVANCED; 28 RIGID; 29 RECESSED; 30 ADVANCED ANUS

FEET & LEGS
REAR HEEL DEEP 9 8 7 (6) 5 4 3 2 1 SHALLOW
BONE FLAT 9 8 (7) 6 5 4 3 2 1 COARSE
REAR SET 9 8 7 (6) 5 4 3 2 1 (SICKLED — DESIRED — STRAIGHT)

LEGS: 31 WEAK PASTERNS; 32 LACKS BONE; 33 CLOSE HOCKS; 34 CRAMPY; 35 THICK THIGHS; 36 COARSE HOCKS
FEET-FRONT: 37 TOES OUT; 38 OPEN TOED
FEET-REAR: 39 TOES OUT ✓; 40 OPEN TOED

MAMMARY SYSTEM
TEXTURE DESIRED 9 8 (7) 6 5 4 3 2 1 FLESHY
FORE ATTACH DESIRED (9) 8 7 6 5 4 3 2 1 WEAK
REAR ATTACH HIGH 9 8 (7) 6 5 4 3 2 1 LOW
MED. SUSPEN. STRONG 9 8 (7) 6 5 4 3 2 1 WEAK
TEAT PLACE F UNDER (9) 8 7 6 5 4 3 2 1 OUT
TEAT PLACE R UNDER (9) 8 7 6 5 4 3 2 1 OUT

UDDER: 41 TOO DEEP; 42 TILTED; 43 HEAVY FORE; 44 FRONT UNBAL; 45 FRONT SHORT; 46 QUARTER; 47 NARR REAR ATT; 48 BULGY FORE; 49 REAR UNBAL ✓; 50 REAR SHORT
TEATS: 51 CLOSE-SIDE; 52 WEBBED; 53 FRONT LONG; 54 FRONT FUNNEL; 55 FRONT NOT PLUMB; 56 BLIND; 57 SIDE-LEAK; 58 REAR LONG; 59 REAR FUNNEL; 60 REAR NOT PLUMB

FINAL CLASSIFICATION — SCORE CARD BREAKDOWN

CLASS	SCORE	GEN'L APP	DAIRY CHAR	CAPACITY	RUMP	FEET & LEGS	MAMM SYS.	FORE UDDER	REAR UDDER
VG	85	VG 2	VG 1	VG 3	GP 1	VG 1	VG 2	EX 1	VG 1

DAY	MONTH	YEAR	CLASSIFIER:	NO.	CALVING DATE MONTH	YEAR	REG. CERT. CANCELLED	CHARGE BREEDER	CHARGE UNIT
15	09	82	SM	9	08	82			

COMMENTS

REV. 03/82 — WORD ABBREVIATIONS REVERSE

Fig. 9.3. Typical classification report.

cise both identifies traits that should be changed and provides a score system to weight these traits vis-à-vis each other. Examples are shown in Figs 9.1–9.3.

North American type classification programmes have used the following ratings for identifying conformation categories:

Category	Abbreviation	Score range
Excellent	EX	90–100
Very good	VG	85–89
Good plus	GP	80–84
Good	G	75–79
Fair	F	70–74
Poor	P	Below 70

The percentage of cows classified in each rating is dependent upon the standards established. Most breeds with type classification programmes tend to have well over 90% of all animals classified in three categories: VG, GP and G. Computer programs are required to summarize the information by sires, age groups, classifiers, time periods, etc.

3.6. Artificial insemination (AI)

AI with fresh semen was first developed in the USSR in the 1930's. The development of deep-frozen semen in the 1960's added a powerful tool, making AI virtually independent of space and time. In its initial stage, AI played an important role in controlling breeding diseases, but nowadays its major function is genetic improvement through selection within populations and gene migration from other populations of the same breed, or from other breeds. AI has helped to increase the reproductive capacity of bulls substantially and to permit much sharper selection. It also permits the exploitation of quantitative genetics in large cattle populations making use of performance recording and computers. Further breed development in dairy cattle has become unthinkable without AI.

Cooperative AI breeding programmes in western Europe operate on the following principles (Kräußlich, 1981):

(1) adjustment of the results of performance recording for systematic environmental influences in order to obtain unbiased genetic proofs in all steps of the programme;
(2) progeny testing of potential AI bulls (test bulls) by random mating with females in herds covered by AI and milk recording (active population);
(3) selection among progeny-tested bulls on basis of their results, use of bulls selected as cow sires and of the top bulls as bull sires;
(4) selection of bull dams among cows of the active population on basis of the results of their genetic proof; and
(5) planned matings of bull sires and bull dams in order to breed test bulls (potential AI bulls) for the next generation.

In 1985, for example, 21.7 million first inseminations were carried out in 11 EEC member countries (excluding Spain), corresponding to 68.6% of all matings (Table 9.2). Breeds with large active populations have a better chance of making genetic progress and becoming competitive than breeds with small active breeding populations. Special efforts are necessary for the preservation of breeds that are not economically competitive at this time, but may be needed in the future. The more specialized the cattle breeds, the more risky is a change in economic conditions for their continued existence, for example, the introduction of the quota system.

Chapter 9 references, p. 219

Deep freezing techniques have permitted the development of a sizeable international trade in semen which has aided the spread of leading dairy and beef breeds; but this bears the risk that production conditions in the importing country may not be suitable for a transfer of genetic material for pure breeding (e.g., climate, feed cost, product : price ratio, meat : milk price ratio).

3.7. Embryo transfer and other reproductive techniques

Embryo transfer (ET) was first used commercially in the 1970's. Breeders use it to improve genetic exploitation of the females. It increases the chances of obtaining a calf of the desired sex from a planned mating of a bull sire with an outstanding cow. Furthermore, ET helps to overcome veterinary barriers in the worldwide trade of genetic materials, by reducing the spread of diseases such as bluetongue, foot-and-mouth disease and enzootic bovine leukosis. Apparently, trypsin-treated embryos bear little risk of transmitting disease, in comparison with live animals and semen (Singh, 1988). The shipment of frozen embryos facilitates the movement of genetic material and further breed development, but it may also contribute to the further narrowing of genetic variance. The cloning of sexed embryos which is currently the subject of intensive research and development will further increase the probability of genetic gains, but also cause further narrowing of the genetic variance.

3.8. Government efforts

Governments assist in breed identification and development through stud herds, the operation of breeding organizations, breeding legislation, the provision of livestock breeding officers, and subsidies. The operation of government stud herds occurs in areas where neither the cattle producers nor the breed organizations have enough 'critical mass' to operate a meaningful breeding programme or where innovations are intended. Government nucleus breeding herds are typically found in developing countries, but also in the centrally planned economies. One of the first nucleus breeding herds was the Simmental herd established by the King of Württemberg at Hohenheim castle in 1844. Some valuable results were obtained with nucleus herds in identifying productivity and in breed formation. Frequently, however, the programmes have suffered from lack of continuity. Some good breeding work was done on the Sahiwal, Red Sindhi and Tharpakar breeds on military farms in India and Pakistan. Furthermore, the creation of national studs for Sahiwals, Boran (zebu) cattle and a number of *Bos taurus* breeds by the Agricultural Development Corporation of Kenya are worth mentioning.

In centrally planned economies such as the German Democratic Republic and Czechoslovakia, governments have commissioned state breeding operations to carry out the breeding programmes and produce genetic improvement for commercial herds. For example, the United Animal Breeding Farms (VVB) of the GDR operate 42 élite breeding stations with about 250–300 élite cows and 6000 herd book cows each. Each élite breeding operation consists of several farms. A new synthetic breed, the SMR, consisting of 25% German Friesian, 50% Holstein-Friesian and 25% Jersey genes was developed by VVB and rapidly distributed throughout the country.

In countries with a family-farm structure, governments usually assist cattle breeding by legislation, provision of extension staff and subsidies. The degree of legislation in cattle breeding has varied from country to country and over time. During the days of natural service, bull licensing was introduced in several European countries in order to accelerate genetic progress (e.g., Great Britain, Ireland, Germany, Austria, Switzerland and Italy). Other countries support the farmers by subsidizing cooperative bull keeping (Denmark and Sweden) and provision of extension staff (Denmark, Belgium, Germany, Austria and Switzerland). Other governments, e.g., Canada, the Netherlands, Australia, New Zealand and United States, restrict themselves to the regulation of the operation of breed organizations.

As artificial insemination has become more important than natural service, governments are inclined to set standards for AI bulls and withdraw from bull licensing schemes in natural service. The EEC, for example, passed such a directive in 1987.

4. SUMMARY AND OUTLOOK

There are only eight dairy and dual-purpose breeds of worldwide importance: the Holstein-Friesian, Simmental, Red and White, Brown Swiss, Red Cattle, Jersey, Guernsey and the Ayrshire. Of national importance are the Montbéliard subtype of the Simmental, Normandy, Pinzgau, Gelbvieh, Illawara Shorthorn and Australian Milking Zebu. For beef, the basis of effective selection still exists for a larger number of breeds, because the more diverse production conditions call for a wider choice. Breeds with worldwide importance are the Hereford, Aberdeen Angus, Charolais, Limousin, Chianina, Simmental, Piemontese, Blonde d'Aquitaine, Belgian Blue, Shorthorn, Brahman and Santa Gertrudis.

The main tools for further breed identification and development are performance records and cooperative breeding schemes supported by artificial insemination and computers.

So far, cattle breeding plans have mainly exploited the genetic variance for the production traits milk and beef. In future, it will be necessary to expand selection to fitness characters such as calving ease and fertility as well as disease resistance. The Scandinavian countries are implementing such programmes which require larger numbers of progeny than the yield traits because of their low heritabilty. In the long-term, however, these traits will have to become integrated into cattle breeding plans to avoid genetic losses through antagonistic gene action.

5. REFERENCES

Bratt, Gunilla, 1988. Utilization of integrated milk, AI and health recording with special aspects to genetic improvement. Paper presented at the 26th session of ICRPMA, Oslo, 3 pp.

Cunha, T.J., Koger, M. and Warnick, A.C., 1963. Crossbreeding Beef Cattle. University of Florida Press, Gainsville, 228 pp.

Dmitriev, N.G. and Ernst, L.K. (Editors), 1989. Animal Genetic Resources of the USSR. Animal Production and Health Paper 65, Food and Agriculture Organization, Rome, 517 pp.

Epstein, H., 1972. Studies on the relationship between the cattle breeds in Africa, Asia and Europe. In: World Review on Animal Production VIII, Food and Agricultural Organization, Rome, No. 1, pp. 26–32.

Faulkner, D.E. and Epstein, H., 1957. The Indigenous Cattle of the British Dependent Territories in Africa. Publication of the Colonial Advisory Council for Agriculture, Animal Health and Forestry, London, 5 pp.

Hammond, J., Johannsson, I. and Haring, F. (Editors), 1961. Handbuch der Tierzüchtung, Vol. 3, Part 1. Parey, Hamburg and Berlin, pp. 207–478.

Hayman, R.H., 1977. The development of the Australian Milking Zebu. In: Animal Production and Health Paper 1, Food and Agriculture Organization, Rome, pp. 55–59.

Hofmann, G., 1980. Angeln — Deine rote Kuh. Verband Angler Rinderzüchter, 352 pp.

ICRPMA (CICPLB), 1988a. Situation de la production laitière et du contrôle laitier dans les pays membres. Résultats 1986, Paris, 117 pp.

ICRPMA (CICPLB), 1988b. Situation des contrôles de performances dans les troupeaux des vaches allaitantes. Résultats 1986, Paris, 8 pp.

Joshi, N.R. and Phillips, R.W., 1953. Zebu Cattle of India and Pakistan. Agricultural Study 19, Food and Agriculture Organization, Rome.

Joshi, N.R., McLaughlin, E.A. and Phillips, R.W., 1957. Types and Breeds of African Cattle. Agricultural Study 37, Food and Agriculture Organization, Rome.

Kräußlich, H., 1981. Rinderzucht. Ulmer, Stuttgart, 562 pp.

MacEwan, J.W.G., 1941. The Breeds of Farm Livestock in Canada. Thomas Nelson & Sons Ltd.

Mahadevan, P., 1966. Breeding for Milk Production in Tropical Cattle. Commonwealth Agricultural Bureaux, Farnham Royal, 154 pp.

Mason, I.L., 1951. A World Dictionary of Breeds, Types and Varieties of Livestock. Technical Communication 8, Commonwealth Bureaux of Animal Breeding and Genetics, Edinburgh.

Mason, I.L., 1977. Maintaining crossbred populations of dairy cattle in the tropics. In: Animal Production and Health Paper 1, Food and Agriculture Organization, Rome, pp. 40–47.

Mason, I.L. and Maule J.P., 1960. The Indigenous Livestock of Eastern and Southern Africa. Commonwealth Agricultural Bureaux, Farnham Royal, 151 pp.

Meyn, K., 1989. So ist die europäische Rinderzucht organisiert. Tierzüchter, 41: 419–421.

Meyn, K. and Wilkins, J.V., 1977. Breeding for milk in Kenya, with particular reference to the Sahiwal Stud. In: Animal Production and Health Paper 1, Food and Agriculture Organization, Rome, pp. 60–66.

Payne, W.J.A., 1964. The origin of domestic cattle in Africa. Empire Journal of Experimental Agriculture, 32: 97–113.

Singh, E.L., 1988. Determining the disease transmission potential of embryos and semen. In: Proceedings, 3rd World Congress Sheep and Beef Cattle Breeding, Paris, Vol. I, pp. 659–672.

Solbu, H., 1988. Disease recording as an integrated part of a dairy herd improvement program. Paper presented at the 26th session of ICRPMA, Oslo, 5 pp.

Wellington, K.E. and Mahadevan, P., 1977. Development of the Jamaica Hope breed of dairy cattle. In: Animal Production and Health Paper 1, Food and Agriculture Organization, Rome, pp. 67–72.

Wilkins, J.V., 1984. Criollo cattle of the Americas. In: Animal Genetic Resources Information, UNEP/FAO, Rome, pp. 1–19.

Winnigstedt, R., Messerschmidt, H., Haring, F. and Sieblitz, K., 1961. Rinderrassen in Nordwesteuropa. In: J. Hammond, I. Johannsson and F. Haring (Editors), Handbuch der Tierzüchtung. Parey, Hamburg and Berlin, pp. 261–338.

Chapter 10

Population Genetics, Molecular Markers and Gene Conservation of Bovine Breeds

C.M.A. BAKER and C. MANWELL

1. INTRODUCTION

This review concerns the intersection of research on biochemical markers with the conservation of genetic resources in livestock. We are not aware of any recent major synthesis of these topics, although certain aspects of some earlier reviews are pertinent (Manwell and Baker, 1970; Gahne, 1980; Braend, 1981; Baker and Manwell, 1983a, Stormont, 1984).

In many ways, the data base for domestic livestock is the best available (see p. 256). Yet it is generally ignored in discussions of biochemical polymorphisms and population genetics (e.g., Wright, 1978; Scudder and Reveal, 1981; Nei and Koehn, 1983). Even more curiously, domestic animals are ignored or relegated to a minor position in recent prominent works on conservation, although the same books devote considerable space to wild animals and to both wild and domestic plants (Hawkes, 1978; Frankel and Soulé, 1981; Schonewald-Cox et al., 1983).

Our intention is to integrate a number of neglected but important topics. One is history, which is necessary for the interpretation and evaluation of other data (Turton, 1974, p. 65; Brothwell, 1978). It is also essential to answer the question: how did the present degree of genetic erosion come about? If we fail to consider the rise and fall of different breeds, changes in agricultural requirements and fashions, and the politics of scientific research and agricultural advice, then we shall fail in gene conservation.

It is equally essential to understand the reasons for gene conservation and the nature of the resources available.

We summarize aspects of genetic diversity in bovines and marker genes that express themselves at a variety of different levels, from molecules to morphology. Practical breeders are usually most concerned with genetic markers which are either readily visible (e.g., colour and pattern) or are controlling some important characteristic (polled vs. horned, double-muscling, etc.). However, all these traits have a molecular basis, even if it is still obscure.

Population structure is examined with emphasis on the integration of biochemical polymorphism data with genetic theory. The overall view is supplemented by case histories to illustrate important points.

Finally, we make recommendations with practical application to conservation.

Information on these topics is scattered widely, and much of it is in 'non-conventional' literature (Manwell and Baker, 1970, p. 323; Turton, 1974). An idea of the type and value of non-conventional sources can be gained from inspecting the useful annotated bibliography by Lauvergne and Laurans (1979). We have tried to compensate for this situation by including more detail from

Chapter 10 references, p. 289

less readily available sources; at the other extreme a standard work may be given no more than a brief reference.

2. HOW DID THE PRESENT DEGREE OF GENETIC EROSION COME ABOUT?

It is often assumed that the spread or decline of a breed is solely or mainly because of its relative merit (Lerner and Donald, 1966; Dickerson, 1969; Mason, 1973; Jewell and Alderson, 1977). In fact, a complicated web of interacting socio-economic reasons is involved and merit may make a relatively small contribution.

The main factors involved are summarized below.

2.1. Socio-economic reasons of long standing

2.1.1. Availability

Marshall (1796, vol. 2, pp. 99–100) ascribed the decline of Gloucester cattle to breeders switching to running and flying herds in order to maximize milk production. The only replacement cows readily available were Longhorns.

In other cases, small tenant farmers relied upon, or were forced to use, bulls provided by landlords (Milburn, 1848; Dixon, 1865b, vol. 1, p. 33; Deaton, 1981, pp. 214–215.

2.1.2. Fashion

Marshall also considered that fashion, manipulated by agricultural writers, was a major factor in the expansion of a few publicized breeds at the expense of locally adapted cattle such as the Norfolk and the Gloucester. He lamented: 'WHAT MISCHIEFS TO A COUNTRY MAY NOT BE EFFECTED BY ILL-FOUNDED FASHIONS, INCONSIDERATELY FOLLOWED' (Marshall, 1818, vol. 3, p. 396. Capitals in the original).

Agricultural writers have continued to display partisan behaviour, which sometimes conflicts with their private opinions. An insight into one such case has been given by Austin (1943, p. 19) who noted that '. . . a journalist could scarcely criticise the leading judges of his time' and that the paper by which that journalist was employed benefited from stud advertisements.

2.1.3. The pedigree mystique

This is the belief that merit resides in the existence of a pedigree, or in a pedigree containing certain animals, rather than in the characteristics of the animal to which the pedigree refers (reviewed by Manwell and Baker, 1970). Concentration on certain pedigree lines to the exclusion of commercial traits can cause a breed to deteriorate (see p. 264).

2.1.4. Relaxed selection in a popular breed

It has been recommended that desirable breeds should expand by 'reduced culling of female progeny' (Dickerson, 1969, p. 191). But this can result in less predictably good performance which, as it is often combined with high prices, eventually causes prospective purchasers to seek alternative stock.

In the 19th century, 'In ordinary herds indifferent milkers are never allowed to have a second calf, while highly-bred shorthorns are too valuable to be put aside on such a plea.' (Bowly, 1868, p. 441). Some 80 years later, the Shorthorn was largely replaced as a dairy cow in Great Britain by the Ayrshire. This breed also spread by keeping a higher proportion of females for breeding stock (Wiener and Yao, 1952), and was in turn replaced by the British Friesian. Friesians made a four-fold expansion between 1935 and 1947, again by registering and keeping more females (Robertson and Asker, 1951b). However, only one-sixth of the genes were derived from the animals in the first (1910) British Friesian herdbook; the rest were from imported sires, which were, of course, highly selected (Robertson and Asker, 1951a).

2.1.5. Limited assessment

Although it is well-known that breeds with a reputation for superior yields usually achieve these under good conditions, comparisons between breeds often emphasize production with little or no reference to other factors. Even when breeds are tested against each other (and often they are not) it is usually under standardized conditions and without allowance being made for less conventional attributes (e.g., see Maijala, 1974; Hickman, 1981, 1984).

2.1.6. Habitat

Loss of habitat is a serious factor in the decline of the remaining wild bovines: Betisoak (Dent, 1983; and see p. 235), gaur, banteng and kouprey (Wharton, 1968) and African buffalo (Sinclair, 1977; Mloszewski, 1983). Destruction of habitat can lead to the failure of feral populations (Baker and Manwell, 1981). It also affects domesticates, especially those which use natural grazing: for example, yak numbers are diminishing because closed borders have made alpine pastures unavailable (Swaminathan, 1981, p. 13).

2.1.7. Genocide

Wild, feral and semi-feral extensively kept animals are often slaughtered on the grounds that it is necessary to protect superior stock from competition or contamination. In this way the American bison almost became extinct, and with it what some have said were the prime target, the Plains Indians (McHugh and Hobson, 1972, Roe, 1972). Texas Longhorns were also eradicated on many holdings to make way for 'better' stock (Dobie, 1941). Now both the bison and the Longhorn are regarded highly for meat production.

At present the Australian Government is involved in a massive slaughter of feral and semi-feral bovines under the B-TEC Program, supposedly to eradicate brucellosis and tuberculosis. Banteng, described as 'apparently free of tuberculosis' may be shot as game under licence (Austin, 1984 a). 'More than 200,000 wild buffalo are to be killed in one of the greatest mass slaughters the country has seen . . . the plan will cost in excess of $200 million' (Austin, 1984b). Tuberculosis is only estimated at 3%, but buffalo are also accused of having adverse effects on lotus and water lilies and on 'the scarce pied goose' (*Anseranas semipalmata*). Yet other reports have described an idyllic coexistence of lilies, buffalo and magpie geese, the last being so plentiful that they were popularly blamed for the failure of the Humpty Doo rice project (Thomson, 1970).

Range cattle are another target, despite objection that this will mean 'the loss of the genetic pool of cattle best suited to the harsh regions they were bred for'; and that suitable replacement females are not available (Brown, 1984).

One of the horrifying aspects of B-TEC is that previous experience seems to have been ignored. As in the American example, there are Aboriginal tribes which exploit free ranging bovines (Austin, 1984a,b; Brown, 1984). In recent American programmes of brucellosis eradication, slaughter of bison was only planned for reactors. Even this met with strong opposition, with there being a significant body of opinion that maintaining isolation was adequate (De Young, 1973). In Africa, it was found that control of rinderpest in cattle led to its disappearance from wild ungulates (Sinclair, 1971). There does not seem to be any published cost-benefit study of B-TEC, although there is an important precedent in Tisdell's (1982) excellent economic analysis of feral pigs in Australia.

Chapter 10 references, p. 289

Mr Tim Emanuel (a descendent of a legendary pioneering family) is quoted as saying: 'The cattlemen of northern Australia have survived drought and fire and flood for over a century but . . . will be destroyed by a group of bureaucrats playing God' (Brown, 1984).

It should not be thought that the rarity of surviving animals necessarily leads to protection. When the American bison was almost extinct, American museums hastened the process by having specimens killed for their collections (McHugh and Hobson, 1972, pp. 246 *et seq.*).

2.1.8. Hybridization

Breeds (and species) can disappear through hybridization. The problem is only mentioned for completeness as it is discussed on p. 228 and 238.

2.2. Socio-economic factors associated with agribusiness

There are two major differences between agribusiness and the preceding 10000 years of animal husbandry. First, in contrast to the traditional emphasis on the husbandry of renewable resources, the prime concern of agribusiness is to maximize present financial returns. Secondly, control of wealth and technology gives agribusiness firms immense power, which they use to influence the socio-economic structure of agriculture to their own advantage. As a result, situations have arisen which have far reaching consequences for gene conservation.

2.2.1. The search for quick profits

The 'charm of the exotic'. The import of foreign stock is often advocated as a means of rapid improvement (Dickerson, 1969); and the availability of foreign breeds is frequently given as a reason why expenditure on conserving or improving national stocks is unnecessary (see papers in Hodgson, 1961; Lerner and Donald, 1966, p. 207; Chapman, 1974, p. 277).

There is also a third, less publicized attraction: profits which result not from genetic merit but from the trade itself. Transport, quarantine and other services are necessary — and profitable. These high costs limit participation — and so guarantee possession of a scarce import with the prospect of lucrative sales of animals or gametes. Countries with export markets for 'superior' stock (often as foreign aid) can improve the balance of payments. Scientific advisers responsible for such decisions earn the approval of the powerful interests which benefit financially.

In this way, crossing is often recommended to 'improve' stock in developing countries: as, for example, the N'Dama (Touchberry, 1967; Trail, 1981) although pure N'Dama respond well to more intensive conditions in larger enterprises (Mortelmans and Kageruka, 1976; Trail, 1981). An insight into how cattle sales enter into the politics of the international meat market is given by Machado (1981). The U.S.A. lent money to Mexico for the purchase of American stock, including seed bulls for small cattle owners, and thus eroded the Mexican Criollos; and powerful U.S.A. interests used their Mexican ranches as a means of importing zebu cattle from Brazil, spreading foot-and-mouth disease in the process.

The danger of genetic erosion from imports is not confined to developing countries. The search for a large beef breed for use in Great Britain ignored the potential of the native South Devon (Mason, 1971) despite attention drawn to the merits of this breed (MacKellar, 1960; Manwell and Baker, 1970, pp. 327–330). Breeders have since told us that when they were asked to send cattle for comparison, it was emphasized that the South Devons should be average animals, and that the information that the exotics in the comparison would be highly selected was withheld. The depreciation continues. A British official report which drew attention to the advantages of muscular hypertrophy illustrated it with the Belgian Blue and White, and ignored MacKellar's description of the same condition in the South Devon (C. Smith, 1984 a; see pp. 248 and 281).

The 'heterosis mystique'. (Medawar, 1960). This is the belief that certain techniques of crossbreeding (or in extreme cases *any* crossbreeding) will invariably produce progeny with performance better than that of the parents or the parental lines.

Hybrid vigour (also known as positive heterosis or nicking) from certain matings is a real phenomenon and has been recognized by stockbreeders for many centuries. But, heterosis is environmentally labile. Even for defined circumstances, there are very few examples where hybrid vigour can be produced reliably, and attempts to do so may end in either no improvement or negative heterosis.

Two aspects of heterosis appeal to agribusiness. One is the possible chance of producing large numbers of uniform stock which yield well above the average commercial level. The other is the probable profits for a firm which has a monopoly of parental lines, whether or not the combination of these produces positive heterosis.

Further discussion of heterosis, including biochemical aspects, is contained in Manwell et al. (1963), Manwell and Baker (1970) and Baker and Manwell (1983a,b).

The 'quick technological fix'. (Weinberg, 1967). Agribusiness is characterized by a desire (common to most people) to solve problems rapidly; the faith that modern technology can provide the solution; and the financial ability to purchase technology. From this position, '... with our present high level of husbandry, local adaptation of cattle is not important in this country nor for that matter throughout much of the world' (Mason, 1973). This is true to a limited extent. Exotic milch cattle (mostly Holstein or Friesian) can yield well in hot regions; but they must be fed well and kept cool, and often have more infertility and higher mortality (Osman, 1981). A scheme to supply fresh milk for Darwin, Australia (at present largely dependent upon dried and frozen imported milk) will involve 1000 cows, '... probably high yielding guernseys or jerseys' supplied by an embryo transplant firm. These will be 'fed on hydroponically grown grass in luxurious air-conditioned quarters close to the city.' The cost was estimated to be 10 million Australian dollars (Ford, 1982).

Even concern with disease resistance is considered '... only partially valid. In the past the advances made in veterinary science appear to have come more quickly than truly resistant individuals could be bred' (Lerner and Donald, 1966, p. 206; see also Mason, 1974). In fact, for many years there has been concern in some medical circles about the consequences of the almost continual exposure of intensively kept livestock to antibiotics, usually just administered as a food additive. It has been feared that this continuous exposure to low levels of antibiotics would select for antibiotic-resistant strains of bacteria (which, then, could not be treated with the usual medical or veterinary antibiotics).

Recently, evidence for a clear linkage between human illness and antibiotics in animal feed has been demonstrated. By using restriction endonuclease digests of bacterial plasmids (as a way of precise 'fingerprinting' antibiotic resistance genes), it was possible to trace one serious *Salmonella* outbreak among humans to 'hamburger originating from South Dakota beef cattle fed subtherapeutic chlorotetracycline for growth promotion' (Holmberg et al., 1984a, p. 617). Especially worrying is the fact that antibiotic-resistant

Salmonella cause a 21-fold higher mortality in man (Holmberg et al., 1984b). These new facts have greatly intensified the drive for legal restrictions to prevent the use of medically or veterinarily important antibiotics in animal feed (Sun, 1984).

Accordingly, Lerner and Donalds's (1966) opinion that concern about disease resistance is '. . . only partially valid' is likely to be out-of-date. Customers are not likely to continue purchasing food from which they might get a fatal disease. Added to the concern about saturated fats and cardiovascular disease (which is believed to have caused some reduction in milk and meat sales in some locations), it will be necessary to market cattle as healthier and leaner. This could well reduce the number of animals finished in feedlots, or at least require improved conditions of sanitation. There is likely to be a much more thorough search for cattle with better genetic resistance to pathogenic micro-organisms, or with better genetically determined growth rates (so as to reduce the dependence on antibiotics and other chemicals as growth stimulants).

The possibility of demonstrating a dramatic technical triumph may deflect effort from more certain methods. An example is the lost breeding opportunities when I.W. Rowlands applied standard techniques of embryo transfer to Norfolk Horn sheep without first learning the physiological idiosyncracies of this rare breed (Jewell, 1971, p. 525; Ryder, 1976, p. 245). The lesson is an important one: subsequently marked differences in response to superovulation stimuli have been found within and between different breeds of cattle (Saumande et al., 1978).

2.2.2. Size of enterprise

In many countries farm size has been increasing, often with the approval, and sometimes with the financial aid of governments (James, 1971, especially chapter 8). This had led to more emphasis on the requirements of larger enterprises: standardized livestock (R.D. Baker et al., 1973, p. 41): and potential for high output, usually associated with high input and often with large body size (e.g., Taylor, 1973; Barlow, 1984).

Small enterprises need not be inefficient. Warriner (1934) found that the standard of living of European peasants was not dependent upon farm size except in extreme cases where overpopulation has resulted in subdivision to the size of inadequacy. Bachman and Christensen (1967) surveyed a number of studies, including that of Japan and Russia, and found no evidence that smallholdings were less efficient than large farms. In Australia, smaller holdings were found to be more economically efficient, whether for crops (Davidson, 1966) or for pastoral purposes (Kelly, 1971).

Similarly, while recognizing the connection between body size and high yield, many scientists distinguish between yield and efficiency, recommending a range of sizes for different conditions (R.D. Baker et al., 1973; Dickerson, 1978; Barlow, 1984).

So why are large farms encouraged? Some justifications include: the need to compensate for rising costs and diminishing returns by adding more units of production; greater efficiency; and to support a higher total population (although a smaller rural one). A more pragmatic reason is that it is easier to sell industrial products and services to larger enterprises (Hunter, 1970). An astounding reason, not generally given, is that many Western countries are embarrassed by the high production of small farms and prefer larger farms because production per acre (and hence total production) is less (Peters, 1968; James, 1971, p. 96). Finally, a component of large farming enterprises, the large breeding unit, has been advocated as the best means of achieving genetic improvement. This last reason has so many ramifications that it is necessary to give it a section of its own.

2.3. The role of genetic theory

Science is hierarchical. Those at the top control publication, research grants and jobs. Regardless of whether or not individual members of the top stratum intend to impose their ideas, most members of the lower strata usually perceive compliance as more rewarding than dissent (Manwell and Baker, 1986). This social structure is responsible for great loss of breed resources under the guise of breeding plans based upon genetic theory.

The theory of population genetics is based largely upon the work of R.A. Fisher and of Sewall Wright, who had some fundamental differences in approach. These are still the source of much discussion but, for the present purpose, a simplified contrast is adequate:

Fisher's model was of a panmictic population with selection acting upon individual characteristics: in large populations genetic drift ('chance') was not important (Fisher, 1930; and see comments by Nei, 1980 and by Wright, 1982). Fisher also worked on the effects of domestication (1931, 1934, 1935). He considered that breeds arose mainly or entirely through selection by man and, because of this, differed greatly from their wild progenitors (see p. 270 and p. 272).

Wright considered that a population was divided into subpopulations, each of which was a separate breeding unit (now known as a *deme*). Within these, selection was thought to act upon superior combinations of traits, which were concentrated rapidly by drift because of small subpopulation size. Selection occurred between subpopulations by means of the spread of the most successful (Wright, 1968, 1969, 1977, 1978, 1982; Nei, 1980). Wright has explained (1982, p. 16): 'The theory was suggested by an analogous two-level process of artificial selection that has been employed in the improvement of livestock, involving (a) the development of superior herds . . . followed by (b) selection amongst such herds as sources of breeding stock, especially males, by breeders in general.' It is now known that this same population structure is found in many species of wild mammals (Wilson, 1975).

Adherents to each theory tended to be of the same national origin as the proponent. However, both American and British texts on animal breeding originally followed Wright's interpretation (Lush, 1945; Nicholls, 1957). But attempts to apply quantitative genetics to farm animals made Fisher's approach more attractive: simplification of the aims of selection to individual traits gave theoretically faster progress; and large populations meant less error variance (Hazel, 1943; Donald and El Itriby, 1945). The expansion of artificial insemination (AI) favoured large populations to meet costs and for testing sires (Edwards, 1959; Lauvergne, 1977). The use of blood grouping for pedigree testing, especially useful in respect of AI, also favoured large sire families as these are necessary for the interpretation of some blood group systems (see p. 252).

Fisher's work was used as a major justification that the average herd size of 15 British breeds of cattle was genetically inefficient. Factors mentioned were: frequent changes of bulls, necessary to avoid close inbreeding, random fluctuations in gene frequency; the difficulty of progeny testing; and that '. . . independent methods of breeding and selection are carried out . . .'. It was suggested: '. . . to minimize these drawbacks and to coordinate the presently independent and conflicting policies of individual breeders . . . breeding plans should embrace whole breeds or localized subdivisions of breeds.' (Donald, 1944; Donald and El Itriby, 1945, pp. 93 and 94).

A warning that genetic erosion was taking place was given by Landauer (1945). Eventually this led to the symposium *Germ Plasm Resources* (Hodgson, 1961). Most participants exhibited no urgency: their main interest was in exotics which might supply new genes, or which could be used to exploit heterosis.

Promulgation of the advantages of large enterprises continued. Lerner and Donald (1966, p. 146) included non-genetic benefits such as technical and managerial staff, market research, risk-spreading and advertising. In addition (p. 186): 'No conglomeration of individual small operators can produce the genetic improvement of which a large concern is capable, unless they band together and become large themselves.' The possible loss of genetic variability was discussed but dismissed as of '. . . no immediate urgency . . . except, perhaps, for chickens' (Lerner and Donald, 1966, p. 208).

These statements were echoed by other influential geneticists such as Fredeen (1977, p. 207). King (1981, p. 230) also considered '. . . exhaustion of genetic variation is not a great problem, except perhaps for egg laying poultry.'

The repeatedly expressed concern for poultry did not result in any practical help. When a public appeal was made for the conservation of stocks held by traditional breeders (Accredited Poultry Breeders' Federation, 1963) it was attacked in the farming press by the 'chief geneticist, Chunky Chicks (Nichols) Ltd, which is the Ross Group subsidiary responsible for all the genetic research in the group' (J.D.H. Archibald, 1963). Only one reply in support of the traditional breeders was published (Baker, 1963).

In such a climate of opinion,

> . . . an animal geneticist, who worries about the conservation on genes, can be considered unrealistic and therefore trust in him can be lost even in present day matters. Another geneticist, who doesn't worry at all, can for his part be relatively sure that he doesn't need to answer for the consequences at the time these became apparent. The same reasoning applies to entire breeding organization . . . (Maijala, 1974, p. 42).

Another disturbing development is that some geneticists have an arrogant attitude that it is they, and not the breeders, who should make decisions. R.A. Barton, Reader in the Department of Animal Science at Massey University has complained that breed societies are only '. . . keeping the Flock or Herd Book, checking on pedigrees, appointing judges and inspectors, issuing prizes and printing propaganda . . . arranging social events and generally maintaining the *status quo*'; and that descriptions of breed type are '. . . colloquial, imprecise, difficult to understand by the novice and may emphasize features of the animal that could be in conflict with commercial realities' (Barton, 1984, p. 4). Breed societies would have to be reorganized with emphasis on the role of '. . . professionally trained animal breeders and others . . .' and '. . . pedigree breeders who are unable to accept the discipline that will be imposed through the revamped breed society will have no alternative but to resign . . .' The outlook for minority breeds is bleak: 'They will either go into recess or join with other similar sized societies . . . there will be a loss of independence but this will be inevitable' (Barton, 1984, p. 7).

Similar criticisms have been made by Gaunt (1984). He, too, recommends that the control of breed societies should be removed from breeders, and advocates a civil servant as the chief paid executive officer. Amalgamation of breed societies is again regarded as 'inevitable.'

Some of these statements may seem extreme, but there is already an example of what can happen. Professor Harald Skjervold of the Agricultural University of Norway has achieved the deliberate replacement of some eight pure breeds of Norwegian cattle with one mongrelized population, based on the native breeds, Swedish cattle, Ayrshires, British Friesians and American and Canadian Holsteins (Epstein and Mason, 1984).

Finally, we present the view of a prominent member of a breed society which took advice from a well-known animal geneticist. After several years it was decided to terminate the arrangement. There was a feeling that experimental considerations took precedence over breed interests, and far from there being any sign of genetic improvement, '... if we'd kept on, he'd have had us in the Rare Breeds' tent.' Since terminating the services of the geneticist, and having made a number of changes as a result of their own perception of the market, this breed society has enjoyed considerable recent success.

3. REASONS FOR CONSERVATION

At one time, it was just accepted that there was a variety of breeds. Their existence was not felt to require any justification, although individual breeders could give good reasons for their particular choice. But now it is necessary to marshal these reasons to counter the immediate interests of agribusiness and of these animal geneticists whose main consideration is large populations on which they can test their theories.

3.1. Intangibles

Economists recognize as *intangibles* a number of factors which are difficult to assess in quantitative terms.

3.1.1. Ethical and moral considerations

Although 'breed' is not a recognized taxon, breeds of livestock have many attributes of natural taxa (e.g., Darwin, 1875; Lush, 1945) and so have the same 'right to exist' (Myers, 1979, p. 46; Ehrlich and Ehrlich, 1982, p. 42). Our own species depends on the continued evolution of domesticates, making it a moral duty to ensure that the necessary variation is retained (Heslop-Harrison, 1976, p. 4). In contrast to many farm crops, 'The gene pool of livestock species is . . . almost entirely domestic, and this emphasises the need to preserve and manage it to best advantage' (Frankel and Soulé, 1981, p. 254).

An arrogant attitude to the germ plasm of non-human animals can easily be extended to people. Thus the attitude that domesticates are merely products of human selection, replaceable at will (see pp. 234 and 242) became confused with the value judgement that some domesticates are degenerate. This view, extrapolated to man himself, constituted Konrad Lorenz's explanation for his support of the Nazi 'eugenics' programme (Haldane, 1962; Nisbett, 1976).

3.1.2. Aesthetic

The appreciation of diversity of form, horn types, colour and colour patterns is shown by the wealth of descriptive language found in groups as widely separated as African tribes (Evans-Pritchard, 1940; Brownlee, 1977); contemporary *aficionados* of the bullfight (Anon., 1974a; McCormick and Mascareñas, 1967); Texas ranchers (Dobie, 1941); Welsh bards (F.G. Payne, 1969); and modern poets (Hopkins, 1967). Such 'fancy points' are often criticized (e.g., Barton, 1984; Gaunt, 1984) but many are cultivated because of some original belief that they are 'really correlated with welfare and purpose' (Van Riper, 1932, p. 90; and see pp. 244 and 245).

3.1.3. Cultural

Ryder (1970, 1976) has pointed out that the cultural importance of many breeds of livestock makes them at least as worthy of preservation as monuments and other buildings.

There is ample evidence concerning human–bovine relationships to support Ryder's claim. (See, for example, references in the preceding section; and papers in Mourant and Zeuner, 1963; and in Leeds and Vayda, 1965). There are also many modern manifestations, ranging from popular literature on rare breeds (Alderson, 1978; Whitlock, 1980) to cattle shows, bullfights and rodeos. Many terms in the '. . . colloquial, imprecise, difficult to understand . . .' livestock vocabulary criticized by Barton (1984) can be traced to proto Indo-European sources (Buck, 1949). Cattle breeders are not unaware of this link: even in modern Australia, 'It is thousands of moons to the cattle-raid of Cooley/But we could still find common knowledge, verb-roots/And noun-bark enough for an evening fire of sharing/Cattle-wisdom . . .' (Murray, 1972, p. 43).

Many cultural practices have significant social and economic functions. Examples have been discussed for cattle in Hindu culture (Harris, 1966; Heston, 1971; Odend'hal, 1972); the water buffalo in the same milieu (Hoffpauir, 1982); cattle in Africa (Seago, 1971; Rutman and Werner, 1973); and for less well-known bovines of local importance such as the yak (Hermanns, 1949; Societé d'Ethnozootechnie, 1976) and the mithan (Simoons and Simoons, 1968). In at least one case there is a sound dietary basis: the cultural co-adaptation of man and cattle when the former suffers from lactose intolerance (Simoons, 1979).

3.1.4. Education

If professionally trained agriculturalists are to attain credibility, they should learn at least a little about their nationally kept breeds, including how these are recognized (Stufflebeam, 1983, p. 36). Teaching in other disciplines, including archaeology, evolution, genetics and zoology, is also facilitated by living examples (Reynolds, 1979; Rudolph et al., 1980).

Public education concerning conservation has been described as '. . . the foundation upon which all our efforts must be built . . .' (Raven, 1976). Considerable interest, involvement and sympathy have been generated by displays of different breeds in Regional National Parks in France (Laurans, 1974; Lauvergne, 1979) and at Farm Parks in the U.K. (J.L. Henson, 1978).

3.1.5. Research

Some idea of the multifarious research possibilities of unusual breeds can be demonstrated by reference to two widely different disciplines.

Archaeology. Butser Farm was established to make empirical tests of theories by reconstructing Iron Age farming practices, and for the general education of the public. Authenticity was greatly enhanced by using surviving breeds of primitive types, including Dexter cattle for draught (Reynolds, 1979). In contrast, lack of a suitable small breed to test the replica of an ard at Lejre made it necessary to obtain and castrate two Jersey bull calves and then wait for them to grow to working age, when their performance was not found to be entirely satisfactory (Coles, 1973, pp. 28–29).

Physiology. The understanding of maternal effects on growth in cattle was advanced significantly by having available for reciprocal crosses the South Devon (bull 2464 lb or 1120 kg; cow 1052 lb or 478 kg) and the Dexter (bull 978 lb or 445 kg; cow 484 lb or 220 kg) (Joubert and Hammond, 1958). In other cases opportunities have been lost. The value of the seaweed-eating North Ronaldsay sheep for studies of copper metabolism (Wiener, 1979) could have been extended by studies on Manx and Scillonian seaweed-eating cattle, but these two breeds are extinct (Train, 1845; Scott and Rivington, 1870).

Other areas. There are many other cases and most scientists agree that research justifies at least some conservation (e.g., Lerner and Donald, 1966, p. 207). But the extent of commitment varies. Landauer (1945, p. 498) believed that stocks should be perpetuated because '. . . the geneticist cannot build with the knowledge of his predecessors unless he possesses the necessary building stones, the mutants . . .' Others have been more capricious. The Zoological Society of London scheme to preserve rare breeds for research was discontinued, some 7 years after it was announced, ostensibly because of a 'disappointing' response, although two projects had been published, and at least one request for material remained unfulfilled (Rowlands, 1964; Ryder, 1971; Zuckerman, 1971). The large firm which maintained the last Lincolnshire Curly Coat pigs for experimental purposes sent the remaining animals for slaughter in 1972 (Jewell and Alderson, 1977).

Health of consumers of animal products. In recent years there has been a widespread feeling that saturated fats contribute to heart and artery disease. Diets with a greater proportion of polyunsaturated fats are recommended, and there has been a reduced consumption of meat and butter. It has long been known that winter butter from stall-fed cows is harder than butter from the same cows on grass with little or no supplementary food. Comparisons within and between species have produced evidence that browsing animals have a higher proportion of polyunsaturated fatty acids in their body fat than grazers or stall-fed animals (Crawford, 1968). Species, breeds and production methods adapted to browsing and to grazing young grass could be beneficial for the health of consumers and the sales of producers. In marginal areas, the use of browsing animals would reduce the temptation to remove trees in the hope of getting more grass, which frequently causes erosion. Browsers include mithan (Simoons and Simoons, 1968), kouprey (Wharton, 1957) and small mountain breeds of Indian cattle (Wallace, 1888, p. 58).

3.2. Demonstrated economic advantage

3.2.1. Economic studies of non-conventional breeds

Unbiassed studies of non-conventional breeds are not plentiful. When they are made, they frequently reveal the economic superiority of the breed for a non-conventional niche. In Africa, there is an increasing amount of data to show that relatively unimproved indigenous breeds do as well as, or better, than highly selected exotics. One set of comparisons involved Hereford, Simmental and Santa Gertrudis with a Sanga herd (the last-mentioned established on *culled* animals); the Sanga yielded considerably higher net income when marketed directly off veld without supplementary concentrates (Hamburger and Ramsay, 1984).

Economic studies of small luxury markets are even less available, but one is provided in Longsworth's (1983) analysis of the Japanese beef industry. In common with other industrialized countries, a significant proportion of home-produced beef comes from the largely Holstein dairy sector. In 1980 this yielded 812 892 beast (p. 110) averaging 75 493 Yen per head net profit (p. 128). Some of the meat went to the expensive 'high quality' market, but much of it did not comply with the Japanese quality requirements of considerable marbling without excessive subcutaneous fat. This is provided by the slower growing, higher food consumption Waygu breeds. In 1980 these yielded 374 147 beast (p. 80) averaging 88 290 Yen per head net profit (p. 128). Practically all of these went for the high quality market.

The pinnacle of the Japanese beef industry is the 6% luxury market for Kobe, Matsuka or Omi beef. This market is very stable. A single animal may fetch 1.7 million Yen, and Kobe beef retails at 3000 Yen per 100 g. (Longsworth's conversion rate is 250 Yen = 1 Australian dollar.) Kobe beef is produced from certain Waygu strains, especially the Tajima strain of Japanese Black. Feeding must be by the traditional 'Ideal' methods, involving individual care, special rations (including beer), exercise and massage. A detailed description has been given by Rouse (1970).

Chapter 10 references, p. 289

Although beef is a very small part of the Japanese national product, and herds of less than five cattle are common among Waygu breeders, these have considerable political influence which they use to protect and improve the Waygu breeds (Longsworth, 1983).

3.2.2. Cost-benefit aspects of conservation

Often no detailed study is available for a particular breed. Then decisions about conservation depend upon the relationship between probable costs and possible returns, another topic for which few data are available.

Charles Smith (1984b,c) has assembled some useful information on the costs of conserving livestock as breeding animals, semen and ova. He has also calculated the level of benefit which would make it worthwile to maintain a breed for future use. For cattle this could be as low as a 0.1% use of stock and a 1% gain in the efficiency of the conserved stock relative to animals in common use, although Smith suggests that it would be more realistic to aim for increased efficiency in the region of 5–10%. Smith concluded that even if the conservation of any particular stock may be a gamble, preservation of several breeds on a national level is justified in terms of the benefit which would accrue in the annual value of national production.

3.3. Economic potential

3.3.1. Yields

Even tests biassed to certain aspects of production have revealed considerable merit in relatively unimproved breeds. Osman (1981) has given the following figures for milk yield: Butana (Sudan) 2253 kg in 240 days; Damascus (Syria) 2974 kg in 283 days; South Anatolian Red (Turkey) 2700–3000 kg in 250–300 days; compared with Friesian yields in Egypt, Iraq and the United Arab Emirates of 2573 kg in 322 days to 3253 kg in 305 days. The Rathi (India) is also said to attain economic levels of milk production (Swaminathan, 1981).

Minority breeds have done quite well in beef performance tests. British White bulls have had 400-day weights up to 575 kg and averaged 475 kg; while the South Devon averaged 544 kg compared with Charolais (565 kg) and Simmental (553 kg) (C.M. Wright, 1984).

3.3.2. Special traits

Many breeds are valued for characteristics which are discussed in the section on markers. Examples are resistance to specific diseases, muscular hypertrophy, high butterfat and colour.

3.3.3. General adaptability

Even in a developed country where a combination of agribusiness and government intervention standardizes many agricultural conditions, variations in requirements occur. It is instructive to consider the choice of breeds for two contrasting farms in the British Isles, summarized from accounts by the farmers themselves.

For a small dairy farm the choice was the Dexter (see pp. 230, 263 and 264). Its small size confers risk-spreading and flexibility and contributes to the ability to find a living on poor land. Dexters can live out all the year round: they are light enough not to poach their grazing and, in contrast to comparably sized Jerseys, have a coat which is good protection against cold, chapped udders and flies. This cuts the overhead cost of housing and the annual cost of straw for bedding. In addition, Dexters qualify for a suckler premium (Hopper, 1984).

On larger, more fertile farms, rising costs for intensive inputs and the difficulty of finding skilled labour have caused a search for alternatives to systems which are becoming financially inefficient. One such farmer, in search of a crossbred cow to breed beeves, explained that the Hereford × Shorthorn cow was 'almost unobtainable'; and that he was 'disillusioned' with the Hereford × Friesian. Of other conventional possibilities he remarked: 'To have put in continental blood would have given us a big, hungry, inefficient cow. Traditional beef blood would be fine in winter but we would get fat instead of milk in summer. Dairy blood would take us back whence we had just come.' The successful solution was the Longhorn × Welsh Black (Close, 1984).

3.3.4. Changing requirements

There are a number of examples where breed characteristics have been appreciated to a different extent at different times. Unimproved beef conformation, unsuitable for changes in early 19th century markets, led to the absorption of Suffolk Dun milch cattle into the dual-purpose Red Poll (Raynbird, 1847, pp. 267, 303 and 308; Chevallier, 1910, p. 48). In the mid-20th century the extinction of the Suffolk Dun was regretted on the grounds that the breed would have been an asset to the specialized dairy farming of that time (Trow-Smith, 1959, pp. 105–107).

In the last decade some dual-purpose breeds have made an attempt to survive by emphasizing beef qualities. This could result in a serious loss in milking capacity, as happened in the (North) Devon, Hereford and Shorthorn in the 19th century (Dent, 1864, p. 427; Dixon, 1865a,b, p. 324). Fortunately at least one breed, the South Devon, has sought to maintain milking capacity by including 200-day weight (known to be a consequence of the milking qualities of the dam rather than the growth potential of the calf) in the selection of breeding stock (J. Pappin, personal communication, 1984). This is a wise strategy. The milk surplus in the EEC has led to a reduction in support for dairying, at a time when costs, especially of imported concentrates, are rising. Analysis of economic factors suggests that in the future it will be most profitable in many cases to produce beef and milk from dual-purpose herds (Pirchner, 1984).

3.3.5. Formation of new breeds

Rastogi (1978) has drawn attention to the circumstance that, despite the number of existing breeds, further breeds arose when new geographical niches became available. He illustrated the point by reference to West Indian cattle: the Jamaica Black (similar to Brangus) the Jamaica Red Poll (Creole, Zebu and Red Poll) and the Croix Sennepol (N'Dama and Red Poll). Similar breeds have arisen in Australia: the Australian Milking Zebu (Red Sindhi, Sahiwal and Jersey) the Belmont Red (Africander, Brahman, Hereford and Shorthorn) and the Droughtmaster (mainly Brahman and Shorthorn). Comparable breeds in the U.S.A. are the Santa Gertrudis (Brahman and Shorthorn) and the Beefmaster (Brahman, Hereford and Shorthorn).

New breeds may also be formed to fill niches created by changes in commercial conditions. Thus R. Pisaturo, already well-known as a breeder of Shorthorns and Charolais, evolved the Mandalong Special. He combined Brahman for '. . . a small calf and a hardy beast', Shorthorn and Charolais for '. . . a well muscled carcass with adequate fat', British White for '. . . milking ability yet hardness and a good carcass in its own rights' and Chianina '. . . to maintain the size' (Bowen, 1983; R. Pisaturo, personal communication, 1983). At least two new breeds have been formed because of changes in farming practice in the U.K.: the Beevbilde (Lincoln Red, Beef Shorthorn and Aberdeen Angus) and the Luing (Beef Shorthorn and Highland).

New breeds of water buffalo include the Buffalypso, a cross of various Indian breeds selected for meat (Rastogi, 1978); and a Bulgarian new breed from 'native' buffalo crossed with Murrah imported from India (Makaveev, 1984).

Chapter 10 references, p. 289

4. GENETIC RESOURCES

4.1. Gene pools

The development of the concept of a gene pool has been traced by Adams (1979). A gene pool is not just a 'pile of genes' but an integrated system. In this, original, sense (which arose from Serebovsky's studies of gene geography) a gene pool is explicity or implicitly associated with a population, e.g., a species or a breed.

Unfortunately this concept has been perverted by some biologists who use the term gene pool for a mixture of populations made or recommended as a means of conservation: e.g., see Boyer's (1965) description of a 'gene reservoir' formed by mixing breeds of chickens with different morphological characteristics; or see Frankel and Soulé (1981, p. 273) who contrast the conservation of individual breeds with '*gene pools* consisting of a number of breeds.' Such a mixture is not an integrated system. Presumably, if it existed long enough, a mixture would evolve to become an integrated system, as, indeed, has happened in breeds formed from crosses (see p. 239 and 275). However, until the latter stage is reached, some other descriptive term seems more appropriate than gene pool. Simmond's (1962) 'mass reservoir' is liable to confusion with gene pool. 'Pile of genes' (Adams, 1979, p. 247) is descriptive and matches R.A. Fisher's philosophy behind the making of a mixture: *that individual genes can be selected at will from the mass.*

Frankel and Soulé (1981, and with acknowledgement of a personal communication from F.H.W. Morley) advocate mixture of breeds on several grounds. Operationally, a mixture is said to be cheaper and easier to maintain than individual breeds, and more breeds can be added with a minimum of extra facilities. Biologically, it is claimed that several advantages would be gained from a large number of interbreeding individuals: less loss of genes from random drift; large effective size; fewer males would be necessary; less inbreeding; and the possibility that new combinations would arise from the mixture in comparison with the 'crossing of only two breeds' which these scientists think is the usual way of developing new breeds.

Frankel and Soulé (1981) made no reference to Jaap's (1965) discussion of genetic problems which can arise from attempts at conservation based on population mixtures. Jaap considered that only a few alleles could be maintained at a frequency over 0.2 at each locus in any one population, and that mixing more than three populations would '. . . reduce the frequency of alleles so low that their future value for selective breeding would be greatly diminished.' For a multi-allelic locus he advocated '. . . many populations . . . to insure having each of the alleles at a desirable frequency for change by selective breeding.'

It is true that new combinations can arise from breed admixture. But this is already a means of producing new breeds which, contrary to the belief of Frankel and Soulé, frequently involve more than 'only two breeds' (for examples see pp. 239 and 275).

It is often inferred or stated that breeds can be reconstituted at will from a mixture. An extreme example is Lerner and Donald's (1966, p. 207) claim: 'Given Holstein and Jersey cattle, it is likely that every other known dairy breed could be reconstructed as closely as need be, and many more.'

Such claims of reconstruction are dubious. How, for example, would Lerner and Donald produce the red, white and roan Dairy Shorthorn from their mixture? There is not even experimental evidence that a breed can be reconstituted from a mixture in which its major known alleles were kept segregating. There is not even an estimate of the probable cost of such an undertaking. There is a real danger that attempts to conserve a 'pile of genes' will only result in a scrap heap.

4.2. Species and interspecific hybrids

Our summary includes wild species and feral populations as well as domesticates. The two former are sources of genetic variation and, managed properly, constitute renewable resources which can be harvested.

The most recent inclusive writings on bovine taxonomy and natural history are by Lydekker (1894, 1898). The present section is based on these, supplemented by references to more modern works on individual species.

4.2.1. Cattle

When used as a collective noun in a wide sense, 'cattle' corresponds quite closely to the presently living and recently extinct species in Lydekker's 'typical or taurine', 'bibovine' and 'bisontine' groups. These have two characteristics in common: all have (or are probably closely related to species which have) a domestic relationship with man; and all the living species can exchange genetic material with each other to a greater or lesser extent.

European or taurine cattle, *Bos taurus* L. *Bos taurus* is unknown as a wild species unless the Chillingham cattle or the Betisoak represent surviving populations. Feral populations seem to be established easily if suitable habitat is available (Baker and Manwell, 1981).

Most (but not all) writers consider that *B. taurus* is descended from the aurochs, *Bos primigenius* Bojanus, a suggestion made by Bojanus (1827) although he regarded the two species as distinct. It is usually accepted that the last aurochs '. . . died in a Polish park in 1627 . . .' (Zeuner, 1963, p. 203). However, Dent (1983) raised the possibility that the Betisoak of the Basque country are a relict population of a separate race or subspecies of aurochs, supporting this idea with an allusion to Gessner. We have found the passage in Topsell (1607, p. 721): 'These [Aurochsen] are found in the wood *Hercynia*, in the *Pyreney* Mountaines, and in *Mazouia* near *Lituania*.' It is not impossible that an isolated population should remain in the Pyrenees mountains in the Basque country where the Betisoak occurs.

Zebu or indicine cattle, *Bos indicus* L. Zebu cattle have their centre of diversity on the subcontinent of India, but the free-living populations found there have been regarded as feral rather than wild (Lydekker, 1894). Feral populations have become established elsewhere, notably in Australia (Kelley, 1959).

The absence of *Bos indicus* as a wild species has led to speculation about its origin. A common theory is that it was derived from the now extinct *Bos namadicus* (Zeuner, 1963, p. 239; see p. 277).

The mithan or gayal *Bos frontalis* Lambert and the gaur, *Bos gaurus* H. Smith. (Zeuner, 1963; Simoons and Simoons, 1968; Wharton, 1968; NRC, 1983). All authorities associate the mithan with Assam and Chittagong. Lydekker (1894, p. 180; 1898 p. 33) also mentions Tenasserim.

Mithan have been domesticated for a long but undetermined time. Their local socio-economic importance is out of all proportion to their relatively small numbers. On a practical level, mithan eat a high proportion of browse and, through the medium of ritual feasts, provide high biological value protein (Simoons and Simoons, 1968). A minor but still important use is the importation of mithan to Bhutan for crossbreeding (Chatterjee, 1926; Hickman, 1982).

The general agreement that mithan and gaur are closely related is supported by evidence from cytology (Fischer, 1969; Winter et al., 1984; see p. 250) and biochemistry (Lalthantluanga et al., 1975; Winter et al., 1984; see p. 272). The nature of the relationship is not clear. The most favoured theory is that the wild gaur is the ancestor of the domestic mithan (e.g., Simoons and Si-

Chapter 10 references, p. 289

moons, 1968). But both Lydekker (1894, p. 34) and Zeuner (1963, pp. 253–255) found the literature confusing. As pointed out by the Ad Hoc Panel (NRC, 1983, p. 26), mithan and gaur look very different in certain respects. This could partly be a consequence of the localized mithan being compared with gaur from a distant part of the latter's geographic range. This comprises the forested parts of the subcontinent of India (with the exception of Sri Lanka) and continues east through the hilly districts into Burma, Malaya and Vietnam (Lydekker, 1894, 1898; Wharton, 1968). The differences between regions, especially between the east and west parts of the range, have led to the recognition of at least two geographic races or subspecies (Lydekker, 1898, p. 26; C.P. Groves and P. Grubb, personal communication to the Ad Hoc Panel, 1983).

The difference in geographic distribution of mithan and gaur adds a further dimension to the problem of relationship. If mithan are domesticated gaur, why did domestication only occur in one very small part of the range of the wild species, especially when over much of the range, domestication of more than one bovine species is common?

Gaur usually live in small groups of 5–6 to 20 animals. Bulls tend to keep apart in twos and threes or, as they age, as singles. Lydekker's description of gaur habitat has been confirmed by Wharton (1968): forest and savanna, with exploitation of grass and bamboo shoots after forest fires.

Banteng, *Bos sondaicus* Müller and Schlegel; *B. banteng* Wagner; or *B. javanicus* d'Alton. (Hooijer, 1956; Meijer, 1962; Halder, 1976; NRC, 1983).

Both domestic banteng, sometimes distinguished as Bali cattle, and wild banteng are considered to be the same species. Domestic banteng occur largely in Indonesia. The wild banteng currently occurs in Burma, the lower parts of Thailand, Kampuchea, Vietnam, Java and Borneo. In parts of this range there is overlap with gaur, but each species is thought to exploit a different niche (Wharton, 1968, p. 155). Like gaur, banteng occur in small herds, described as 10–30 in Manipur and 8–20 in Burma. Each herd had 2–3 young bulls, but as these matured they were driven off by an old bull (Lydekker, 1898).

Formerly banteng were also reported in the Malay Peninsula (Lydekker, 1898, p. 43). There is a small feral population of banteng in northern Australia, descended from 20 Bali cattle introduced in 1849 and subsequently abandoned (McKnight, 1976; see p. 270).

Bali cattle are locally important. They are particularly valued for working ability and adaptation to poor food. They produce lean meat (Subandriyo et al., 1979). Some data have been collected for characteristics of feral banteng in Australia (Kirby, 1979; NRC, 1983).

Banteng have the reputation of being able to manage on infrequent water (Lydekker, 1898, p. 45; Halder, 1976). They have been observed to drink seawater and the feral Australian banteng are said to graze seaweed on coral reefs at low tide (NRC, 1983).

The kouprey, *Novibos sauveli* Urbain. (Coolidge, 1940, 1955; Wharton, 1957, 1966; Bohlken, 1961; Pfeffer and Kim-San, 1967; NRC, 1983). The kouprey has primitive taxonomic characters which have led to suggestions that it is a relict of the Miocene. The few surviving animals are in Kampuchea and possibly in bordering parts of Laos, Thailand and Vietnam. Wharton (1957) suggested that the kouprey was a domesticate of the Khmer civilization, over 800 years ago. It is not known whether the remaining free-living herds are feral or truly wild.

Kouprey usually occur in small groups of up to 20. The habitat is similar to that of the banteng and the two species may overlap.

Domestic yak, *Bos grunniens* L. and wild yak *B. mutus* Prezewalski. (Hermanns, 1949; Societé d'Ethnozootechnie, 1976; NRC, 1983; see p. 272). Yak are adapted to the cold and extremely high altitudes of the Himalayas, ranging from 14 000 to 20 000 feet (4000–6000 m) above sea level for summer grazings. Wild yak occur at the highest levels in isolated districts. Herds usually consist of about 10 cows and followers including young bulls. Old bulls may be solitary or occur in groups of up to four. When pasture is available, larger herds of up to 100 animals may be observed.

Lydekker (1898, p. 54) described the semi-domesticated yak of Rupshu and other high plateaux as 'practically indistinguishable' except that they were somewhat smaller than and not always the dark blackish colour of wild yak. Both wild yak and the domesticates from high altitudes are said to be unable to live at low altitudes.

On the lower levels (down to about 6000 feet or 2000 m) domestic yaks extend into Mongolia. These are smaller and have considerable variation, including colour, colour patterns and polling. Even yak from the lowest levels have only a limited ability to adapt to life in India, and then only for short periods; and '. . . it is such alone that are exhibited alive in Europe' (Lydekker, 1898, p. 55). Contrary to the impression given by the Ad Hoc Panel (NRC, 1983, p. 32) yak taken to North America earlier this century did not adapt to low altitudes easily and bred more successfully when taken to higher altitudes (White et al., 1946). However, yaks were kept successfully by the Duke of Bedford at Woburn.

In their limited area in the Himalayas yaks provide for almost every human need and pervade almost every aspect of human culture (Phillips et al., 1945; Hermanns, 1949).

The inability of yak to live and work efficiently below a certain altitude and the similar inefficiency of *B. indicus* at higher altitudes has given rise to systems of crossbreeding and back-crossing to provide bovine hybrids capable of work in the intermediate altitudes. A measure of the importance of these animals is that there are special names which indicate the sex and species of ancestors, sometimes for several generations (Hermanns, 1949; Downs and Ekvall, 1965). In a few districts similar crosses are made between yak and mithan (Simoons and Simoons, 1968).

Wisent or European bison, *Bison bonasus* L. (see pp. 250 and 270–272).There is no record that the wisent was ever domesticated, although calves can be tamed and the herd in the Białwiecz Forest has been regarded as 'managed' for many years (Vasey, 1851). The last truly wild bison lingered in the Caucasus until early this century.

Lydekker (1894, 1898) describes the normal habitat of wisent as woodland. Animals lived in groups of 15–20 in summer but would form larger herds of 30–50 in winter. Old bulls were solitary but joined herds for breeding.

American bison or 'buffalo', *Bison bison* L. (McHugh and Hobson, 1972; Roe, 1972; see pp. 250 and 270–272). American bison originally consisted of two or possibly three subspecies (Krumbiegal, 1980). Lydekker (1898, p. 84) considered the abundance of plains bison unique among the ungulates, and ascribed this to the periodic migrations when huge herds were formed. However, there was still evidence for an underlying deme structure. For parts of the year the bison were dispersed over a wide area in small bands, which would coalesce for breeding and migrations. Even the big herds would form smaller groups when feeding (Lydekker, 1894, p. 197; 1898, p. 86).

There is evidence of sporadic attempts to domesticate bison. Roe (1972, p. 706) thought herds may have been managed by Amerindians in Mexico. Several writers mention that calves could be tamed, and these writers give examples of isolated instances of quondam domestication in colonial times (Vasey, 1851; McHugh and Hobson, 1972; Roe, 1972). The major contribution to livestock production to date seems to be through hybridization with taurine cattle.

4.2.2. Interspecific hybrids

Hybridization is possible between all species of cattle, although in most cases for which information is available the F_1 male is sterile (Gray, 1972; Scheifler, 1974). It has been claimed that crosses between *B. taurus* and *B. indicus* are completely fertile (Zeuner and Mourant, 1963; Epstein and Mason, 1984; Gray, 1972). However, when pedigree records are kept, and a control is available, there is evidence that limited hybrid breakdown can occur (J.M. Rendel, 1980).

Cattle hybrids are valuable because they provide information about the processes of evolution and because of their utility. We have chosen the latter aspect as the basis of our present discussion.

Introgressive hybridization with reciprocal gene flow and maintenance of the identity of parental species. Simoons and Simoons (1968, p. 24) have drawn attention to '. . . the remarkable series of domestic bovine hybrids that occurs in the Eastern Himalayas and marks that as the foremost area of bovine hybridization in the world.' The following examples illustrate the chances for two-, three-, or even four-way gene flow.

Hybrids between yak and zebu, yak and taurine cattle and mithan and zebu are contrived deliberately and involve the movement of one species into the zone of the other. Hybrid cattle are often named with reference to the species and sex of their ancestors, but a stage is reached when one species predominates and the individual is considered a member of that species (Hermanns, 1949; Simoons and Simoons, 1968; Societé d'Ethnozootechnie, 1976; NRC, 1983).

Mithan and gaur overlap in their range. Some (but not all) mithan owners are indifferent to, or encourage, hybridization. The hybrid females are known to be fertile although there does not seem to be any concrete information about the fertility of the hybrid males (Gray, 1972).

There are also reports of three-way hybrids involving yak, mithan and zebu.

So far, there is little evidence as to the amount of introgression which persists in any of these cases. However, the Simoons (1968) have drawn attention to where physical characteristics suggest introgression.

Introgressive hybridization with limited one-way gene flow from one species into another. This has happened many times. What (if any) part of the gene pool of the absorbed species has persisted is not known.

Probably the best-documented example is the deliberate grading up of taurine cattle with *B. indicus* to produce Brahman cattle. *B. indicus* has also been absorbed into *B. taurus*. It is possible that this was the fate of indicine cattle imported to England in the 18th and early 19th centuries (Baker, 1984); and it is known that the Illawarra evolved in Australia from imports of African and Indian humped cattle graded up with British breeds, mainly the Ayrshire and the Shorthorn (McCaffrey, 1909; see p. 275 and 284).

It was found in 1932 that at least half of the remaining wisent had in their pedigrees not only American bison but '. . . traces of the silver grey cattle of South Russia . . .' (Mohr, 1949). Scheifler (1974) has explained that this cross was made to save the wisent as a species.

Introgressive hybridization and the evolution of new forms. In nature, a hybrid population capable of exploiting a new ecological niche may evolve into a distinct new type and ultimately achieve a relatively integrated gene pool, although segregation of blocks of traits is common. This process is regarded as a major means of plant evolution (Anderson, 1949). In animals, the only method of speciation for which good proof exists is by hybridization (Scudder, 1974).

There is evidence that some species of domesticates have a hybrid origin (Manwell and Baker, 1976; see p. 272). Hybridization is also suspected or known to have occurred in the more recent evolution of some types of domestic cattle.

There are three cases of suspected introgression from *B. indicus*: humped yellow cattle of China; humped cattle of the Middle East; and humped cattle of Africa. These, and especially the last, have been the subject of considerable debate (Epstein, 1971). It is generally accepted that the present humped African cattle of zebu type are derived from a migration of *B. indicus* in historical times; but many observers recognize the humped sanga cattle as different (Vasey, 1851; Lydekker, 1894; Epstein, 1971). This has raised questions concerning the persistence of an original North African species or subspecies of cattle, and the possible influence of an early migration and introgression of *B. indicus* (Epstein, 1971; see pp. 276 and 277).

Introgression has occurred between *B. indicus* and Bali cattle, possibly with a further contribution from *B. taurus* in some cases. The best known example is the Madura breed, thought to have evolved over some 1500 years (Rouse, 1970; Payne and Rollinson, 1976). It is probable that similar introgression has occurred in other parts of Southeast Asia (Namikawa et al., 1984; see p. 247 and 277).

Introgression has been manipulated to produce breeds from interspecific hybrids of cattle. Examples include: taurindicus breeds, such as Braford and Droughtmaster, derived from crosses of *B. taurus* and *B. indicus*; taur-sanga breeds such as the Bonsmara and Drakensberger, derived from *B. taurus* and sanga; and three-way crosses between *B. taurus, B. indicus* and sanga, such as the Renitelo and the Belmont Red. Crosses between bison and *B. taurus* have produced Cattalo and Beefalo (see p. 282). Investigations have been made into crosses involving yaks in North America (White et al., 1946). In Russia it is claimed that by the fifth generation of crossing yak with taurine cattle, male hybrids are fertile and the hybrids can be bred *inter se* (Scheifler, 1974).

Breeders of élite taurindicus cattle in Australia have told us that at present these involve some careful compensating matings to balance adaptability with high production and to maintain a constant type.

4.2.3. Buffalo

It is convenient to use buffalo as a collective noun for Lydekker's bubaline group. There are no records of hybridization between the cattle and buffalo groups, and hybridization between species of buffalo is very limited (Gray, 1972).

Domestic water buffalo and arnee or wild water buffalo, *Bubalus bubalis* L. (Epstein, 1971; Cockrill, 1974, 1975, 1976; Fahimuddin, 1975; Caldwell, 1977; see pp. 241, 251, 252 and 278). Wild buffalo are native to India and Southeast Asia. They live in swampy areas in large herds. Lydekker (1898, pp. 123 and 126) did not consider that there was any real difference between the 'typical' water buffalo of India and other types.

In fact, there are at least two main groups of domestic water buffalo: the river type of India and the swamp type of China and Southeast Asia. It is thought that there were at least two major centres of domestication (corresponding to the distribution of river and swamp buffalo, respectively) around 2500–3000 BC (Fahimuddin, 1975). Water buffalo of the Middle East and Europe are basically the river type, although they have diverged sufficiently to be named separately. It is debatable whether Middle Eastern water buffalo are derived from indigenous stocks or imports (Zeuner, 1963; Epstein, 1971; Fahimuddin, 1975). European water buffalo are regarded as imports, although Lydekker (1898, p. 123) warned: '. . . there is a Plistocene [sic] European form to which it is just possible their ancestry may be traceable.' An import of water buffalo to Italy occurred around AD 600 (Lydekker, 1898, p. 125; Zeuner, 1963). They throve in malarial districts and became sufficiently important to have a big annual fair at Foggia in Apulia (Vasey, 1851). More recently, water buffalo have been imported to Latin America.

Feral herds of buffalo establish easily if there is suitable habitat. They occur in the original range of the species, Papua-New Guinea, Guam, Australia and Latin America (Lydekker, 1898; Caldwell, 1977; see p. 223).

The tamarao, *Bubalus mindorensis* Heude. Tamarao are small animals, about 1 m at the withers, which are related to water buffalo and anoas. Tamarao are native to Mindoro in the Philippines. The species has not been domesticated but has been tamed (Lydekker, 1898, pp. 128–130; NRC, 1983).

The anoa, *Anoa depressicornis* H. Smith (see p. 251). Anoas are about the size of the tamarao. There are two or three species of anoa: lowland, *Anoa depressicornis*; and upland *A. quarlesi* (sometimes thought to be two species, *A. quarlesi* and *A. fergusoni*). All anoa are native to the Celebes (Sulawesi) (Groves, 1969; Amano et al., 1982b). Anoa have been tamed but not domesticated (NRC, 1983). Lydekker (1898, p. 135) states: 'The flesh, especially that of calves, is tender and well flavoured . . .'

African buffalo, *Syncerus caffer* (Sparrman). Sinclair, 1977; Mloszweski, 1983; see pp. 251, 271 and 272). *Syncerus* is often placed between *Bison* and *Bubalus*. We have placed *Syncerus* at the end of the bubaline group because it has not been domesticated and because there has been little work on markers in this species. Thenius (1980) also places *Syncerus* in this position.

Until comparatively recently, the African buffalo was found over much of the African continent, with marked regional differences which have caused taxonomic confusion (Lydekker, 1898, especially p. 96; Sinclair, 1977). In areas where the African buffalo had not been reduced in numbers, all the species or subspecies occurred in large herds of 50–300 animals, although old bulls were solitary (Lydekker, 1894, 1898). There do not seem to have been any attempts at domestication or even large-scale ranching, although African buffalo have many suitable qualities (Sinclair, 1971, 1977; Mloszewski, 1983). All recorded attempts at hybridization seem to have been within the genus (Gray, 1972).

4.2.4. Other Bovinae

Although Lydekker did not include *Boselaphus, Taurotragus* and *Strepsiceros* among the 'oxen', these genera are usually included in the Bovinae (e.g., see Thenius, 1980). There are sporadic instances of the eland, *Taurotragus oryx* Pallas, being kept as a domesticate since at least the 19th century (Wallace, 1896; Sinclair, 1971). Matings of eland with Africander and taurine cattle (naturally and by AI) do not seem to have resulted in authenticated living offspring (Gray, 1972).

4.3. Breed groups

Breeds do not occur at random within a species, but in groups, many of which are subdivided hierarchically into further groups. There are too many groups to list in the space of this review. Much of the information about breed groups is scattered throughout the older literature on animal breeding, mainly in continental works. *A Dictionary of Livestock Breeds* (Mason, 1969) provides many convenient summaries. A four-page linear arrangement of over 200 breeds into 48 taurine and indicine groups is given in an appendix to a recent paper (Baker and Manwell, 1980).

The traditional definition of breed groups is by geography and morphology; relationship within a group usually exists or is implied. The geographical and morphological criteria are supported by biochemical criteria (Baker and Manwell, 1980; Manwell and Baker, 1980, see p. 275–277).

Despite some breeds with equivocal positions (largely because of crossbreeding) there is a remarkable concensus regarding the composition and characteristics of the major breed groups. Some traits are sufficiently distinct for workers to suggest that they indicate separate specific rank, as in the case of *Bos brachyceros* and *B. frontosus*. Although it is debated whether these constitute valid taxa, the names are still convenient for common use.

Water buffalo groups consist of the two major types, river and swamp; and some authorities add Mediterranean. Each contains hierarchical subgroupings (Mason, 1969; Cockrill, 1974).

4.4. Breeds

4.4.1. Source of information

There are so many breeds that it has only been feasible to use individual names when giving illustrative examples. In *A Dictionary of Livestock Breeds*, water buffalo occupy about 5 pages and cattle a little over 76 pages (Mason, 1969). More breeds appear in lists compiled for individual countries (Mason, 1979; Maijala et al., 1984). In at least one country: 'New breeds and strains are being identified every day, such as Siri cattle in Sikkim, Kashmire Black in Kashmir Valley, Annapurna cattle in Kerala . . .. Some of these . . . have special qualities' (Bhat, 1981). Unfortunately very little is known about breeds of yak, although these are known to exist (NRC, 1983).

For many (but far from all) breeds there is also descriptive literature. There is not space here to consider even all the major works in English. Many, including comparatively recent books are out of print. Some of the most recent books which we have found useful are the volumes on *World Cattle* and *The Criollo* (Rouse, 1969, 1970, 1973, 1977); Epstein's (1971) monograph on African livestock, which has a wider scope than the title suggests; the recent discussion of modern breeds by Briggs and Briggs (1980); and the recent major works on the water buffalo (Cockrill, 1974, 1976; Fahimuddin, 1975). These, with Mason (1969), provide many references to older literature. A further source is *Animal Breeding Abstracts*, where information concerning individual breeds can be traced through the livestock index.

4.4.2. Definitions of breeds

Although there is considerable overlap of the many definitions of what constitutes a breed, it is possible to discern two categories.

(1) Animal-oriented definitions recognize that breeds differ by the totality of average differences observed in many qualitative and quantitative traits. The differences may be subtle and overlap, but they have a genetic basis and, taken together, provide a unique description. Often it is stated that the distinctions between breeds do not differ in kind (although they may differ in degree) from the criteria used to distinguish between species. The differences are ascribed to various factors, including natural selection, artificial selection (i.e., selection by man) and genetic drift (e.g., Darwin, 1875; Lush, 1945; Nichols,

Chapter 10 references, p. 289

1957; Johansson and Rendel 1968; Rouse, 1969; Chapman, 1974; Briggs and Briggs, 1980).

(2) At the other extreme, definitions emphasize the role of man, either as a manipulator of genetic material or in conferring formal (and sometimes arbitrary) recognition that a particular population constitutes a breed (e.g., Lerner and Donald, 1966; Whitlock, 1980). The view that man had an important role in the creation of breeds is often underlain by the idea that 'man-made animals' can be distinguished from wild species in the archaeological record (Zeuner, 1963; Clutton-Brock, 1981, especially pp. 19 and 50–51).

4.4.3. Origins of breeds

Breeds of livestock are usually regarded as the result of man-mediated genetic modification. However, the Asiatic elephant (*Elephas maximus* L.) is classified into breeds, although for 2000–3000 years the most common pattern of exploitation has been of continuous recruitment from wild populations (Baker and Manwell, 1983b). Elephant breeds are of two types. One is analogous to a *landrace*: a primitive or incipient breed associated with a geographical region and distinguished by a set of common traits, determined by selection for the common environment. This situation supports the recurring belief that one origin of a landrace is from indigenous wild stocks (Marshall, 1818; Rouse, 1969). The other type of elephant breed may occur as one of several breeds in a region, or be found in a number of regions. It is defined by its members being within an agreed range of variation for certain points, including 'fancy' points. This type of breed is usually associated with an advanced stage of domestication and selection by man. But it could arise from the population structure of elephants, which is based on small demes (Baker and Manwell, 1983b).

The natural formation of breed-analogous populations raises several matters. It is likely to occur in other species with the same population structure, which from Lydekker's (1898) descriptions probably includes most species of cattle. The possibility of a natural origin of breeds means that some indigenous breeds may represent ancient survivals. Finally, even though deme formation and evolution of breed-analogous types is not a feature of all species, breed formation by man represents the exploitation or imitation of a natural situation rather than a new conceptual achievement.

4.5. Marker genes

4.5.1. Taxonomic traits and breed points

Marker genes have two aspects. One is as systems to be studied in their own right in the context of biochemistry, genetics and animal breeding. The other aspect is the application of marker genes to a series of interrelated problems. At one end of the spectrum are academic investigations which use genetic markers to define populations in studies of taxonomy, systematics and population structure. At the other extreme is the use of marker genes to identify useful traits and their source. This application is the one of predominant interest in farm practice and is formalized in the drawing up of breed points.

In many cases a marker 'gene' is really a marker trait with an incompletely identified genetic basis. For example, Lauvergne (1981) has drawn attention to morphological traits, such as shape of horns or tail, which are associated with certain populations but for which little or no genetic information exists. These traits are not without value, especially when related to a single population. However, caution is needed before phenotypic marker traits observed in several populations are assumed to be genetically identical and before markers are used to assess genetic relationship.

Gene identity. Phenotypic resemblances may suggest genetic identity but a number of possibilities exist. As these (and the genetic techniques for distinguishing between them) are described by Hadorn (1961) we give only a summary.

Apparently identical phenotypes can be caused by different alleles or by genes at different loci. This may be obvious from mating experiments as in the case of the different types of white coat colour in cattle (Ibsen, 1933; Lauvergne, 1966). Less easy to interpret are situations when crossing between mutant types or into another stock alters phenotypic expression. This may be due to non-identity; but it can also occur when identical genes are transferred into different genetic backgrounds. In particular, there may be a difference in *expressivity* (the degree of manifestation in the individual); or in *penetrance* (the frequency with which a trait is expressed relative to the known number of carriers of the gene in a population). Environment can influence penetrance and expressivity, as for example, the level of nutrition affects the identification of muscular hypertrophy (MacKellar, 1960). Finally, a resemblance may be caused by *phenocopy*: the mimicking of a phenotype known to be caused by a particular genotype by environmental action on another genotype.

Marker genes as evidence for relationship. Even if there are good grounds for believing that the same marker allele occurs in two (or more) populations, care must be taken before making assumptions about relationship. There are at least five reasons for possession of the same marker (Baker, 1965; Manwell and Baker, 1970, pp. 294–295): common descent from the same ancestor; descent of one from the other; introgressive hybridization (from one to the other, between the two, or into each from yet another source); independent mutation; and parallel or convergent evolution. All these possibilities should be examined in conjunction with other information. Pedigree or other historical evidence is probably the most satisfactory, but other factors such as geographical location can be useful (Baker, 1982, 1984).

4.5.2. Marker systems available

Although this review is concerned primarily with systems for which there is reasonably reliable biochemical and genetic information, other systems are discussed. Our reason is twofold: ultimately all markers have a biochemical basis in the genetic code, and depend upon biochemical pathways for phenotypic expression; and all markers can be informative, especially when a number are used together.

There are too many markers to consider each individually in the space available to us here. As a compromise we try to give some idea of the range available, and to use some markers to illustrate particular points. Reviews of cattle genetics occur in several places (e.g., Gowen, 1927; Shrode and Lush, 1947). Johansson and Rendel (1968) include a section on biochemical polymorphisms and have photographs of colour patterns and of genetic abnormalities but give few references. All these reviews (and others) are arranged primarily by genetic system. There seem to be very few examples of sustained research upon a particular breed or population of cattle. Among the exceptions are Gowen's (1933) papers on the Jersey; the series of reports on the Belgian Blue and White (Ansay and Hanset, 1979) and the integrated morphological, cytological and biochemical studies on cattle in Southeast Asia (see pp. 247, 251, 277 and 278). More surprisingly, there appear to be few attempts to synthesize scattered investigations upon individual breeds, even in monographs. For example, 60 years of genetical research, including several studies of breed structure, were completely ignored in a recent supposedly definitive history of Hereford cattle (Heath-Agnew, 1983).

Chapter 10 references, p. 289

Colour and pattern. In addition to general reviews of cattle genetics which include colour and pattern, there are several works devoted to this topic (Ibsen, 1933; Lauvergne, 1966; Olson and Wilham, 1982). Many geneticists criticize selection for colour as they think it impedes selection for production. Yet colour markings can provide economic advantages. Attractive skins can realize good prices for furnishing and ornament. Identification of individual animals can be more precise. Some markings, such as pied or belted, make it easier to locate cattle on extensive grazings on a variety of seasonal backgrounds. Such considerations could be important under pastoral conditions (Marshall, 1818, vol. 1, p. 94).

A natural extension of identification is the use of colour and pattern (and other traits) as a trademark. This usually occurs as *character displacement* to prevent confusion of one breed with another. There is a parallel in nature where closely related species tend to differ more in the region of overlap than when each is in a region of its own.

In livestock, character displacement is particularly marked at times of breed expansion when naive observers use easy visual cues for identification rather than the complex of traits employed by experienced breeders. Two processes seem to be involved:

(1) Consumer preference for a particular colour which they associate (often erroneously) with breed 'purity'. Prentice (1942) has described how American demand greatly diminished the original range of colour and pattern of Jersey cattle. However, many variants still exist on the island of Jersey and in South Australia, both places where the Jersey is unlikely to be confused with other breeds.

(2) Selection by breeders against a trait which has become associated with another breed, as happened with white face in British breeds. Originally, although individual British breeds might be characterized by a high frequency of certain traits, there was also considerable heterogeneity. White face occurred in Longhorns, Shorthorns, and South Devons, and in Welsh and Scottish cattle as well as in the Hereford. The latter also had a variety of markings, including mottle faced and grey (Youatt, 1834). The rise of white face in the Hereford is traditionally traced to a bull, kept as a sire in the mid-18th century because he had this marking, then regarded as unusual by his breeder (Rowlandson, 1853). By the end of the century 'bald' (i.e., white) face was regarded by some as '. . . characteristic of the true Hereford breed' (Marshall, 1796). Breeders of other British cattle gradually selected against white face. By the 20th century, the once-accepted occurrence of white face in many breeds had been forgotten. This led to speculation that the Hereford might have got its white face from one of the continental breeds characterized by this marking (Heath-Agnew, 1983). But the contemporary accounts cited above suggest an indigenous origin is more likely. There is proof that white face (and colour sided) can arise independently on more than one occasion from observation of these markers in water buffalo in Sulawesi (Amano et al., 1981).

As white face in the Hereford is dominant it has been useful to indicate that crossbred calves have beef breeding for the benefit of those not skilled in distinguishing between beef and dairy stock. Crossbreds often have some degree of facial mottling, emphasizing that a pure white face means a pure Hereford. This economically useful mark is physically harmless in temperate climates similar to that of the Hereford's origin, but it is not adapted for continual exposure to high intensity sunlight. The complete lack of pigment around the eyes contributes to cancer eye, which is a cause of carcase rejection in American and Australian slaughterhouses (Gardiner et al., 1972).

There are also occasions when colour may be perceived as adaptive for certain environments. The dark skin and white hair of British White cattle have been among the reason for choosing the breed to resist conditions as diverse as the Canadian prairies, where sun reflected from the snow can injure ventral surfaces (Anon., 1974 b) and Australia, where the main problems are insolation and heat (Anon., 1984).

Many animal scientists would agree that 'Natural selection has played but a small part in deciding the colours of our domestic breeds' (Mason, 1973, p. 241). However, evidence is beginning to accumulate that cattle colours may have an intrinsic survival value. In both Kenya and Transkei, statistically significant associations between colour and environmental factors have been reported. The associations were not always simple but involved altitude, heat stress and availability of water (Finch and Western, 1977; Siegfried and Hofmeyr, 1979).

In addition to the breeds and species mentioned, variation of colour has been observed in yak and American bison.

Finally, we wish to draw attention to the use of the distribution and frequency of colour and pattern to define native breeds. This project could be persued by individuals at many localities at very little cost. As data for different geographic regions accumulate, synthesis can lead to further insight, as in the review of work on coat colour in populations of cats, *Felis catus* L. (Todd, 1977). Even though the genetics of bovine coat colours are not fully understood, the methodical recording of the distribution and abundance of phenotypes has been found helpful in the definition of breeds and populations of cattle and water buffalo (Amano et al., 1981; Namikawa et al., 1982). The technique can also be used for other physical characteristics.

Hair. Hair survives many conditions, including digestion. Even when colour, shape and size are altered, the structure of the medulla, pattern of cuticular scales, and the shape of cross-section of single guard hairs can be used to identify taxa (Dziurdzik, 1975). It is possible to distinguish between *B. taurus* and wisent: F_1 hybrids and the first and second back-cross to cattle have both parental types and a new hybrid type not found in the parental species (Dziurdzik, 1978). *B. primigenius* hair has a structure different from that found in *B. taurus* of modern, mediaeval and Roman times, thus supplying a useful marker in archaeological investigations (Ryder, 1980).

Most studies are confined to gross morphologic differences in pelage. Differences have been reported between *Bison bison, Bos taurus* and their hybrids (Peters and Slen, 1964); and between *B. taurus, B. indicus* and their hybrids (Hayman, 1965). Hair type also varies within and between breeds of taurine cattle and is thought to have some association with adaptive traits: e.g., the fine short hair of Jersey cattle with tick resistance (Johnston and Bancroft, 1918); and woolly coats with poor heat tolerance (Bonsma, 1955).

Skin. Although studied primarily from the standpoint of thermoregulation, the morphology of sweat glands and hair follicles has taxonomic utility. Species of Bovinae exhibit a similar basic skin structure, but can be distinguished from each other to some extent (Jenkinson and Nay, 1975). An extensive survey of taurine, indicine, sanga and banteng cattle revealed breed characteristic patterns. These showed considerable consistency within breed groups although exceptions occurred. Of particular interest is the finding that the Jersey differed from most British and European cattle by a high frequency of skin type I, generally characteristic of humped cattle. Chillingham cattle were also towards this end of the range of British breeds, but the paucity of Chillingham samples did not allow any firm conclusion to be drawn. A particularly interesting exception was that the Belted Galloway differed from the Galloway, confirming the former's position as a separate breed and not just a variety (Jenkinson and Nay, 1972, 1973). Criollo breeds had a high frequency of a skin type which was not found in European cattle apart from the few

Chapter 10 references, p. 289

Iberian breeds studied (Jenkinson and Nay, 1973). This recalls the suggestion of a separate race or subspecies of aurochs made by Dent (1983; see p. 235).

Although skin thickness is of commercial interest, it is not prominent in most modern discussions of breeds. The older literature reveals that breed differences did occur. It is also known that the muscular hypertrophy syndrome includes a thinner skin than is normal for the breed (Lauvergne et al., 1968). It has been observed that both water buffalo and African buffalo have thicker skins than cattle (Jenkinson and Nay, 1975).

Horns and polling. Horn size, colour and shape are mentioned frequently in descriptions of cattle, but little attention has been paid to the inheritance of these traits. It is not clear how much selection pressure is applied. Horns can be trained, and the practice is common for show animals. Wallace (1888) was told that the shape of Jafarabadi water buffalo horns owed their shape to selection for fighting by butting. Schwabe (1984) has drawn attention to contemporary horn training in the Nile Valley which can be traced back at least 4500 years.

In many texts it is conventional to refer to polled as completely dominant to horns. In some breeds this appears to be so: e.g., the polling gene which was eliminated from the Pinzgau in the 1950's (F. Pirchner, personal communication, 1984). In other breeds the expressivity of horns in the heterozygotes varies. Many have scurs. At one extreme these are small scales, no more than half a centimetre in diameter, and virtually invisible, giving a polled appearance. At the other extreme, scurs can be quite large and even become attached to the skull, giving the impression of a normal horn (Dove, 1935). It is not clear whether complete and incomplete dominance represent different genes for polling, or whether the expressivity varies because of different genetic backgrounds.

Attempts have been made to trace migrations of cattle from the occurrence of the polled gene. Wilson (1909) thought that the geographical distribution of polled breeds in the British Isles indicated a Scandinavian origin. But historical accounts reveal that polled cattle were once common in many other parts of the country, Young (1771) mentions them in County Durham and Derbyshire as well as in Norfolk and Suffolk. One variety or breed of Longhorn was 'either entirely destitute of horns, or had merely rudimentary processes of loose horns' (Dickinson, 1852). Polled cattle were found among both North and South Devons (Baker, 1984); some present-day breeders of South Devon cattle are using scurs to identify carriers of the gene for polling in a project to re-establish polled strains (Mumford, 1981). Polled cattle often occur among Welsh Blacks, but the trait is traditionally selected against as many farmers associate it with small size (the late Miss P. Taylor, personal communication, c. 1964). Thus it seems that polling is indigenous to the British Isles.

Both polled yaks (Lydekker, 1898) and polled water buffalo have been reported. The latter are said to have defects of the genitalia (Caldwell, 1977).

Other aspects of external morphology. Reviews on cattle genetics include a number of other inherited external traits in otherwise normal cattle. There are very few genetic studies of normal conformation, including aspects such as distribution of body fat and udder size and shape. However, one such trait has recently become the subject of much research and extension effort: size of testes.

Sociobiologists have drawn attention to the advantage of large testes, producing large amounts of sperm, for species in which males have to compete for females at the time of mating. This applies to bulls on range and, especially, to those used for AI. Research on bulls revealed a correlation between scrotal measurements and semen production, and that these traits had moderate to high heritability. These findings have been promulgated enthusiastically, at least in Australia, where judges give much prominence to testicle size when giving reasons for their placings. In fact, the measure needs applying with care. First, there are breed differences. It has been recommended that comparisons should not be made between breeds or with some general standard, but within breeds (Latimer et al., 1982). Secondly, there are indications that in hot climates selection for a large scrotum may be counterproductive and lead to early sterility (Bonsma, 1955).

Traditionally, size of cattle has been measured by weight, and sometimes by height at the withers, although less data are available for the latter measure. A further concept of size which has been popularized recently is 'frame score', based on standard measurements of live animals. Frame score is used mainly to describe size, but it can also define shape. Such measurements can yield genetic information. Gowen (1933) analysed data collected by the American Jersey Cattle Club for standardized measurements of 6000 cows and 300 bulls from 15 states. The genetic structure of the breed was revealed as a series of groups, each of a definite and homogenous type maintained by assortative mating. Considerable variation existed between herds.

Otsuka et al. (1982) used the standardized measures of the Waygu Cattle Registry Association to define 16 Indonesian cattle breeds and the banteng. Two breeds stood out: the Ongole (*B. indicus*) on size and shape; and the Grati (Javanese × *B. taurus*) on size. The Mishima, banteng, Bali and Philippine breeds were somewhat more alike to each other than to the group which had zebu influence only. Bali cattle and the banteng were similar to each other in shape, but the banteng was larger.

Amano et al. (1980, 1981) made similar measurements of swamp and river buffalo. The former was consistently smaller in both Indonesia and the Phillippines. Nine river (Murrah) × swamp (Carabao) hybrids at Central Luzon State University were smaller than pure swamp water buffalo of the same age.

Skeletal traits. Although measurements of living animals provide some idea of skeletal structure, the skeleton itself is required for more precise taxonomic information. When Bojanus (1827) described *B. primigenius* he used a whole skeleton (less a few missing caudal vertebrae). More usually, the skull is the main or sole part examined because it survives well and is taxonomically informative. Much of the literature in this area can be traced from papers by Grigson (1980) and by Hayashi et al. (1982).

The distinction possible between types of Southeast Asian cattle by measurements made on live animals has been extended by craniometric studies (Hayashi et al., 1982). The most important finding is that Bali cattle and banteng have a complete overlap in skull shape. They differ in size, the banteng being larger and having more sexual dimorphism in respect of size. Frequently archaeologists use size as a criterion to assign bones either to a domesticate, or to the species thought (with varying degrees of certitude) to be the wild progenitor. The Bali cattle–banteng comparison is the most convincing case, and the best demonstration we know that the use of reduced size as a criterion of domestication is valid.

Epstein (1971) has pointed out that bifid processes to the last thoracic vertebra are a marker of zebu cattle or zebu introgression. Yamane and Kato (1936) found this marker in *Bos indicus*. Taiwan cattle also had bifid vertebrae, but the expressivity varied and, in the animals examined, was less than in *B. indicus*. Korean cattle resembled the Friesian in lacking bifid vertebrae. An F_1 male from a Friesian bull and a Zebu cow had slightly bifid vertebrae. Bettini and Masina (1972) found that this marker occurred in about a third of the Modica breed, which had been suspected of having ancient unrecorded introgression from zebu cattle. The Modica also has α-lactalbumin

Chapter 10 references, p. 289

A, a milk protein variant associated with humped cattle. However, bifid vertebrae found recently in England have been identified as part of a *B. taurus* skeleton (Stallibrass, 1983; Grigson, 1984). This raises some questions about the occurrence of bifid vertebrae: Are they a primitive trait from a common ancestor, fixed in humped cattle by selective advantage, but lingering in non-humped species and breeds; a common trait which varies in expressivity; or do they occur sporadically through mutation? Yamane and Kato (1936) examined the thoracic vertebrae of wild and domestic *Bos javanicus* and found that they were different from both *B. taurus* and *B. indicus*: The figures suggest that, in *B. javanicus*, the process has a hole, as if it had bifurcated and then rejoined at the tip.

Wriedt's paradox: Great sires and lethal factors. The literature on cattle genetics contains many references to developmental abnormalities which can have lethal or semi-lethal consequences. Hadorn (1961) still has the best discussion of many fundamental aspects of the genetics and physiology of lethal factors, and includes a section on economic losses. The clinical approach to the problem has been reviewed by Schäper (1936) and by Leipold et al. (1972); and Lasley (1963) discusses some of the practical consequences.

Much of the original genetic treatment of lethal factors stems from the work of Wriedt (1930). An important feature of his studies was the repeated observation that many lethal traits could be traced to sires which were famous. Thus arose 'Wriedt's paradox': that great sires, chosen for beneficial characteristics and exploited for their ability to transmit those characteristics, should also transmit lethal factors. Two explanations are possible. The more facile is that the continued use of a sire and his male descendants caused inbreeding, which revealed the genetic load of undesirable recessives. This explanation is true to a certain extent, although not in such simple terms (see p. 280). However, it was accepted in its superficial sense and the general response was that there should be selection against carriers to expunge lethal factors. This approach was doomed to failure. Not all traits were easily identified as simple recessives, and expressivity in heterozygous carriers and even homozygotes could vary. In the extreme case of a simple recessive, the most that selection could do was to limit the spread of the allele.

The second explanation of Wriedt's paradox is that, from an evolutionary standpoint, it is unreasonable to dismiss any trait as undesirable when it is so frequent that there is likely to be some selective advantage, at least for the heterozygote. The circumstances connected with some lethal or semi-lethal factors support this hypothesis. One example is the *comprest factor* in American Hereford cattle (Lasley, 1963). This appeared at a time when selection emphasized early maturity and blocky type, both characteristic of the comprest heterozygote. However, matings from comprest × comprest resulted in lethal or semi-lethal dwarf types. There was a change to selection against comprest animals, partly because of the lethal factor, and partly because it was found that 'normal' Herefords made more economic gains.

Muscular hypertrophy or *double-muscling* affords an example of how a potentially lethal factor can be exploited continuously. Until quite recently, most scientists regarded muscular hypertrophy as undesirable. Most farmers had the same opinion of some of the extreme manifestations of the syndrome, but butchers regarded some expression as desirable. Two possible solutions emerged (Manwell and Baker, 1970, pp. 327–330): to stabilize expressivity so that the less desirable aspects in the homozygote were avoided, as appears to have occurred in some breeds (Lauvergne et al., 1968; King and Ménissier, 1982); and to exploit the commercially significant hybrid vigour available from planned crossbreeding. Rouse (1969) has described how the latter approach was used by French farmers who, in defiance of the then official policy, produced terminal crosses from Charolais sires homozygous for muscular hypertrophy. Partly as a result of the persistence of breeders there is now a considerable body of opinion that muscular hypertrophy can be beneficial in the right circumstances.

Wriedt's paradox has two lessons for animal breeders. One is that no trait should be discarded before there has been a careful assessment of its positive aspects and how these can be used. The second lesson is the warning that uncritical selection for extreme types will create problems.

Milk and butterfat. The economic structure of milk production has resulted in records which characterize many dairy and dual-purpose breeds in terms of average yield of whole milk, butterfat and, in recent years, various other solid components. Unfortunately, the emphasis on sales and processing has caused other aspects of milk to be neglected. Our attention has been drawn to butterfat by an observation that, in arid-land beef production, dairy-cross cows (frequently recommended as milky dams) dehydrate and cease production; but that South Devon cross cows keep milking and maintain some condition (Edwards, 1983). In seeking reasons for this observation it occurred to us that South Devons have a high average butterfat of 4.5%. High butterfat is a well-recognized physiological adaptation to difficult environments in many species. High milk solids reduce the water requirement for lactation; and fat gives most energy and most metabolic water per unit weight. In marine mammals, which have acute problems of osmoregulation for the dam, and an urgent necessity for fast growth in the offspring, milk fat can exceed 40% (Duke, 1979). Thus bovine butterfat is of interest not only for direct human consumption but in terms of adaptation, stock rearing and beef production.

The data available for cattle support the role of butterfat in adaptation to difficult environments. Water buffalo are said to average 7.64%, with a higher average of 9.65% in the Carabao (Caldwell, 1977 pp. 123 and 127) and up to 13% in the Bhadawari (Swaminathan, 1981). Estimates for the yak vary from 12% or more with 7.6–9% in F_1 hybrids (Kalia, 1974) to 6.5% (NRC, 1983, p. 31). Mithan are credited with 10.5% butterfat (Winter et al., 1984; Hickman, 1982). Data for butterfat in the zebu include an 'overall' average of 6.5%; and averages of 4.9% for the Red Sindhi and 3–6% for the Sahiwal (Barrett and Larkin, 1974) though Caldwell (1981, p. 123) gives an overall average of 4.97%. Taurine dairy and dual-purpose breeds average from about 3.5% for Friesians to 4.5–5% for Channel Island cattle.

There are many other aspects of milk which should be investigated for adaptive value including size of fat globules (large in the yak, water buffalo and Jersey, and small in the zebu and Ayrshire); presence of carotene (as in the Jersey and Guernsey) vs. vitamin A; and variants of individual milk proteins (see pp. 274 and 275).

Resistance to parasites and diseases. The case of the tick, *Boophilus microplus*, in Australia provides an illustration of limitations of the 'quick technological fix'. Zebu cattle are resistant to this tick. Taurine cattle are usually considered susceptible, but varying degrees of resistance have been found in individuals of many breeds, most commonly Jerseys and Jersey grades. Johnston and Bancroft (1918) suggested that such animals should be used to breed for tick resistance. The idea was suppressed in favour of treatment with pesticides. Over 50 years later, the evolution of ticks which are resistant to most chemicals has caused the realization that the solution to the problem in taurine cattle is selection for tick resistance (Wharton et al., 1970).

Trypanosomiasis resistance is thought to be confined to a few West African taurine breeds: the Dahomey, the Muturu, the N'Dama and the West African Dwarf Shorthorn (Stewart, 1938; Gates, 1952; Chandler, 1958; Mortelmans

Chapter 10 references, p. 289

and Kageruka, 1976; Murray et al., 1979; Trail, 1981). The Nuba, a small humped breed of the Sudan, which lives in a tsetse pocket in the Nuba mountains, is also said to be resistant (Mills, 1953). The choice of breeds contributes to greater overall efficiency: the N'Dama has been found suitable for large enterprises; and the Dahomey does better on small family farms where cattle are allowed freedom to roam in the forest (Mortelmans and Kageruka, 1976). Meyn (1984, p. 4) notes that trypanotolerant cattle are also resistant to dermatophilosis, 'a disease which has wiped out development projects . . . with so-called adapted breeds to the tropics, such as Brahman and Droughtmaster.'

Resistance to rinderpest is not a clearly marked phenomenon but, in West Africa, humped African cattle are said to have more resistance to rinderpest than taurine breeds (Stewart, 1938). A similar observation has been made concerning the Angoni (Oliver, 1966). Lydekker (1898, p. 76) reported a belief that wisent were immune to rinderpest; but this could have been lack of close contact with carriers as wisent had 'great antipathy to *Bos taurus*' and did not mix with taurine cattle (Vasey, 1851, p. 43).

Bovine leucosis is a relatively new but economically important cause of loss. Reliable breed data are not easy to find, but the disease is often associated with Holsteins, in which the incidence can be as high as 29% (Bernoco et al., 1984). In contrast, a study of 32 246 Brown Latvian cows sired by 121 AI bulls revealed an incidence of only 1.45%, with a range of 0.00–8.33% for individual half-sib groups (Karlikov et al., 1979).

Chromosomes. Hsu (1979) has described how it was only in the 1960's that the accurate determination of numbers and gross morphology of mammalian chromosomes became possible. More recent advances in staining techniques have added the ability to reveal differences in chromosomal DNA: C-banding for highly repetitive sequences; Q-banding or G-banding for A–T-rich regions; R-banding for G–C-rich regions; and a combination of R- and G-banding to define chromosome ends, improving distinctions between chromosomes as telocentric or acrocentric, or between chromosomes as acrocentric or submetacentric (Hsu, 1979, pp. 121, 125, 127; Gustavsson, 1980).

An overview of current information for the Bovinae follows:

Data are available for all species of cattle except wild yak and kouprey. The others are very similar in the number and gross morphology of their chromosomes (Hsu and Benirschke, 1967–1977; Fischer, 1969). All have $2n = 60$ with 58 acrocentric autosomes except the gaur and mithan. The latter two species have $2n = 58$, with 54 acrocentric autosomes and one pair of submetacentric autosomes (Fischer, 1969; Winter et al., 1984).

There is some variation in descriptions of X chromosomes, which different authors may describe as acrocentric or submetacentric in the same species. As most authors also liken *B. taurus* X to that of other species, the problem may be one of subjective classification of centromere position.

The major morphological difference between cattle species is the Y chromosome. American bison and wisent both have an acrocentric Y (Basrur, 1969; Betancourt et al., 1974). So does *B. indicus* in most of the breeds studied (Gupta et al., 1974). However, Hadžiselimovic (1971) reported that the dwarf zebu of Sri Lanka had a small submetacentric Y chromosome. This could be explained as an unrecorded introgression from *B. taurus* in colonial times. Alternatively, it might be that the acrocentric Y of *B. indicus* represents the evolution of an isolating mechanism which would be less important on Sri Lanka than on the mainland where *B. indicus* overlaps with other species of cattle.

B. taurus, domestic yak, gaur, mithan, banteng and Bali cattle all have a submetacentric Y chromosome (Makino, 1944; Fischer, 1969; Popescu, 1969; Matsuda et al., 1980; Namikawa et al., 1983a; Winter et al., 1984).

The difference between *B. taurus* and *B. indicus* in the Y chromosome has made this a convenient marker. Among African cattle, the Kouri (usually classed as taurine) has the *B. taurus*-type submetacentric Y (Petit and Queval, 1973). The *B. taurus* Y also seems to be characteristic of sanga cattle (Halnan and Francis, 1976; Meyer, 1984; Harris et al., 1984). Makino (1944) found a submetacentric Y in both Holsteins and Taiwan cattle, although the latter breed is often regarded as a zebu because of its hump. Korean cattle (also suspected of some indicine ancestry) likewise had the taurine Y; but two out of the thirteen bulls examined had the atypical autosome numbers of 57 and 59 (Senn, 1972). The Chianina, suspected of having introgression from *B. indicus*, yielded only *B. taurus* Y chromosomes in the karyotypes of 13 bulls (Eldridge and Blazak, 1977. In the Brahman and the Ibagé (a taurindicus breed derived from bulls of both species) individual bulls may have either the *B. taurus* or the *B. indicus* Y (Eldridge and Blazak, 1977); Pinheiro et al., 1980).

Some 20 years ago a 1 : 29 chromosomal translocation was found to occur as a polymorphism in Swedish cattle (Gustavsson and Rockborn, 1964; Gustavsson, 1969). Since then, other chromosomal polymorphisms have been found in taurine cattle (Popescu, 1981) and some occur in sanga breeds (Harris et al., 1984; Meyer, 1984). Improved techniques have led to the discovery of further morphological differences: in the size of homologous chromosomes of yak and taurine cattle (Popescu, 1969); and in the C- and G-banding of several species (Gupta et al., 1974; Gustavsson, 1980; Halnan et al., 1981).

In water buffalo, $2n$ may be 50, a number associated with river breeds, or 48 a number associated with the swamp type (Hsu and Benirschke, 1967–1977; Amano and Martojo, 1983). However, Sri Lankan swamp buffaloes have $2n = 50$, suggesting that this population is derived from Indian river buffalo which have acquired swamp habits (Bongso and Hilmi, 1982). Taiwan water buffalo and the Australian feral population both have $2n = 48$. Swamp and river buffalo will hybridize and the progeny have $2n = 49$. Both parental types have similar sex chromosomes, with X the largest acrocentric and Y the smallest acrocentric. The smaller number of autosomes in the swamp buffalo is thought to be due to fusion of what in the river buffalo are separate autosomes 4 and 9 (Bongso and Hilmi, 1982; Amano and Martojo, 1983).

Hsu and Benirschke (1967–1977) show the karyotype of *Anoa depressicornis depressicornis* as $2n = 48$. However, Amano and Martojo (1983) found considerable variation of chromosome number among different types of anoa. All resembled the water buffalo in having the largest and smallest acrocentric chromosomes as X and Y respectively. A pair of lowland anoa, *A. depressicornis* were; male, $2n = 36$; female, $2n = 38$. Six mountain anoas, *A. quarlesi* (four males and two females) were all $2n = 46$. Three mountain anoas, *A. fergusoni* (one male and two females) were all $2n = 47$. Fischer and Hohn (1976) give the karyotype of as one female tamarao *Anoa mindorensis* $2n = 46$. It lacked an acrocentric pair of chromosomes present in *A. depressicornis*.

In the African buffalo, differences have been found between *Syncerus caffer caffer* ($2n = 52$) and *S. c. nanus* ($2n = 54$). The chromosomes of the other bovinae are morphologically different from the species mentioned previously (Hsu and Benirschke, 1967–1977).

Blood groups. The two most recent reviews on bovine blood groups known to us are those by Stormont (1977) and by Bell (1983). Except where stated otherwise, our information in this section comes from these two reviews and from their references.

In cattle blood grouping the red cells of individuals are screened for lysis by standardized antisera plus complement. There has been little work on the

Chapter 10 references, p. 289

structure of the red cell antigens apart from the long-term studies of Thiele and his colleagues (Thiele and Urbaschek, 1966; Thiele et al., 1979). However, is is possible to obtain a large amount of information by the isolation of specificities by techniques such as absorption and blocking (Denniston, 1976) and by using serial dilutions.

There are ten recognized blood group systems in cattle. These range in complexity from L (with two alleles and two blood types) to B (with over 600 alleles and over 60 000 blood types). In the B and C systems specificities segregate in blocks, called phenogroups, certain of which are associated with particular breeds.

Interpretation of blood typing is not simple: '. . . for many . . . systems, especially most of those involving a single marker (like J and L of cattle) . . . in the absence of progeny tests, the genotypes cannot be ascertained by inspection of the blood groups alone. Genotypes can, however, be reasonably inferred in such blood group systems as B, C and S of cattle . . . but usually only in those breeds which have been thoroughly analyzed . . .' (Stormont, 1977, p. 576). For example, Fiorentini et al. (1980) found it difficult to identify B phenogroups in East African zebu cattle because the large number of B factors made it difficult to find suitable pedigrees among 146 animals, including 36 dam–offspring pairs. E.L. Henson et al. (1983) experienced similar trouble with the B and C systems of Gloucester cattle because, although 80% of the breed was sampled, this was only 125 animals; and there was a lack of large and complete families due to the use and turnover of relatively large numbers of bulls in an attempt to keep inbreeding low.

Another complication is the standardization of reagents. Most workers prepare their own, often by different methods, and Bell (1983, p. 135) warns that individual papers should be consulted on this point. The International Society for Blood Group Research holds periodic tests to determine the equivalence of reagents and blood types. While this maintains a high standard of reliability: 'It is a rare event when all laboratories now participating in the cattle comparisons come out with the same results with any reagent going by the same name . . . as I recall, in the last cattle comparison tests (1975) only one reagent gave consistent overall results for all the laboratories' (Stormont, 1977, pp. 582–583).

Despite these drawbacks compared with simpler screening methods, blood groups continue to be used. The large number of specificities in the B and C systems makes them very useful for pedigree exclusion and breed identification. The large laboratories engaged in this work have access to the pedigree records of the breeds they serve. There is a high investment of time and money in the technique, but at least some of the expense is offset by fees. Another reason is that immunological systems are known to have a role in disease. This may be direct (as in neonatal isoerythrolysis in foals, or adverse reactions to blood transfusions as in dogs and cats) or exist as a correlation between blood group factors and disease (as in pigs and poultry).

Most blood typing with bovine species has used anti-taurine reagents: e.g., wisent (Gasparski, 1965); African buffalo (Osterhoff and Young, 1966; Osterhoff et al., 1970); banteng and Bali cattle (Bailey, 1968; Amano et al., 1982a,b; Namikawa et al., 1983,a,b,c); water buffalo (Makaveev, 1970; Amano, 1974); yak (Sorokovoi et al., 1982); and gaur and mithan (Winter et al., 1984). A common finding is that many anti-taurine reagents react with red cells of other species, but the reactions are not necessarily identical with those found within *B. taurus* and may occur only in some individuals of other species. Standard anti-taurine reagents also gave non-standard reactions with African cattle (Osterhoff, 1966; Braend, 1979; Fiorentini et al., 1980).

The use of anti-taurine reagents seems to be largely a matter of convenience and expense, as species-specific reagents can be made. Work on *B. indicus* breeds in India was based on reagents made using Hariana and Kuamoni Hill cattle (Ram and Khanna, 1961). Murrah water buffalo reacted with 16 of the 35 reagents (Ram et al., 1964). Swamp buffalo have naturally occurring haemolysins (Amano, 1978). Reagents have also been produced from hetero- and alloimmunization of swamp buffalo. Cells from river buffalo did not react with the anti-swamp reagents, but cells from hybrids between swamp and river buffalo did (Amano et al., 1983).

Bovine lymphocyte antigens (BoLA). BoLA systems are a relatively new set of markers. Much of the current information is contained in the reports of the International BoLA Workshops (Spooner et al., 1979; Anon., 1982). Frequency data are available for a few popular breeds (Caldwell et al., 1979; Oliver et al., 1981) and for the Gloucester (E.L. Henson, 1981; E.L. Henson et al., 1983). The work on the Gloucester drew attention to two drawbacks to the BoLA system. First, BoLA gene frequencies are calculated on the assumption of Hardy–Weinberg equilibrium. But equilibrium was not found for two out of six other loci for which inheritance was codominant, suggesting that, at present, BoLA is a more reliable phenotypic marker than an accurate measure of gene frequencies. Secondly, the Gloucester had a high frequency of 'null' alleles, which the authors thought might be because the antisera were obtained by skin grafting among Friesian cattle. If this is the case, care will be needed in the use of standard BoLA reagents to define unusual breeds.

Allotypes. Cattle allotyping on an organized basis is another fairly recent development. The field has been reviewed by Faber and Stone (1976) who define an allotype as '. . . an inherited variant . . . detected by immunologic methods . . . not ordinarily distinguished by the usual physical and chemical methods'; excluding particulate antigens. Allotypes have been used with other biochemical polymorphisms to measure genetic distance (Kidd et al., 1980).

Allotypes have also been reported for water buffalo (Ianelli, 1978).

Monoclonal antibodies. Monoclonal antibodies produced from interspecific hybridomas are highly specific reagents and can be manufactured reproducibly. Thus they are a powerful research tool (Harris, 1983). Monoclonal antibodies also have great potential for the better standardization of routine blood typing. The sale of reagents would make participation in blood typing research possible for workers who do not have facilities for the production of antisera. Although monoclonal antibody techniques have been available for nearly two decades, most reports of work involving farm livestock are recent (Longenecker, 1982; Metinier and Grosclaude, 1984; Tucker, 1984).

Polymorphism of mitochondrial DNA. In mammals the mitochondrial DNA is a closed circular double helix of approximately 16 500 nucleotides in length. It is a remarkable genetic system, with certain characteristics which may make it useful as a molecular marker in studies on bovines. As a cytoplasmic subcellular component, mitochondria are believed to be inherited only through the female line (e.g., see studies on mitochondrial DNA of mules and hinnies: Hutchison et al., 1974). The sperm apparently does not contribute mitochondrial DNA to the egg that it fertilizes.

There is general agreement that mitochondrial DNA evolves at a much faster rate than nuclear DNA. For example, cattle (*B. taurus*) and American bison (*Bison bison*) are members of closely related genera, capable of forming fertile female hybrids. Yet, when cattle and bison mitochondrial DNA's are compared (by digesting them with a restriction endonuclease, HaeIII, which cleaves any polynucleotide where the specific sequence GGCC occurs), they differ in half of their HaeIII-digested fragments (Potter et al., 1975). Presumably,

Chapter 10 references, p. 289

they differ in about 10% of their total nucleotide sequence. (Use of the Upholt–Nei–Li formula gives a divergence estimate of 17%, but that formula does not allow for unequal nucleotide frequencies, nor unequal nucleotide substitution probabilities; in most, though not all, instances the Upholt–Nei–Li formula overestimates the amount of divergence, under certain conditions a GG/CC restriction enzyme digest comparison will result in an 88% overestimate: see pp. 118 and 119 in Tajima and Nei, 1982.)

The most remarkable finding concerning mitochondrial DNA in bovines is the individual variation observed by Hauswirth and Laipis (e.g., 1982) in a maternal line of Holstein cows. There is a polymorphism of mitochondrial DNA, with two genotypes L_S and L_L. (These differ by a single nucleotide substitution which results in an extra HaeIII restriction site in the L_S genotype and, therefore, an electrophoretically distinct pattern where the L_L polynucleotide is replaced by two polynucleotides, L_S and K^1.) The remarkable observation is that the maternal lineage appears to have switched back and forth between L_L and L_S at least three times. Since ova carry at least 100 mitochondria, such oscillation between essentially fixed states (and without any individuals being clearly with *both* L_S and L_L mitochondria), cannot have occurred at random. Hauswirth and Laipis (1982, p. 4686) claim that in 'dairy herds maintained for breeding studies . . . calf switching is extremely rare (approximately 1 switch in 500 births)'. They do not consider other types of pedigree mistakes and, unfortunately, their paper includes no data on pedigree checks, using blood groups or protein polymorphisms.

If the Hauswirth and Laipis (1982) results are not the result of errors in pedigree recording, then there is a new genetic phenomenon to be explained. Perhaps on some occasions the rule of maternal inheritance can be violated. There may be some kind of nuclear control which specifically mutates a single base position, but that is without precedent.

If the results are real, they serve warning about the necessity to consider extranuclear DNA in gene conservation programmes. Unusual results have also been observed for chloroplast DNA in barley and these have specific implications for genetic conservation (Clegg et al., 1984).

Mitochondrial DNA specifies only a few of the protein subunits which occur in mitochondria. However, those protein subunits include components of cytochrome oxidase and ATPase, multisubunit enzymes which play a major role in energy production in the mitochondrion. Certain bovines are known to differ in their energy requirements and thermal tolerance, e.g., *B. taurus* versus *B. indicus*. It will be of interest to see if such energetically differing species or breeds differ most in their mitochondrial DNA.

Protein polymorphism. Over 7 years ago, we wrote:

> The literature on genetic variation of enzymes and other proteins in domesticated species is now too large to be handled inclusively in a review of this length. Yet, there are many gaps in this literature, especially for rare or 'native' breeds. It is urgent that researchers attempt to fill these gaps in view of the rapid disappearance of many local breeds of farm animals. Such information is vital both in analysing the evolution of domesticated species and in conserving 'gene banks' for the future. (Baker and Manwell, 1983 a, p. 367)

Our views have not changed. The review just quoted was prepared to complement other reviews which had appeared a few years previously. Our present aim is to concentrate upon population structure and evolution. There is a general consensus of opinion that successful conservation depends upon an understanding of these topics for the organism to be conserved; and that one of the most efficient ways of understanding both population structure and evolution is through the study of polymorphism, especially of proteins (see Frankel and Soulé, 1981 and papers in Schonewald-Cox et al., 1983).

Protein polymorphisms are usually detected by electrophoresis: the separation of charged molecules in solution by exposure to a voltage gradient. The migration of each molecular species depends upon a number of factors, especially its net charge, the strength of the voltage gradient and the nature of the medium in which electrophoresis is occurring. There are many detailed reviews on various types of electrophoresis and its application to molecular markers in population genetics and biochemical systematics; for researchers who are entering this field, we would recommend two quite different books: Ferguson (1980) and Harris and Hopkinson (1976). The latter provides a useful compilation of recipes for staining different enzymes for electrophoresis and extends the earlier compilation of Shaw and Koen (1968). Techniques for milk (including a tabulation of various gel and buffer combinations) are available in the contributions of various authors in *Milk Proteins* (McKenzie, 1971). For serum proteins, the best complete source is still the monograph by Schultze and Heremans (1966). Recent special aspects of electrophoretic techniques are discussed by us elsewhere (Baker and Manwell, 1983a, pp. 368–385).

'Protein' polymorphism is a convenient term for the variation observed after routine screening. But, close to half of all known proteins have a subunit structure, or at least show some tendency to aggregate into components of different molecular weights. Where proteins have a relatively stable subunit structure, this is referred to as a quaternary structure. There are two types of situation, each with an important different implication in terms of using proteins as phenotypic markers of genetic loci:

First, quite a number of proteins are made up of basically identical subunits (homomultimers), all coded from the same genetic locus. If there is a protein polymorphism, segregating in a Mendelian manner, then heterozygotes will have at least some of their protein molecules as 'hybrid molecules' (or heteromultimers). Whether or not such 'hybrid molecules' are actually visualized as 'hybrid zones' after electrophoresis depends upon the *stability* of the quaternary structure.

Secondly, quite a number of proteins are basically made up of two different kinds of polypeptide chain, each coded by a *different* locus, e.g., the α and β-chains of typical mammalian haemoglobin, which has the quaternary structure $\alpha_2\beta_2$ (a biquaternary protein with a tetrameric molecular species). Thus, genetic variants can be at *either* locus. Detection of a protein polymorphism of adult cattle haemoglobin does not, in itself, tell us whether the α or the β locus (known to be on different chromosomes) is involved. So far, as a result of polypeptide chain separation and further characterization (especially amino acid sequence determination), all but one of the known variants of bovine adult haemoglobin reside in the β-chain (see p. 272).

Amino acid sequencing reveals differences not detectable by electrophoretic techniques, such as the β-caseins B and B_Z. A further application is that whether the differences are electrophoretically detectable or not, the amino acid sequence is closely related to the DNA sequence and can be used to trace the evolutionary history of a protein and its variants — although when this is extended to the evolution of animals it must be remembered that not all proteins evolve at the same rate (Jope, 1976; Manwell and Baker, 1976). Neither chain separation nor amino acid sequencing is at present suitable for routine screening; both these techniques, and the more recent DNA sequencing, are useful in solving particular problems. Sequencing of amino acids and DNA are both very expensive.

Information about individual proteins and references to other literature are available elsewhere (Manwell and Baker, 1970; Baker and Manwell, 1983a,b). The rest of this section will be devoted to an assessment of the data which are available for cattle.

The products of some 50 marker loci of cattle can be resolved by electrophoresis:

Ignoring the loci coding for embryonic haemoglobins in cattle (for which we know of no polymorphism data), four to five loci code for the globin chains of the respiratory pigment haemoglobin: α-, β-, γ- and myoglobin; and, in some species there is a second α-chain locus which has arisen by gene duplication.

There are some eight serum proteins: slow α_2-macroglobulin (which combines with a number of different proteases to cause their inactivation); post-transferrin 1; post-transferrin 2; the iron-binding protein transferrin; coeruloplasmin (a copper transport protein which has a role in iron metabolism and also has enzymatic activity as an oxidase on certain aromatic amines); post-albumin (= vitamin D-binding protein); other protease inhibitors which migrate in the albumin–prealbumin region; and serum albumin.

Milk contains seven markers: α-lactalbumin; β-lactoglobulin; α_{S1}-, α_{S2}-, β- and $\varkappa$-caseins; and lactoferrin; plus some serum proteins, mainly transferrin and serum albumin. With the exception of two or three polymorphic proteins of leucocytes and erythrocytes which have not yet been fully identified, the remaining 25–30 markers are all enzymes.

Not surprisingly, most effort has been placed upon systems which are sampled easily and repetitively, such as blood; and upon proteins that are easy to resolve. There are also some puzzling gaps, such as the paucity of data for α-lactalbumin and for serum albumin in *B. taurus*. It is not clear how much of this gap in the record is the failure to publish data on monomorphic loci, or a failure to screen loci which were claimed in early reports to be monomorphic in North European cattle breeds.

Another factor which causes disproportionate emphasis on certain loci is that some loci are more useful than others in parentage testing. Thus there is an emphasis on loci which have a high probability of excluding parentage. However, there are also many studies reporting gene frequency data for milk proteins, which from their sex-limited expression are less useful for parentage exclusion than proteins which occur in both sexes.

Possibly the main reason for different emphasis upon certain marker loci is the attitude of individual workers and laboratories. For example, Belgian cattle breeds have been surveyed for more enzymes of red and white cells than have the British breeds.

A recent survey of the literature revealed approximately 1000 papers reporting on protein markers in cattle, representing over 200 different breeds (Baker and Manwell, 1980). Many breeds had gene frequency data from more than one location. Since then, many more reports have appeared. Thus, for cattle there is probably the largest data base of published gene frequencies for molecular markers aside from those for man, mouse, and *Drosophila*, equalled or exceeded by very few other species.

In common with other species, the patterns observed after electrophoresis of cattle proteins usually allow the easy identification of both homozygotes and heterozygotes, the latter often (but not always) having a pattern recognizable as a combination of the parental types. Thus it is permissible to make assumptions concerning inheritance in non-pedigree populations. Cattle are again unusual in the extent to which these assumptions are often tested repeatedly against pedigree information.

Furthermore, individual variants of cattle proteins are well-characterized. Many are screened frequently in parentage tests. Laboratories engaged in parentage testing participate in comparisons arranged by the International Society for Animal Blood Group Research. There is also some exchange of samples between individual researchers, to provide a cross-check on identification of variants; however, as mentioned previously, disease risks have limited such an exchange between workers in some countries.

It is inevitable that there is a time lag in the characterization of new variants, especially if these are rare; but, in cattle the identity of more individual variants can be regarded with greater confidence than in any other species except horses, sheep, pigs, poultry, mice and man. Cattle also compare especially favourably with other species in the number of proteins and variants which have been sequenced (Manwell and Baker, 1976).

The size and reliability of the cattle data base mean that, in conjunction with suitable genetic techniques, it can be used to explore genetic structure of bovine populations at all levels, from individual herds to species. Although the data base for water buffalo is not as large, it is also of sufficient size to yield some useful information.

5. POPULATION STRUCTURE

5.1. The importance of population structure in conservation and animal breeding

Population structure is another topic which is worthy of study both in its own right and as a source of information for practical application. A number of interrelated aspects are: determination of size (and effective size: see p. 263); analysis of age structure and determination of generation interval; the distribution of variation within and between populations; the identification of centres of origin and centres of diversity; to monitor inbreeding; and to trace gene flow.

Studies of population structure are advocated frequently. Miller (1977) considered that data on biochemical polymorphisms 'should provide the primary means of judging whether a breed in question is sufficiently unique in its genome to justify preservation.' Three examples he suggested were: identification of rare alleles; estimation of genetic distance; and simple comparison of breeds for frequencies of alleles at single loci. Maijala et al. (1984) drew attention to the 'need to analyse the trends in genetic relationship, expected homozygosity and marker gene frequencies . . . to get some indication of the rate of gene loss.' Hickman (1984, p. 20) advocated a more positive role: 'IF A BIRD'S-EYE-VIEW OF THE BASIC POPULATION STATISTICS OF INDIGENOUS BREEDS COULD BE ESTABLISHED, THEN CONSERVATION PROBLEMS COULD BE PREDICTED AND PERHAPS AVOIDED.' (Capitals in original.)

5.2. Consequences of population stratification

5.2.1. Differences in gene frequencies in different samples from the same breed

Gene frequencies for the same protein marker may differ significantly between different populations of the same breed. This has led some workers to suggest that protein polymorphisms are not suitable for the characterization of breeds or for use in studies of relationships between breeds (e.g., A.L. Archibald, 1981). In fact, the variance for the frequency of an allele may vary considerably between breeds (and breed groups) as is shown graphically by Baker and Manwell (1980). This suggests that the observed differences may reflect the way that individual breeds are divided into subpopulations (e.g., herds), and that the distribution of variation between and within herds differs in different breeds.

5.2.2. Heterozygote deficit

Observation of a deficit of heterozygotes usually raises questions as to the cause. If errors in classification are ruled out, there are at least five genetic causes:

(1) Heterozygote disadvantage, also referred to as negative heterosis or contracomplementation.
(2) Assortative mating. This is most likely for a visible characteristic.
(3) Wahlund effect: stratification of the population into distinct groups differing in gene frequency, usually associated with inbreeding relative to the total population (Wahlund, 1928).
(4) A 'null' or 'silent' allele.
(5) Unrecognized sex linkage.

These causes are all discussed in more detail elsewhere (Manwell and Baker, 1970, chapter 1). We have listed them here because it is important to identify the true cause of the observation. This is especially the case in an applied situation, as failure to identify the true cause could lead to wrong decisions.

5.2.3. Heterozygote excess

An excess of heterozygotes may also be due to a variety of causes. Indeed, it appears that for most mechanisms capable of producing a deficit of heterozygotes, there is an opposite mechanism which can generate an excess:
(1) Heterozygote advantage, also called (positive) heterosis or overdominance.
(2) Disassortative mating.
(3) Robertson effect: differences in gene frequency between sires and dams can give an excess of heterozygotes (Robertson, 1965).
(4) Fixed heterozygote formation.
(5) Sampling from a population with an appreciable proportion of individuals with an extra chromosome could lead to an apparent excess of heterozygotes, if the marker locus occurs on that particular chromosome.

These causes are also discussed elsewhere (Manwell and Baker, 1970) and it is important to try and differentiate between them if an excess of heterozygotes is observed.

5.3. Pedigree

Many (but not all) measures of population structure are based on pedigree data. These are readily available for some breeds and are recorded in herd books. The main reasons for keeping these is to help the selection of animals known or believed to have certain attributes and to determine the identity of individual animals so that purchasers could be confident of getting the animal or bloodline of choice. Breeders have always used markers such as colour and pattern to aid identification, so there was a rapid integration of biochemical markers as an aid to checking parentage.

Parentage testing is based on exclusion of relationship when an animal has a genotype inconsistent with that of a putative relation. In simple cases, one putative parent and the offspring may share a rare marker not present in another putative parent; or it may be possible to disprove parentage because the putative parent and offspring are homozygous for different alleles at the same locus. Usually it is necessary to screen an adequate number of alleles from several loci. The choice of markers is made partly because of their biochemical suitability, discussed by us elsewhere (Baker and Manwell, 1983a, pp. 386–387) and partly on the exclusion value of certain loci. This differs with the occurrence and frequency of alleles, which is not the same in all breeds.

The probability of exclusion has been treated in detail by Jamieson (1965). For a diallelic locus with codominant inheritance, the exclusion value can be calculated from the simplified expression $pq\,(1 - pq)$, where p and q represent the frequencies of the two alleles. In Jersey cattle, the gene frequencies for haemoglobin (Hb) are: HbβA = 0.59 and HbβB = 0.41. Substitution of these gives $pq = 0.59 \times 0.41$ and so $0.24\ (1 - 0.24) = 0.18$; i.e., haemoglobin alone can be expected to detect 18% of the parentage errors in the Jersey. Different gene frequencies give different rates of exclusion. Jersey frequencies of alleles for carbonic anhydrase (CA) are A = 0.30 and B = 0.70. The probability of exclusion for these values is 16%.

For a multi-allelic locus with n codominant alleles, Jamieson gives the formula:

$$P_n = \sum_i p_i (1 - p_i)^2 - \sum_{i>j} (p_i p_j)^2 [4 - 3(p_i + p_j)]$$

He has also presented a very useful simple method of calculating the value by hand (Jamieson, 1978). As this reference is not easily obtained, we repeat it here. The Jersey population of the U.K. is triallelic for transferrin (Tf) and has the frequencies: A = 0.70; D_1 = 0.13; and D_2 = 0.17 (Jamieson, 1966) so we will use these data.

First Jamieson (1978) expands the formula to give:

$$P_n = \Sigma p - 2\,\Sigma p^2 + \Sigma p^3 + 2\Sigma p^4 - 3\Sigma p^5 - 2(\Sigma p^2)^2 + 3\Sigma p^2 \Sigma p^3$$

where p = the gene frequency. From the expansion it is obvious that the major part of the calculation is to obtain the powers of the gene frequencies and to sum these. Jamieson arranges this step as follows:

	p	p^2	p^3	p^4	p^5
Allele p_1(TfA)	0.70	0.49	0.34	0.24	0.17
p_2(TfD_1)	0.13	0.02	0.00	0.00	0.00
p_3(TfD_2)	0.17	0.03	0.01	0.00	0.00
Σ	1.00	0.54	0.35	0.24	0.17

Substitution of these values in the expanded formula gives:

$$P = 1 - 2\Sigma p^2 + \Sigma p^3 + 2\Sigma p^4 - 3\Sigma p^5 - 2(\Sigma p^2)^2 + 3\ \Sigma p^2 \Sigma p^3$$

$$P = 1 - (2 \times 0.54) + 0.35 + (2 \times 0.24) - (3 \times 0.17) - (2 \times 0.54^2) + (3 \times 0.54 \times 0.35) = 0.25,$$

i.e., the probability of exclusion using the transferrin locus alone is 25%.

For loci with more than three alleles the procedure is identical except that there is an additional row for each additional allele, $p_4 \ldots p_n$.

The probability of exclusion E, for a set of $\varkappa$ polymorphic loci, is calculated from the formula:

$$E = 1 - \prod_{\varkappa} (1 - P).$$

First the probability of exclusion for each locus is subtracted from 1. For the three loci used here, this gives Hb: 1 − 0.18; CA: 1 − 0.16; and Tf: 1 − 0.25. The resulting values are multiplied together and the product again subtracted from 1 to give the total probability of exclusion if all three loci are used

$$E = 1 - (0.82 \times 0.84 \times 0.75)$$
$$= 0.49 \text{ or } 49\%.$$

As Jamieson (1967) has demonstrated with worked examples, the utility of a locus increases with the number of alleles to a certain point (roughly around five alleles, but depending on their frequencies). Above this it is more efficient

Chapter 10 references, p. 289

to test several loci, each with a moderate number of alleles, than one permultiallelic locus. In practice, most cattle parentage testing laboratories combine loci to obtain probabilities of exclusion which are close to 100%.

The acceptance of AI by breed societies was facilitated by the availability of parentage testing, and the development of embryo transfer seems to be following a similar course. In the U.S.A., breed societies impose conditions concerning the typing of parents and progeny; and some societies only permit the use of two bulls in one programme if it is possible to exclude the progeny of each from the progeny of the other (C. Stormont, personal communication, 1984). In South Africa, similar precautions are enforced by law; yet, despite prior knowledge that checks would be made, in 707 cases there were 1.6% parentage errors (Meyer et al., 1984).

Embryo transplants involve another aspect of parentage testing. For cattle, sharing a uterus may result in early foetal anastomosis of the circulatory system. In addition to the danger that a heifer twin to a bull may be a freemartin, exchange of red cell primordia can occur. This results in red cell chimaerism, in which the phenotype of red cell markers is some combination of the animal's own genetically determined phenotype and the phenotype of its twin (see Baker and Manwell, 1983a,b; Stormont, 1984). In one such accidental case, the true identity of a Simmental bull, born by embryo transfer to an already pregnant cow, was only established after very careful investigations (Kraay et al., 1978). Schröffel et al. (1983) deliberately transferred embryos to previously inseminated cows and obtained ten pairs of uterine twins in which one of each pair was the natural offspring and the other a fosterling. In all cases the erythrocyte markers of the natural progeny predominated over the phenotype of the foster sibling, and in many cases the phenotype of the latter was suppressed completely. These experiences suggest that careful planning is necessary to ensure that calves born by embyro transfer can be identified with confidence. The matter will be especially critical in the conservation of rare breeds by frozen ova and embryos, as later rejection of an animal through inadequate means of identification might mean loss of rare genetic material. Serum proteins are more useful markers in such situations as they do not exhibit chimaerism. Also, colour-marked host cows can be used.

5.4. Does pedigree matter?

Some scientists criticize breeders for their concern with pedigree, and for the use of parentage exclusion tests to eliminate incorrect pedigrees. It is claimed that the herd book is 'to ensure parentage more than to compare performance . . .' (Seidel and Seidel, 1981, p. 68) and has 'little or nothing to do with the genetic improvement of the breed . . .' (Barton, 1984, p. 4).

However, genetic improvement depends on the accuracy of progeny tests, heritabilities and mating plans, all of which depend on the accuracy of pedigrees (Baker and Manwell, 1983a, p. 385; Stormont, 1984, p. 4). Pieper and Geldermann (1984) found that of 2113 cattle used in milk performance testing, 256 (12.1%) were not the progeny of their recorded sires. The rate of paternity error varied between sires and had an effect on the ranking of sires by heritability of performance traits and differences in breeding values. Graml (1984) noted the argument that incorrect pedigrees would have little effect on genetic progress if large enough numbers were tested. He also noted that testing is expensive. Graml's calculations show that without parentage control, and especially for traits with low heritabilities, a disproportionately greater number of animals need to be tested; with parentage control the number can be reduced accordingly. A comparison of the costs of performance testing with the costs of parentage control suggested that a critical level (in favour of parentage control) was reached with 5% incorrect pedigrees.

This raises the question: how many pedigrees are incorrect in practice? For Swedish cattle, the range reported is from 12% of the cases where parentage checks were requested (Rendel and Gahne, 1961) to population levels of 8% (Rendel, 1957) and an 'average' of around 4% (Rendel, 1958a). Ashton (1958) found 3% errors in screening British cattle for purposes other than parentage testing; but McCoubrey et al. (1983) suggest that the level may be as much as 13% for sires and 6% for dams. Stormont (1984) said that, over 30 years of parentage testing in the U.S.A., most errors were in the range of 2–10%, but that there had been especially high errors in the early years of the introduction of 'exotic' European breeds to the U.S.A. There had been '. . . a dramatic reduction in the percentage of error in all cattle breed registries . . .' but the average still remained around 5%. Stormont's experience was paralleled by the experiences of delegates who discussed parentage exclusion at a recent meeting of the International Society for Animal Blood Group Research. The discussion produced additional data: 13% error for Irish cattle; and a 10% average for Germany (against the average of 12.1% already cited for sires under test by Pieper and Geldermann, 1984).

A special case is parentage testing of range cattle, where exclusion rates may rise to 58%. This high percentage is not caused by error, but is the result of routine screening to determine the parentage of cattle bred naturally in herds where there is more than one bull (C. Stormont, personal communication, 1984). In addition to its value in determining pedigree, parentage exclusion testing of range cattle is an important management tool. For example, one set of trials revealed that individual herds might have from 65% to 100% of the calves sired by one-third of the bulls (Lehrer et al., 1977). Parentage exclusion also allows the breeder to assess the reproductive performance of cows by identifying cows whose living calves were stolen; cows who steal calves to replace dead offspring: and cows which have reared their own calves.

The inescapable conclusion is that the attention of breed societies to registering correct pedigrees is worth the cost and effort. The opportunity of increasing efficiency and reducing numbers under test is favourable to breeds rejected as inefficient on account of their small numbers by some animal geneticists (see p. 228).

It has been suggested that publication of herd books should be replaced by computer storage of pedigree data (Barton, 1984, p. 6). This would limit access and prevent the maximum utilization of herd book records. Studies of herd books have contributed to the formulation of genetic theory (Wright, 1982), and to revealing social factors which were important in breed history (Perry, 1982). We would also like to draw attention to the potential of herd books as research material when funds are limited. Tracing pedigrees by hand may be slower and less glamorous than using a computer, but this in no way detracts from the value of the results.

5.5. Wright's *F*-statistics

As Wright (1969, p. 173 *et seq.*) has presented a detailed discussion of the development and use of F-statistics only a brief description is necessary. The *fixation index, F*, is a measure of the correlation expected between uniting gametes. It is best understood by references to three extreme hypothetical cases. Under panmixia (random mating) $F = 0$. However the same gene frequencies observed under panmixia can also occur in the extreme case of heterozygote deficit, when a population consists of a number of homozygous (fixed) lines and $F = 1$; or in the extreme case of heterozygote excess, when a population consists of nothing but heterozygotes (as in a balanced lethal system) and $F = -1$. In many practical situations, F has been found in the range 0.00–1.00: i.e., the population is subdivided.

Chapter 10 references, p. 289

The relation of F to a particular situation is used to define population structure:

F_{IT} is the correlation between gametes which unite to produce individuals (I) relative to the gametes of the total population (T). It is often just called F and defined in the narrow sense of the *coefficient of inbreeding,* in which case it may also be relative to a famous ancestor. F_{IT} is usually a positive value. A negative value may occur if there is no systematic subdivision of a population and consanguineous matings are avoided.

F_{IS} is the average, over all subdivisions of a population, of the correlation between uniting gametes relative to the gametes of one individual subdivision (IS). F_{IS} is usually positive, but may be negative if consanguineous matings are avoided.

F_{ST} is the correlation between random gametes within subdivisions (S) relative to the gametes of the total population (T). F_{ST} always has a positive value. It is related to the other two terms by the equation

$$F_{ST} = (F_{IT} - F_{IS})/(1 - F_{IS}).$$

Further hierarchical subdivisions can be accommodated if necessary.

5.6. *F*-Statistics, herd books and breed structure

Wright's theory of F-statistics grew out of a study of herd books and has been applied to breed structure. Many of these investigations have been discussed by Vu Tien Khang (1983). Her review reveals that individual authors have differed in their approach, sometimes considerably, but that most studies have been based on two measures used by Wright: the coefficient of relationship and the coefficient of inbreeding.

The *coefficient of relationship, R,* is the probability that two individuals with a common ancestor will have a gene in common. The basic relationship is that between parent and offspring, where meiosis ensures that the genes in common will be 50%. As pointed out by Lush (1945, p. 243) all other relationships are chains of the parent–offspring relationships which link two individuals. In the absence of inbreeding, the calculation of relationship is simply the summation of these chains. For two individuals, X and Y, the coefficient of relationship, R is

$$R_{XY} = \Sigma[(½)^n],$$

where n = the number of meiotic segregations between X and Y via the common ancestor. If X and Y are ½ sibs, with the same sire, A, the path is X–A–Y, $n = 2$ and $½^n = 0.25$. If X and Y were full sibs and also had the same dam, B, there would be another path X–B–Y, $R = 0.25$. Summing the two pathways gives $0.25 + 0.25 = 0.5$ as the relationship between full sibs. More distant relationships involve longer pathways. Thus two cousins, X and Z, with one common grandparent, D, would be connected X–A–D–C–Z and $½^4 = 0.0625$.

If any of the animals are inbred, allowance must be made for this, using the coefficient of inbreeding, F. The formula for the coefficient of relationship between X and Y through their common ancestor, A then becomes

$$R_{XY} = \Sigma[(½)^n(1 + F_A)]/\sqrt{[(1 + F_X)(1 + F_Y)]}.$$

The *coefficient of inbreeding* is the second of the two basic measures used to analyse population structure. It can be calculated in one of two ways. The most simple is that the inbreeding of the offspring, O, is equal to half the relationship between sire, S, and dam, D, corrected for the inbreeding (if any) of the sire and dam.

$F_O = (R_{SD}/2)(\sqrt{[1 + F_S)(1 + F_D}).$

If the relationship between the sire and dam is not known, F is calculated in a similar manner to the coefficient of relationship, but with the difference that n refers to the number of segregations in each path between sire and dam

$F_X = ½ \Sigma [(½)^n(1 + F_A)].$

Usually R and F are related to some base such as a famous ancestor or a certain period. Values for individuals can be combined to give average values for subpopulations (lines or herds) and for total populations (breeds). However, the amount of work involved is such that usually a sampling method is used. Tracing a single random line back from each parent was found to yield an estimate comparable with that obtained from 64 full pedigrees for Bates' Duchess line of Shorthorns (Wright, 1977, Vol. III, p. 537).

Studies on a number of breeds of cattle have been summarized by Wright (1977) and by Vu Tien Khang (1983). Wright also used F-statistics to analyse the genetic history of several breeds. A common pattern was of a hierarchical structure with certain sires, families or herds exerting considerable influence on the breed as a whole. A similar finding has been made recently for the Bonsmara and the Drakensberger (Van Zyl et al., 1984).

Most of the breeds studied have been large or, like the Welsh Black, with at least local importance. In view of the frequently expressed concern about the danger of inbreeding in small populations, it is regrettable that there is not a similar series of studies on rare breeds. One such investigation, that of the Dexter (Young, 1953) was missed by both Wright and Vu Tien Khan, so we summarize some of the findings. During the years of the study (1900–45) the size of the breed, measured by the total number of registered females, fluctuated: the minimum was 79 and the maximum was 1119. The average herd size was 10–12 females, but there was a persistent core of larger herds which accounted for some 22% of the breed. Analysis of the pedigrees of the 86 heifers registered in 1947 did not reveal any stratification into prominent lines. The relationship of the heifers *inter se* was only 2.6% and their average total inbreeding was only 2.4%. It is interesting to compare these values with data from Wright (1977, chapter 16). Values for inbreeding were: Shorthorn (U.K. 1920) 26.0 ± 2.8; Hereford (U.K. 1930) 8.1 ± 0.8; Aberdeen Angus (U.K. 1939) 11.3 ± 1.1; Holstein (U.S.A. 1931) 4.0 ± 0.5; and Brown Swiss (U.S.A. 1929) 3.8 ± 0.6. *Inter se* relationships at the same dates were: Shorthorn, 39.5; Hereford, 8.8; Aberdeen Angus, 13.3; Holstein, 3.4; and Brown Swiss, 4.3. The Shorthorn breed in 1920 had an average relationship to the bull Favourite (252), calved 1793, of 55.2%.

In a recent study of the Kerry, OhUigin and Kelly (1984) calculated the inbreeding coefficients of all 15156 pedigree animals recorded in a period exceeding 100 years (i.e., from before the first herd book in 1887). The mean inbreeding of the current population of about 200 head is 14%.

5.7. Population size

5.7.1. Effective size

The *total number*, N, of animals in a population is not usually the same as the *effective number*, N_e: i.e., the number of animals which are effective in leaving offspring. The concept of N_e has been useful in population genetics; but under certain conditions, effective numbers derived from different fundamental approaches can differ (see Wright, 1969, chapter 8). For most work on breed structure four situations are important (Wright, 1977, pp. 540–541).

Chapter 10 references, p. 289

5.7.2. Sex ratio

For a given number of breeding males, N_M, and a given number of breeding females, N_F, in a breed,

$$N_e = 4\ N_M\ N_F/(N_M + N_F).$$

In most breeds of domestic livestock, where there are relatively few males and large numbers of females, N_e approaches $4N_M$. Using Edwards' (1959) British Friesian figures of 2 million females (N_F) bred to 200 sires (N_M) and substituting these in the formula gives $N_e = 799.9$. The simpler calculation is $N_e = 4N_M = 800$.

5.7.3. Differences in number of offspring that reach sexual maturity

Some sires leave many more male descendants as sires than contemporaries. Where the variance of the number of offspring which reach breeding maturity is σ^2_κ

$$N_e = 4N/(2 + \sigma^2_\kappa).$$

5.7.4. Temporal variations in population size

Many populations pass through bottlenecks and then expand again. If time, t, is measured by the number of generations, and the number of breeding individuals each generation is N_i.

$$N_e = t[\sum_i (N_i)^{-1}]^{-1}.$$

This formula means that the effective population number is proportional to the harmonic mean (the reciprocal, $1/x$, of the sum of reciprocals of a set of numbers). Young's (1953) data for the Dexter are arranged in 5-year intervals (the average generation interval for cattle). The number of registered females expanded as follows: 1905, 79 (reciprocal 0.0127); 1910, 200 (0.0050); 1915, 337 (0.0030); 1920, 528 (0.0019); 1925, 1,119 (0.0009). The sum of the reciprocals is 0.0235, and the reciprocal of the sum is 42.55. For five generations, $N_e = 5 \times 42.55 = 213$. Thus, although the expansion appeared large, the effective size was considerably less. This exemplifies the well-known fact that a bottleneck accelerates the rate of genetic change.

The Dexter (Young, 1953) and the Kerry (OhUigin and Kelly, 1984) have an interesting parallel in fluctuations in population size. Allowing for time lag, both had a period of expansion associated with the First World War, followed by a period of decline and then another period of expansion associated with the Second World War. This supports the role of local breeds as efficient producers without recourse to unlimited supplies of imported concentrates.

5.7.5. Population size and inbreeding

Wright (1977, p. 541) noted that the theoretical rate of change of inbreeding, ΔF_{ST} per generation, is $1/(2N_e)$. Thus

$$N_e = 1/(2\Delta F_{ST}).$$

As an example, Wright used 12 generations of Shorthorns. In 1810, $F_{ST} = 0.128$; and in 1875 $F_{ST} = 0.241$, and $\Delta F_{ST} = 0.113/12 = 0.0094$ per generation. From this, $N_e = 1/2 \times 0.0094 = 53$. As $N_e = 4N_M$, this meant only about 13 sires per generation.

In contrast, the Dexter only accumulated a total inbreeding of 0.024 in the six generations studied to 1947 (Young, 1953). So ΔF_{ST} was 0.004 per generation, and $N_e = 1/(2 \times 0.004) = 125$; and $N_M = 31$ sires. Thus a very small breed like the Dexter may accumulate less inbreeding and have a higher N_e than a highly popular and expanding breed such as the Shorthorn was in the 19th century. Indeed, an N_e of 125 for a breed with only 551 registered females compares favourably with the N_e of only 800 for the 2 million British Friesians bred to 200 sires. The long-term effect of such AI schemes on population structure is not yet known, but reports are beginning to appear which associate loss of blood group polymorphism with AI (Kaczmarek and Dorynek, 1979; Kästli, 1979; Trela et al., 1979).

5.7.6. Effective number of herds

F-Statistics are not always convenient for measuring the extremes of reproductive inequality that are illustrated by the Shorthorn in the previous section. An alternative approach is that of Robertson (1953) who has described hierarchical structure in terms of the *effective number* of herds, $\mathcal{H}$. The effective number of herds is related to different ancestral groups, e.g., herds producing sires, $\mathcal{H}_s$, which is the equivalent of the effective number of males. However, going one step further back gives one $\mathcal{H}_{ss}$, the effective number of sires of sires; and, the process can be reiterated to give 'sires of sires of sires', $\mathcal{H}_{sss}$, etc.

For example, for 200 Ayrshire heifers born in 1947, chosen at random from the herd book, Robertson (1953) found that 50 herds contributed only one sire each, 12 herds contributed two sires, ... all the way to one herd at the extreme end which contributed 28 sires. For this Ayrshire sample $\mathcal{H}_s = 122$, $\mathcal{H}_{ss} = 25$, $\mathcal{H}_{sss} = 14$, and $\mathcal{H}_{ssss} = 14$. A similar trend occurs for some other breeds. In other words, *there are effectively three different levels of structure*, the values of $\mathcal{H}$ being roughly the same after $\mathcal{H}_{sss}$ is reached. Robertson (1953) emphasizes how the number of herds which have any permanent effect on the breed as a whole is comparatively small, in the cases surveyed at that time (four dairy cattle breeds, two beef cattle breeds, and one breed each of pigs and goats) $\mathcal{H}_{sss}$ (and higher $\mathcal{H}$'s) are 30 or less.

To calculate $\mathcal{H}$, one first calculates the reciprocal, C, the probability that, if two animals are chosen at random from the breed records, they will have sires bred from the same herd. For the initial step, the sires, C_s is calculated from the formula:

$$C_s = \frac{\sum_i [n_i (n_i - 1)]}{(\sum_i n_i)(\Sigma n_i - 1)}$$

where n_i is the number of sires from the i-th herd. The sampling variance of the estimate of C_s is 'very roughly' (Robertson, 1953, p. 334):

$$\frac{4\sum_i n_i^3}{(\sum_i n_i)^4}$$

The reciprocal of C_s is $\mathcal{H}_s$. In turn, C_{ss} is calculated by counting the sires of sires, and so forth.

A special value of Robertson's (1953) $\mathcal{H}_s$, $\mathcal{H}_{ss}$, $\mathcal{H}_{sss}$ ... system is that it distills into a small set of numbers (three being adequate in most cases) a representation of the asymmetry of the opportunities of sires to contribute to the next generation. In addition, the set of numbers provides a measure of any change in breeding pattern over the last few generations.

Chapter 10 references, p. 289

5.7.7. Effective number of alleles

Some workers have expressed the variation of biochemical polymorphisms as the *effective number of alleles:* the reciprocal of the probability that two randomly chosen homologous genes in a population are identical by descent. The probability is equal to the expected frequency of homozygous individuals in the population, or to the inbreeding coefficient (Kimura and Crow, 1964). Thus, using the Jersey gene frequencies HbβA = 0.59 and HbβB = 0.41, the expected frequency of homozygotes is $(0.59^2 + 0.41^2) = 0.5162$; and the effective number of alleles = 1/0.5162 = 1.9372.

There is some confusion of terminology. Kimura and Crow (1964) use *n*; but Kimura and Ohta refer to the effective number of alleles as $\underline{n}_e$. Neimann-Sørensen (1956) called this term N_a. He applied N_a to the permulti-allelic B blood group system in the Danish Red and obtained a value of 6.3, which was half the estimated N_e of 12. But Nei (1975, p. 118) uses $\underline{n}_a$ to refer to the *average number of alleles:* the reciprocal of the mean frequency of alleles existing in the population.

5.7.8. Gene migration

Migration, *m*, is the observed proportion of a deme which is replaced by immigrants who are reproductive. A general formula is:

$$F_{ST} = 1/(1 + 4N_e m).$$

Migration can also be calculated in terms of genes (Wright, 1969, pp. 27–28; Adams and Ward, 1973). The procedure is simple in principle, but there are many complications, especially in the estimation of the interaction of migration and selection. Adams and Ward (1973) have a helpful short discussion of the matter and a variety of statistical tests.

Migration is obviously of interest in animal breeding, from the level of the migration of bulls between herds, to the widespread importation of 'exotic' breeds and the formation of new breeds. There are relatively few studies of such situations. The recorded contributions of the Shorthorn to the Swedish Red Pied (Rendel, 1958b) and to the Norwegian Red (Braend, 1975); and of the Ayrshire to the Trønder (Braend et al., 1964) were verified by the use of biochemical polymorphisms. Osterhoff (1966) found that the Drakensberger has frequencies between those of the Friesian and the Afrikaner for the blood group factors L, M, C and SA_2, thereby supporting the tradition that the Drakensberger arose from the other two breeds. However, most studies do not report their findings in terms of *m*.

5.7.9. Immigration load

Wright (1977, p. 485) introduced the concept of immigration load: the amount by which immigration pulls down the mean selective (adaptive) value of the local population. Immigration load is measured by the balance between immigration and local selection against the introduced genes.

Kästli (1979) has been following the recent admixture of Red Holstein-Friesian genes on the Simmental breed in Switzerland, using the bovine blood group B system. After 8 years of massive introgression, using AI, only six typical Red Holstein B-group alleles attained a frequency over 1%. Of particular interest is that she has included in her studies a comparison of purebred Simmental in 1970 versus 1980, thereby having a control experiment to see if there has been any change in the gene frequencies of alleles at this permulti-allelic polymorphism in an unintrogressed population.

It was found in comparing the B-group allele frequencies for 1970 and 1980 in the purebred Simmentals that there was only an 80% correlation, suggesting that considerable differences can arise, either from drift or selection

(Kästli, 1979). These studies emphasize the importance of having data for more than one point in time in studying gene migration — especially for a permultiallelic locus where, as many alleles will be at low gene frequencies, stochastic fluctuations will be large.

Recently Aupetit (1985) has investigated the possible contribution of Shorthorn bulls used on French breeds in the nineteenth century. Twenty-two French breeds and the Shorthorn were screened for transferrin, β-casein and eleven blood groups; the gene frequency data were used to calculate genetic distances by four methods. With the exception of the Maine Anjou (a synthetic breed formed from crosses between Shorthorn and Mancelle) the Shorthorn was not close to the French breeds. This suggests that, if there had been a significant gene flow from the Shorthorn, there had also been selection against Shorthorn traits, at least in respect of the biochemical polymorphisms studied.

5.8. Nei's gene diversity

The usually valid assumptions concerning the control of electrophoretically revealed polymorphisms made it possible to investigate the genetics and genetic structure of non-pedigree populations. Wright's *F*-statistics can be applied to analyses of protein polymorphism data, using variances of each allele (Wright, 1968, pp. 178 and 343, 1978, p. 87; Nei, 1977). However, this is not a convenient method and others were devised. The most widely used is the series of measures devised by Nei (1973, 1975).

Nei introduced the concept of *gene diversity* (or 'expected heterozygosity'), H, defined as the probability that two randomly chosen alleles from a population are non-identical. (Nei chose the term diversity because in a non-random breeding population the 'heterozygosity' thus defined is not related to the frequency of heterozygotes.) H is calculated using *gene identity* (or homozygosity), J, defined as the probability that two randomly chosen alleles from a population will be identical; thus, $H = 1 - J$. For example, in Jersey cattle on the island of Jersey, the frequencies of the Hbβ alleles are A = 0.38 and B = 0.62. $J = (0.38^2 + 0.62^2) = 0.5288$; and $H = 1 - J = 0.4712$.

Gene diversity is the building block used for the definition of other aspects of population structure. Unlike *F*-statistics, H is not affected by departure from random mating, or by the number of loci or alleles. Any number of individuals can be used, although if there are only a few a large number of loci should be screened (Nei, 1978). Any number of hierarchical subdivisions can be accommodated. Finally, as H is defined by gene frequencies from the sampled generation, no assumption (and no information) is required about the pedigree of individuals or about selection and migration in the past (Nei, 1975).

Population structure is analysed by seven measures, which can be illustrated by the Hbβ locus of Jersey cattle. This breed has migrated from the island of Jersey to many countries, but for simplicity we only consider a 'total' world population of Jerseys in three countries. Each has a different frequency of the HbβA allele: Australia: 0.49; Canada, 0.42; and Jersey, 0.38. Thus the total population has an average of $(0.49 + 0.42 + 0.38)/3 = 0.43$. The *total gene identity*, $J_T = (0.43^2 + 0.57^2) = 0.5098$; and the *total gene diversity*, $H_T = 1 - 0.5098 = 0.4902$.

The gene diversity of the Isle of Jersey subpopulation has already been calculated as 0.4717. The same calculation for Australia and Canada gives $H = 0.4999$ and $H = 0.4872$ respectively. The *average diversity within subpopulations*, H_S, is obtained by summing the individual values and dividing by the number of subpopulations: $1.4583/3 = 0.4861$.

The diversity among subpopulations, $D_{ST} = H_T - H_S = 0.4902 - 0.4861 = 0.0041$.

The *diversity of the subpopulations relative to the total population* is called

Chapter 10 references, p. 289

the *coefficient of gene differentiation*, G_{ST}. It is equivalent to, and for diallelic loci equals, Wright's F_{ST}:

$G_{ST} = D_{ST}/H_T = 0.0041/0.4902 = 0.0083$.

The *average minimal difference between populations*, $\bar{D}_M = sD_{ST}/(s - 1)$ where s is the number of subpopulations. In the present example, $\bar{D}_M = 3 \times 0.0041/(3–1) = 0.0062$.

The *interpopulational gene diversity relative to the intrapopulation gene diversity* is $R_{ST} = \bar{D}_M/H_S = 0.0062/0.4861 = 0.0127$.

These calculations confirm what is obvious from the raw gene frequencies: that haemoglobin is variable in the Jersey and that there are only small differences between the total population and the subpopulations and among the subpopulations. The values do form a basis for comparison with other breeds which might differ more markedly in gene frequencies between countries. As the calculations were only made for one locus, it is possible that if enough loci were included, greater differences might be found.

To extend the system to more loci only requires working out the gene diversity for each population for each locus and then obtaining an average H for each population over all loci. The Jersey on the island of Jersey has the following gene diversities for individual loci: Hbβ = 0.4172; transferrin = 0.4032; carbonic anhydrase II = 0.4488; and amylase I = 0.4902. Summed and divided by the number of loci, these yield $H = 1.8134/4 = 0.4534$. Similar average gene diversities over the same loci are obtained for each subpopulation. For each locus the average gene frequencies over all populations are used to calculate a separate H_T for each locus (e.g., H_T for Hbβ = 0.4902); and the average of all these is the H_T for all loci.

The data base compiled from the literature has gene frequencies for Jersey cattle in ten countries. Unfortunately they have not all been screened for the same proteins. The greatest overlap is for Canada, Denmark and Jersey, each of which have gene frequency data for the same nine loci. The values obtained over all loci were: $H_T = 0.3921$; $H_S = 0.3600$; $D_{ST} = 0.0321$; $G_{ST} = 0.0762$; $\bar{D}_M = 0.0471$; and $R_{ST} = 0.1308$ (Baker and Manwell, 1984). A further hierarchical subdivision into lines or herds would be of interest, but there are very few publications which list gene frequency data for individual herds. As pointed out by Powell (1983), when a population contains a lot of variation, the differences between subpopulations may appear small.

Nozawa (1979) and Braend (1981, p. 262) has tabulated the percentage of polymorphic protein loci and the average heterozygosity (gene diversity) for several species of farm livestock, including cattle. The former values are from 14 to 40% and the latter range from 0.029 to 0.109. These values agree well with the values assembled for wild species by Nevo (1978).

5.9. Other measures

5.9.1. Departure from Hardy–Weinberg equilibrium

When phenotypic frequencies equivalent to genotype frequencies are available, these can be used to provide a measure of the difference between the observed number of heterozygotes, H_{obs}, and the expected number of heterozygotes, H_{exp}, calculated under the assumption of the Hardy–Weinberg equilibrium. Statistically significant departures from equilibrium can suggest situations of interest, which may require careful investigation (Manwell and Baker, 1970; see also pp. 257, 258 and 271).

H_{obs} and H_{exp} can also be used to estimate the average level of inbreeding, using the formula:

$F = 1 - (H_{obs}/H_{exp})$.

This, of course, assumes that a deficit of heterozygotes has arisen from inbreeding. Conversely, a negative value of F can arise if deliberate outbreeding is practised (see p. 261).

5.9.2. Proportion of polymorphic loci

A locus is usually defined as polymorphic if the most common allele has a frequency equal to or less than 0.99; however, some authors prefer to use a cut-off at the frequency of 0.95. When comparing different groups for genetic variability it is common to do so in terms of the proportion of polymorphic loci, P_{Poly}, relative to the number of loci examined. This measure is not used much for domestic mammals as monomorphic loci are only reported rarely.

6. POPULATION STRUCTURE AND PRACTICAL CONSERVATION

6.1. General findings

In wild species of animals, and in wild and domestic plants, it is commonplace to analyse population structure in terms of proportion of polymorphic loci, gene diversity and Hardy–Weinberg equilibrium, applied to gene frequency data for protein polymorphisms. This approach is considered to be a useful tool for applying to problems of genetic conservation (Brown, 1978; Frankel and Soulé, 1981; Schonewald-Cox et al., 1983). The occurrence and frequencies of variants are used to define the subdivisions of a population and thus enable conservation in terms of distinct gene pools. There is some evidence that patterns of variation may be correlated with environmental conditions. Nevo (1978) surveyed literature data for 243 species of animals and concluded that genetic polymorphism is often connected with ecological heterogeneity, and varies non-randomly between loci, populations, species and habitats. Brown (1978, p. 153) in a study of the literature on plant protein polymorphisms, found that the local genetic structure of populations varied 'dramatically' over the range of a species. He also noticed that alleles which had a localized occurrence of high frequencies could represent a substantial fraction of the species variation. There are hints that this may also be the case for Hb B and Tf E in cattle (Baker and Manwell, 1980).

Gene frequencies may also be used in the selection of breeding stock in an attempt to maintain identified variation. Studies on polymorphism can provide a measure of any loss of variation arising from inbreeding, bottlenecks, or directional selection; obviously, the more polymorphic loci which are monitored, the more accurate the measure.

6.2. Bovine species and bottlenecks

There are three main causes of bottlenecks: *founder effect,* where a few individuals found a new population; reduction in the size of an existing population; and inbreeding. A common opinion is that reduced size means reduced variability, and even dedicated conservationists may feel that very small populations have a poor chance of survival and thus low priority for the limited resources available. This attitude makes the consequences of a bottleneck of great practical as well as theoretical importance.

The theoretical aspects of bottlenecks have been considered in detail by Nei et al. (1975) and the practical implications for conservation have been summarized by Powell (1983). Four major points emerge

Chapter 10 references, p. 289

(1) A decrease in heterozygosity becomes marked only if a bottleneck is severe.
(2) Gene diversity may actually increase because there is more chance of alleles with low frequencies becoming concentrated in a small population.
(3) The severity of decrease will depend on subsequent population growth. If this is rapid there is little loss. Slow expansion allows more loss by genetic drift.
(4) If a population survives, mutation can give rise to new variants which may substitute for some of the lost variants.

There are few satisfactory tests of these points. As pointed out by Nei et al (1975), small populations mean samples of few individuals, which for accurate results means that each individual should be screened for polymorphism at many loci. Ehrlich (1983) found that in butterfly populations which had been through narrow bottlenecks (some of less than 20 individuals) polymorphic loci tended to maintain the same predominant alleles in roughly the same frequencies.

There are three recent examples of bottlenecks in bovine populations. One is the feral Bali cattle of Australia, currently numbering about 1000, which are the descendants of 20 animals imported in the mid-19th century. Bailey (1968) examined 30 serum samples from these animals. His findings can be compared with those of Namikawa et al. (1980) who screened 114 Bali cattle from the island of Bali. All Bailey's samples had the same transferrin type, similar to D_1 of *B. taurus* and *B. indicus*. Namikawa et al. (1980) found that transferrin was polymorphic. The frequencies of the four alleles were: A = 0.004; D_1 = 0.739; D_2 = 0.212; and E = 0.044. Bailey found two types of serum albumin: A, which was similar to A of *B. taurus* and had a frequency of 0.2167; and 'D'. The latter was slower than *B. indicus* serum albumin B. Namikawa et al. also found two variants of serum albumin: A = 0.013 and B = 0.987. A slow zone, 'C', was not found in pure Bali cattle, or in Bali-type cattle in other islands, but was found in Madura and Jawa local cattle. Bell et al. (1981a,b) found that eight cows from the Australian population were monomorphic for α-lactalbumin and κ-casein but polymorphic for β-lactoglobulin, α_{s1}-casein and β-casein. There do not seem to be any reports concerning milk protein polymorphisms in the island of Bali.

It would be premature to draw too many conclusions from the protein polymorphism found in Australian Bali cattle. Samples have been taken from only a few individuals and only a small number of proteins have been investigated. However, the data do confirm that considerable variation can be present after a small bottleneck. It is possible that the transferrin variants in lower frequencies in the island of Bali either were not present in the founders of the Australian population, or were lost after arrival.

The other two bovine species bottlenecks are in the American bison, which dropped from an estimated 30 million to a few hundred (McHugh and Hobson, 1972) and the wisent, which went through a bottleneck of 12 animals (Slatis, 1960). Neither of these species has much biochemical polymorphism compared with other species of cattle. Braend and Stormont (1963) in a discussion of their investigation of the American bison, put forward three possible reasons: a small sample (113 individuals screened for haemoglobin and transferrin): 'the possibility that bison evolved with little or no genetic variation in such traits'; and a bottleneck. Each merits consideration.

While it is still true that further work on both species of *Bison* is desirable, the numbers screened have been large compared with other species where screening much smaller numbers revealed polymorphism of the same proteins (Braend and Stormont, 1963; Gasparski, 1972; Stormont, 1984).

It is now known that the level of polymorphism does vary between populations and between species (Manwell and Baker, 1970; Nevo, 1978). There is some evidence to suggest that domesticates are more polymorphic than closely related wild species (Manwell and Baker, 1976; Baker and Manwell, 1976). This has been supported by the finding that domestic Japanese quail, *Coturnix coturnix japonica*, have a gene diversity of 0.167 compared with 0.086 for two populations of wild quail of the same species (Kimura et al., 1983). The situation within the genus *Gallus* is not as straightforward (Hashiguchi et al., 1982). Domestic fowl *Gallus gallus* had the highest proportion of polymorphic loci. They also had higher gene diversity than most jungle fowl, but the highest gene diversities were found in green jungle fowl, *G. varius*, and in the Indonesian population of red jungle fowl, *G. gallus*. Six banteng were found to have a higher value for gene diversity than three populations of Bali cattle (thought to be domesticated banteng) when these were compared for nine polymorphic protein loci (Namikawa et al., 1983b). As the banteng were zoo animals, it is not clear how many populations were represented.

Large herds can result in higher rates of inbreeding (Chesser, 1983, pp. 71–72). This might account for some of the low polymorphism of proteins in American bison, but wisent would appear to have had a more pronounced deme structure under natural conditions (Lydekker, 1898). *Syncerus caffer* also occurs in large herds (Sinclair, 1977). One hundred and ninety-one individuals from two herds were found to be monomorphic for haemoglobin, transferrin and serum albumin. There were also high frequencies of some morphological traits such as wry tail, which raised the possibility of inbreeding (Osterhoff et al., 1970).

In describing the numerical decline of the wisent, Lydekker (1898, pp. 74–77) noted that some observers suggested inbreeding as a cause. However, Lydekker considered that other factors were more important, such as disturbance, loss of habitat, liver fluke picked up in the Białowieza swamps, and slaughter during wars and revolutions.

Slatis (1960) analysed the pedigrees in the herd book for evidence of inbreeding depression, measured by early death. He found no correlation with calculated coefficients of inbreeding, even after making allowance for non-selective deaths by slaughter during the Second World War and from foot and mouth disease in 1953. He also calculated the probability of each animal receiving a hypothetical lethal gene, *l*, from each ancestor which its parents had in common. There was some correlation between the probability of having *ll* and early death, but some highly inbred animals were apparently free from lethal genes.

Templeton and Read (1983) suggested that the findings of Slatis (1960) might be used as a basis for breeding plans in a small population. The strategy was to inbreed deliberately but at a slow rate and to eliminate inbreeding depression. This of course is very similar to the cattle breeder's strategy of 'line breeding' (Lush, 1945, p. 299). Templeton and Read reported that their breeding plan was successful with a small herd of Speke's gazelle, founded on only four individuals.

6.3. Inbreeding and pedigree: theory versus experiment

Very little advantage seems to have been taken of biochemical polymorphisms to check the inbreeding calculated from pedigrees. We have made one such attempt, summarized below (Manwell and Baker, 1982):

Data available for cattle include not only a large data base on molecular variation but also some measures of average inbreeding from pedigrees. Seven ancient polymorphic loci were chosen to avoid the non-equilibrium limitation.

Using Wright's $F = 1 - H_{obs}/H_{exp}$, one observes that this F-statistic is not significantly different from the average F based on pedigree data for transfer-

Chapter 10 references, p. 289

rin, carbonic anhydrase II, amylase I and α_{s1}-casein. However, there is a statistically very highly significant negative F for β-lactoglobulin. From the literature on associations between production characters and proteins there is evidence for both positive and negative heterosis associated with this milk protein polymorphism. There are also F's significantly less than the average F-pedigree for β- and κ-caseins.

As predicted by theory, the expected heterozygosity of most proteins decreases as average inbreeding increases. However, transferrin behaves anomalously, the expected heterozygosity *rising* from 0.54 at zero inbreeding to 0.61 at a 10% average inbreeding (regression analysis: $t_{19} = 3.366$; $P = 0.003$). As the analysis described in the previous paragraph indicates, this is *not* from any increased heterozygote advantage *per se* at the *Tf* locus. There is a kind of frequency-dependent selection where, as a population of cattle becomes more inbred, the gene frequencies of the major transferrin alleles approach equality. Such maximization of phenotypic diversity might offset to some extent any increased infertility or reduction in resistance to disease as occurs with increased inbreeding.

OhUigin and Kelly (1984) calculated that the inbreeding of the Kerry is now 14%. Dr Kelly has kindly supplied us with gene frequency data for the whole population. We have calculated H_T for each locus: transferrin, $H_T = 0.6339$; amylase I, $H_T = 0.4855$; and carbonic anhydrase II, $H_T = 0.4270$ (see also p. 263).

7. PHYLOGENETIC PATTERNS

7.1. The evolutionary significance of amino acid sequence data

There are two complementary reviews on the significance of amino acid sequence data for studies of the evolution of domestic animals (Jope, 1976; Manwell and Baker, 1976). Hence we shall give a brief summary based on previous work and concentrate on more recent findings.

Manwell and Baker (1976) noted that the common pattern for nearly all intraspecific genetic variants of protein is a difference of one amino acid substitution. Where variants differed by more than one amino acid substitution, they could be linked by an intermediate variant. In contrast, some protein variants of domestic animals differ by more than one amino acid substitution and in many cases intermediate variants are not known. One plausible explanation is that two taxa have diverged from the ancestral type and then hybridized to give rise to the domestic form.

The globin chains β^A and β^B of cattle differ by three amino acid substitutions (which entail at least four nucleotide substitutions). Counting from the N terminus, and giving β^A first, the differences are 15 glycine → serine; 18 lysine → histidine (a mutation which involves changes in two nucleotides); and 119 lysine → asparagine. Recently Namikawa and his colleagues have found a variant Hb Bali (originally called HbX) with an electrophoretic mobility between the mobilities of HbA and HbB. The allele Hbβ^{Bali} has a frequency of about 80% in Bali cattle (Namikawa et al., 1980; 1983b,c). This variant differs from β^A by the substitution of the 18th amino acid, lysine in Hbβ^A with histidine in Hbβ^{Bali}. This is one of the substitutions separating β^A from β^B, so β^{Bali} is clearly an intermediate. Namikawa et al (1983c) discuss their findings in relation to other sequenced artiodactyl haemoglobins and conclude that the most probable explanation is that the mutation 18 lysine → histidine arose in a common ancestor of the lines which evolved to β^{Bali} and, by two subsequent mutations, β^B.

There are many other variants of cattle haemoglobin. Two more, $C_{Rhodesia}$

and D_{Zambia} have been sequenced and appear to have evolved from β^A by one and two substitutions respectively. Most other variants have not yet been sequenced, including HbI which seems to be a characteristic marker of sanga cattle (Meyer, 1984). Where the globin chains have been separated, most variants have been found to be in the β-chain. However, the mithan has an electrophoretically undetectable mutation of the α-chain (Lalthantluanga et al., 1975). A further dimension to haemoglobin variation is that some species have duplicated α-chains or electrophoretic patterns which suggest this arrangement: e.g., *Bison bison* and possibly *B. bonasus* (Harris et al., 1973), water buffalo (Ranjekar and Barnabas, 1969) and *Syncerus caffer* (Osterhoff et al., 1970).

The situation regarding the yak is not yet clear. Lalthantluanga and Braunitzer (1981) found two types of α-globin chain and two types of β-globin chain in the haemoglobin of a single yak. This finding could be interpreted as either duplication of α- and β-chains; or as some combination of chain duplication and polymorphism. Gene frequency data do not clarify the matter. Mkrtchyan (1975) found the following phenotypic frequencies: of 205 Altai yaks, A = 0, B = 3, X = 1 and AB = 201; χ^2 144.07; and of 377 Mongolian yaks, A = 8, B = 25 and AB = 313; $\chi^2 = 318.91$! Zhanchiv (1978) screened the haemoglobin of 107 Mongolian yaks: 61 from the 'desert–steppe zone' were typed as A = 40, B = 1, and AB = 20; and, 46 from the 'forest–steppe zone' were typed as A = 45, B = 0 and AB = 1.

Thus, the data of Mkrtchyan (1975) are most easily interpreted in terms of a duplicate haemoglobin locus which has spread throughout nearly all of the population of yaks which had been screened. However, the data of Zhanchiv (1978) are more in line with the results of sampling from typical cattle populations, where there is a simple genetic polymorphism segregating out. It remains to be established whether or not the differences between Mkrtchyan (1975) and Zhanchiv (1978) are the result of technical problems in preparing stable haemolysates and in electrophoresing haemoglobin, or the result of significant differences among yak populations in the degree of gene duplication and the amount of genetic polymorphism (perhaps the consequence of different degrees of admixture of wild and domestic yaks, or introgressive hybridization with other bovines).

There are also milk proteins which differ from each other by more than one amino acid substitution without there being a known intermediate. The common variants β-lactoglobulin A vs. B and κ-casein A vs. B both differ by two amino acid substitutions. Mahé and Grosclaude (1982) found that α_{s2}-casein A of *B. taurus* differed from α_{s2}-casein C of the yak by 33 glutamate → glycine, and 130 threonine → isoleucine. Bell et al. (1981a) believe that the β-lactoglobulins E and F, both found in Bali cattle, differ from each other by the substitutions 50 proline → serine and 129 (or 130) aspartate → tyrosine.

The extension of work on milk proteins from *B. taurus* to other species of cattle is yielding interesting results, although so far the numbers of individual animals are small: about 200 yaks and 107 hybrids (Grosclaude et al., 1976, 1982) and a maximum of 8 Bali cattle (Bell et al., 1981a,b). Several new variants (in addition to the two described above) have been identified. The challenge is now to obtain more information to clarify bovine phylogeny and also to establish the role of different variants in calf nutrition, especially in difficult environments. In the latter context, for example, it has been suggested that the carbohydrate moiety of β-lactoglobulin Droughtmaster could add considerable water of hydration, which could be an advantage in the arid Australian environment (Manwell and Baker, 1970, p. 332).

7.2. Measurement of genetic distance

The first comparisons between populations on the basis of protein polymor-

Chapter 10 references, p. 289

phisms involved little more than a locus by locus consideration of a few breeds screened for a few loci. Measures of genetic distance facilitate interpopulation comparisons as a single number summarizes the differences at many loci observed between each pair of populations. Pairwise genetic distances can be used in the comparison of a large number of populations and to determine the degree of relationship between populations.

Various measures of genetic distance have been reviewed by C.A.B. Smith (1977). He concluded that many gave results which were in close agreement with each other. However, other studies have revealed that agreement may only be close when evolutionary time is short; and that some measures make assumptions which are not true of natural populations, such as random mating, gene frequencies between 0.05 and 0.95, and the absence of mutation, genetic drift and hybridization (see discussions by Balakrishnan and Sanghvi, 1968; Heuch, 1975; Nei, 1976).

7.2.1. Standard genetic distance

Probably the most frequently used measure is the *standard genetic distance* of Nei (1972, 1975, 1976). This is based on the concept of codon differences but uses gene frequency data from biochemical polymorphisms. Nei's standard distance accommodates gene frequencies between 0.00 and 1.00 and makes no assumptions about evolutionary forces. In addition to the theoretical advantages, there are two pragmatic reasons for using Nei's standard distance: the wide application by many workers makes it easy to compare the results of different studies; and it is easy to calculate.

The *standard genetic distance* is:

$$D = -\log_e I$$

where I, the *gene identity,* is:

$$I = J_{XY}/\sqrt{(J_X J_Y)}.$$

The J's (see also p. 000) are simply the sum of the cross-products (J_{XY}) and the sums of the squares (J_X and J_Y) of the corresponding gene frequencies in the two populations, X and Y, being compared. In other words, I is essentially the correlation coefficient between the gene frequencies in the two populations.

The identity, I of the Jersey and the Guernsey in respect of the Hbβ locus is calculated from their respective gene frequencies: Jersey, A = 0.59 and B = 0.41; and Guernsey, A = 0.87 and B = 0.13.

$$I = (0.59 \times 0.87) + (0.41 \times 0.13)/\sqrt{(0.59^2 + 0.41^2) \times (0.87^2 + 0.13^2)}$$

$$= 0.5666/\sqrt{(0.5162 \times 0.7738)} = 0.8965$$

The mean value is then calculated over several loci as follows:

Locus	J_{XY}	J_X (Jersey)	J_Y (Guernsey)
Hb (data shown above)	0.5666	0.5162	0.7738
Tf (data not shown)	0.4571	0.5529	0.5322
AmyI (data not shown)	0.5730	0.5854	0.5624
Σ	1.5970	1.6551	1.8691
Means	0.5323	0.5517	0.6206

$I = 0.5323/\sqrt{(0.5517 \times 0.6206)} = 0.9097$

$D = -\log_e I = 0.0946$

(Because of its similarity to the correlation coefficient, the gene identity, I, can be easily calculated on many pocket calculators, especially those programmable versions which yield the basic statistics for two variables. Nei's group have computer programs available to calculate the variance of genetic distances.)

Estimates of genetic distance should be made over a large number of loci (ideally 30 or more) with equal effort applied to both monomorphic and polymorphic proteins. Nei (1975, p. 178) points out that where few loci are used the estimates of genetic distance may 'deviate considerably' from the real value; but that the estimates can still be useful for comparing the relative values of genetic distance between populations within the same species.

7.2.2. Gene substitution

One check on the relative values obtained for an interbreed comparison is to see if the magnitude and ranking of relationships are similar when they are calculated by another method (Blokhuis and Buis, 1979; Manwell and Baker, 1980; Baker, 1982; Aupetit, 1985). Gene substitution is another measure which it is easy to calculate. For each locus, the average gene substitution is half the sum of the differences between two populations for the frequencies of each allele at that
locus: $\Sigma_i|X_i - Y_i|/2$.

For the Jersey and the Guernsey, the gene substitution at the transferrin locus with three alleles A, D and E would be (with the Jersey frequency first in each case): A(0.6638 vs. 0.3717 = 0.2921) + D(0.3351 vs. 0.6277 = 0.2926) + E(0.0011 vs. 0.0006 = 0.0005)/2 = 0.5852/2 = 0.2926.

To obtain an average value over a number of loci, the values for the individual loci are summed and divided by the number of loci.

7.3. Genetic distance and the uniqueness of breeds

Many authorities consider that one of the central problems in gene conservation is how to identify uniqueness, Miller (1977) suggested that biochemical polymorphism could help in three ways: by revealing rare alleles, by the simple comparison of breeds for the frequency of alleles at single loci, and by estimation of genetic distance. Devillard (1981, p. 104) was more sceptical and asked 'Est-il possible d'en donne une mesure relativement objective et globale? En particulier, le polymorphisme biochemique est-il, ou non, un bon indicateur de cette originalité? Comment mesurer la 'distance genetique' entre deux races?'

If the conditions of screening many polymorphic and monomorphic loci are fulfilled, genetic distance can be an excellent means of distinguishing between populations, but *only* in respect of the loci included. Failure to find differences does not mean that differences do not exist. In some methods there is also a danger that an average distance over all loci could mask differences at individual loci. Nei's method obviates that danger, as the comparisons of individual loci are part of the normal calculations.

Another important question is: are the differences significant? Our approach is to use contingency tables to test every pairwise comparison of breeds at each locus for the null hypothesis that the gene frequencies could be sampled from identical populations (Manwell and Baker, 1980; Baker, 1982; Baker and Manwell, 1984). On this basis it is possible to distinguish between closely related breeds compared for only a few polymorphic loci. Breeds which have arisen by, or been influenced by, crossbreeding may also be distinct. For example, the Illawarra, the Canadian and the Swedish Red and White (which have all received contributions from the Ayrshire and the Shorthorn) differ

Chapter 10 references, p. 289

significantly from the parental breeds and from each other at one or more of four loci (Baker and Manwell, 1984).

7.4. Phylogenetic trees for major breed groups

We have discussed the construction of phylogenetic trees in two recent papers (Manwell and Baker, 1980; Baker and Manwell, 1983a). Hence this section will be devoted to the results of existing studies.

Trees were constructed by two methods from data available in the literature for ten major groups: north European (N); Pied Lowland (L); European Red (R); Channel Island *brachyceros* (C); Upland *brachyceros* (U); *primigenius–brachyceros* mixed (M); *primigenius* (P); zebu, *Bos indicus* (Z); African humped with zebu admixture (A); and African humped sanga (S). Considerable confidence can be placed in these trees. Despite the migrations of man and cattle, these breed groups show a surprising degree of coherence (Baker and Manwell, 1980). The data used in the trees were tested for the statistical significance of each pairwise comparison of breed groups, both for individual loci (Baker and Manwell, 1980) and for mean values over all loci (Manwell and Baker, 1980, especially pp. 155–156). Furthermore, the two very different methods of construction yielded essentially identical phylogenetic trees, strong evidence that the underlying data set are of good quality and that the resulting phylogenetic trees are robust to different generating procedures. Our results contrast with some studies where a computer is used to generate

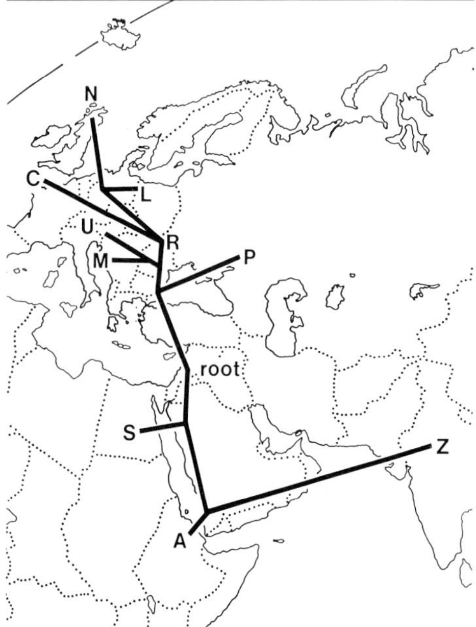

Fig. 10.1. Superposition of the phylogenetic tree for ten major cattle breed groups onto a map of Europe, western Asia and northern Africa. The phylogenetic tree was calculated by a modification of the Fitch–Margoliash minimal average deviation method (see Manwell and Baker, 1980). The *relative* lengths of branches, and the branching pattern, are determined entirely from gene frequency data. The superposition involves an arbitrary scaling of the entire tree. The location of the tips of the branches is partly arbitrary in that the branches can rotate about nodes; however, once the tree is scaled and the first branches placed in appropriate geographical positions, the location of the remaining nodes and branches becomes increasingly constrained by the mathematical analysis of the original gene frequency data. Thus, the degree of genetic divergence is proportional to geographic distance. It is of interest that the root of the tree (located purely by mathematical means) is close to Çatal Hüyük in Turkey in the Near Eastern 'fertile crescent', the oldest known major cattle culture and a probable centre of domestication. The one-letter abbreviations for the major breed groups are explained in the text (p. 275).

a large number of phylogenetic trees from which the 'best' are selected (e.g., Kidd, 1969). When a large number of possible trees are nearly equally probable for a given data set, the final choice becomes rather arbitrary, allowing subjective factors and preconceived ideas to influence what purports to be a rigorously deduced, quantitative measure.

The distances between the ten major breed groups are proportional to the geographic distances between their centre of origin, and by rotating the branches the tree can be superimposed on a map (Fig. 10.1). The locations of the northern European (N) and *primigenius* groups are a compromise in terms of their geographic distribution, but the latter can be accommodated by rotating each of the branches in an arc: from southern England to Scandinavia for northern European cattle, and from Podolia in the U.S.S.R. towards Italy for *primigenius* cattle.

Bos indicus zebu cattle (Z) are very distinct from the taurine breed groups. In the phylogenetic tree the Indian cattle are at the end of the longest branch (Fig. 10.1). The sum of the gene substitutions between all other nine major breed groups is 35.79, as compared with figures of 14.57–23.09 among the other groups. The value of 35.79 is equivalent to the range of distances which Nei (1975, p. 185) cites for differences between mammalian species, thus supporting the validity of the Linnean species *B. indicus* (Francis, 1970; Naik, 1978; Manwell and Baker, 1980; Namikawa et al., 1984).

Recently our conclusions have been criticized on the grounds that: 'Manwell and Baker (1980) do not discuss the taxonomic position of the African zebu which on their chart [sic!] is almost halfway to the European breed but in appearance can be almost identical with the Indian zebu' (Epstein and Mason, 1984, p. 25). In fact, we wrote (Manwell and Baker, 1980, pp. 160 and 161):

> 'The largest deviation in the superposition of phylogenetic tree to geography (Fig. 5) is for the African Humped cattle. The shortness of their arcs can be explained in two ways:
> 1. Their centres of origin are in northeastern Africa. Migration to the present locations of many Sanga breeds in southern Africa is a recent phenomenon, consequent to human migrations which occurred largely in the last two thousand years (Bisschop, 1937; Epstein, 1971).
> 2. Hybridization of *Bos indicus* with *B. taurus* or Sanga breeds. As Epstein (1971) details thoroughly, hybridization among diverse African cattle breeds is extensive . . .'

The Sanga type of African Humped cattle are intermediate between *B. taurus* and *B. indicus*, plus having certain unique characters of their own. Part of this intermediate condition may be secondary gene flow consequent to migration of *B. indicus* into much of Africa in the last two thousand years. However, as Braend (1979) suggests in discussing the humpless West African Dwarf Shorthorns, some similarities may represent convergent evolution in adapting to the rigours of a tropical environment.

It is hoped that the phylogenetic situation of African cattle will be clarified further. For example, do sanga cattle represent, at least in part, the survivors of the taxon variously referred to as *Bos primigenius mauritanicus* P. Thomas 1881 and *Bos opisthonomus* Pomel 1894? Another topic of interest is the position of the West African Humpless cattle and the suggested migration of *brachyceros* cattle to West Africa (Mills, 1953).

Additional trees for breeds considered autochthonous have been constructed for Austria (Kidd and Pirchner, 1971), Iberian cattle (Kidd et al., 1980) and for Italy (Astolfi et al., 1983). Singh and Bhat (1981) have investigated the relationship between breeds of *Bos indicus* (see p. 284).

The cattle of eastern and southeast Asia represent a particular problem as at least three species are involved: *Bos taurus, B. indicus* and *B. javanicus*. Investigations on breeds involving these species have been proceeding for a number of years (Namikawa et al., 1980, 1982, 1983a,b,c and references therein). Recently the relationships of a number of breeds throughout the

Chapter 10 references, p. 289

region have been defined using three polymorphic protein loci and nine blood groups for which all the populations in the study had been screened (Namikawa et al., 1984). Genetic distance was calculated in two ways to give two trees; and the 59 gene frequencies from all loci were examined by principal components analysis based on a variance–covariance matrix constructed from the basic data.

Both trees agreed well in having two major branches. One branch led to the further branching of the taurine breeds. The other branch bifurcated into Bali cattle on the one hand, furthest from the taurine cattle, and indicine and mixed breeds. The purest indicine breeds were closest to the Bali cattle. Principal components analysis confirmed this arrangement. It may be remembered that this coincides with the suggested evolution of the Hbβ alleles (p. 272); but that skeletal measures and craniometrics (p. 247) both placed taurine cattle closer to Bali and mixed cattle, with *B. indicus* in an isolated position. Such data confirm the distinctness of *Bos indicus*.

Namikawa et al. (1984) found that the Asian breeds could be divided into six groups: imported European taurine breeds (actually the Pied Lowland group); East Asian native taurine breeds (Japanese and Korean); Taiwan–Philippine breeds (of mixed origin); Thai–Malaysian–Indonesian breeds (of mixed origin); indicine breeds; and Bali cattle. It was concluded that the major factor for the diversification among the mixed groups was migration and gene flow rather than isolation of subdivided populations.

In another study Namikawa et al. (1982) used 15 electrophoretically identified loci, six of which were monomorphic, to compare breeds of Indonesian cattle and banteng. Three populations of Bali cattle were close to each other and to the banteng. The Ongole (*B. indicus*) and an Ongole-derived breed were separate from *B. javanicus*. Madura cattle gave evidence of a considerable number of Bali genes and also had the highest gene diversity.

A phylogenetic tree has been constructed for water buffalo and anoa, using 23 electrophoretically identified loci (Amano et al., 1982b). Seven Indonesian populations of swamp buffalo were clustered in two subgroups. A population of river buffalo was apart from the swamp populations. Amano et al. (1982b, 1983) suggested that this might indicate domestication from separate populations. Not many anoa were available but the two lowland anoa, *Anoa depressicornis*, were distinct from the 11 mountain anoa, *A. quarlesi* and/or *A. fergusoni*, although the distance was less than between the swamp and river buffaloes.

Further work involving more populations of river and swamp buffalo, screened for the same 23 electrophoretically identified loci and for blood groups confirmed the differences between the swamp and river groups (Amano, 1983). It was found that the transferrin A allele and the albumin X allele were both confined to the swamp buffalo, and that some of the blood typing reagents produced from swamp buffalo gave no reaction with river buffalo. The breeds of swamp buffaloes surveyed formed three subgroups; Taiwan–Philippine–Okinawa, Malaysia–Thailand, and Indonesia.

7.5. The uniqueness of breeds and breed membership

Occasionally it is necessary to decide whether an animal really belongs to a certain breed. There are few published accounts of this problem but most of them involve show animals (Baker and Manwell, 1983a,b; Stormont, 1984). We also know of unpublished cases which involve numerically small breeds or imports for which there was a sudden demand. A common feature of such cases is that the dam is no longer available. Sometimes the problem may be solved readily when the animals in question have a marker which does not occur in their supposed breed, as in the case of the 'pedigree' Holstein who turned out to be part Jersey (Stormont, 1984). The solution is not always so easy. In these cases one method is to use the phenotypic frequencies of whole breeds for single loci to calculate breed phenotypes, both for single loci and for combinations of loci (Hines, 1977). The probability that an animal is a purebred member of a certain breed is calculated by comparing its phenotype with the frequency expected for the same markers within the breed generally. But care is needed to distinguish between crossing and interbreed variation, especially for combinations only expected in low frequency.

These problems may arise in the course of breed conservation, but a more common situation concerns non-pedigree animals. There may be no herd book or pedigree records at all; or there may be a herd book, but only a small number of registered animals. In either case decisions may be needed as to how non-pedigree animals of purportedly pure breeding can be recognized.

One example of such a decision is provided by Osterhoff (1966). Since 1950 a group of cattle had been recognized as a single breed, the Nguni, largely on the basis of type. But doubts remained: the animals were very heterogeneous for colour and pattern, having at least seven whole colours, three mixed colours and eight colour patterns; and there were two separate populations owned by two separate tribes, the Zulu and the Swazi. These two cattle populations were found to have identical gene frequencies for seven blood group factors, which supported the decision to regard them as a single breed.

We know of at least two cases where protein polymorphism data could have helped to resolve problems. One concerns the Blue Albion which, because its colours have led some people to suspect it is derived from recent Friesian–Shorthorn crosses, has not been accepted by the Rare Breeds Survival Trust (Alderson, 1981, p. 55). However, the Blue Albion is associated with Derbyshire, and the earliest reference to the cattle of this county is that they were black (Markham, 1615, Book 2, p. 105). Nearly 200 years later Beevor (1788) wrote of his 'Derbyshire black and white bull'. Young (1771, vol. 1, p. 183 and vol. 4, pp. 40 and 73; 1804, p. 184) noted two types of Derbyshire cattle: the long-horned Derbyshire, similar to the Lancashire and a good milker; and the polled (and sometimes spotted) Derbyshire. We know from other sources that Longhorn stock were common in the Pennines and the adjoining districts, and that at least one other polled breed of Longhorn was known (Marshall, 1818, vol. 1; Dickinson, 1852). Thus the Blue Albion could be one of the last remnants of the Pennine Longhorn breeds. If subsequent crossing has occurred, this need not alter the claim to breed uniqueness. For example, the Belgian Blue and White is known to be based on crosses of Shorthorn and Pied Lowland cattle, but its breed status is unquestioned. Furthermore, crossed-in genes may be lost, either by chance or as immigration load (Kästli, 1979; Namikawa et al., 1983a,b; see also p. 000).

The other case involved a breeder who claimed that he had a relict herd of Glamorgan cattle, generally thought to be extinct. The Rare Breeds Survival Trust rejected these cattle because of the lack of pedigree data.

In both cases, screening the cattle for 30 or more electrophoretically detected loci could have helped to resolve the question of breed identity (and also prevented some bitter arguments). Even if no obviously diagnostic loci were found for either group, there are statistical procedures which will identify of origin of a population with an accuracy of over 90% (Powell, 1983).

8. CASE HISTORIES

8.1. Introductory comment

Concentrating on marker genes, we present four very different case

---

Chaptér 10 references, p. 289

histories to provide a more integrated view of the issues that arise at the intersection of gene conservation and cattle breeding. These four case histories illustrate the value of molecular markers when their study is integrated with historical, cultural and practical information.

8.2. Såtenäs Hero

The interest of practical breeders in breed structure arises from a wish to concentrate desirable traits but to avoid deleterious effects often thought to be associated with inbreeding. Hence, breeders will stress relationship to a famous animal–up to a point. They also take steps to avoid or reduce inbreeding. A traditional method is for a breed to diverge into distinct lines (sometimes called families or tribes) to allow a 'change of blood' (e.g., Tanner, 1858). The case history of the Swedish Red and White bull 134 Såtenäs Hero reveals the genetic consequences of such a policy and illuminates three other situations: the reconciliation of inbreeding due to small numbers with successful conservation (p. 271); Wriedt's paradox (p. 248); and, what Close (1984) considers to be a paradox of rare breeds.

It is expected that the higher the relationship of individuals to a famous sire the more resemblance there will be in gene frequencies to that sire's particular genotype. Rendel (1963) examined this expectation in the Swedish Red and White cattle breed. The coefficient of relationship to the bull 134 Såtenäs Hero (who had been used extensively five to six generations previously) was compared with changes in gene frequencies at nine blood group loci. Groups of animals with the highest coefficients of relationship to Såtenäs Hero were distinguished by significantly different gene frequencies at seven of the nine loci. The coincidence was so marked that, although Såtenäs Hero had not been blood-typed (he died in 1943), his phenotype could be reconstructed. As Braend (1981) has pointed out, it is of particular interest that Såtenäs Hero had the two phenogroups of the B blood group system, B O_3 Y_1 A^1 $E^1{}_3$ and b, which are probably identical with the same phenogroups in the Shorthorn, which was used to improve the Swedish Red and White.

In addition, Rendel's (1963) study of the influence of Såtenäs Hero revealed that the level of inbreeding in the Swedish Red and White was not solely due to the widespread use of this sire. The coefficient of relationship to Såtenäs Hero increased with the coefficient of inbreeding in groups of bulls with F_i values of up to 0.069 – but, groups of bulls with higher coefficients of inbreeding actually had a slightly lower coefficient of relationship to Såtenäs Hero.

Evidence from studies on blood groups of a similar avoidance of too much inbreeding towards a famous sire was observed by Maijala and Lindström (1966) in the Finnish Ayrshire, though not in the Finnish breed of cattle.

Rendel (1963) pointed out that, whether or not inbreeding to Såtenäs Hero increased homozygosity in the population, would depend on his genotype at each locus. If he were heterozygous, the frequency of the two alleles should approach 0.5 as relationship of the population to Såtenäs Hero increased. (Although Rendel did not say so explicitly, this assumes either neutral alleles or a special case of balancing selection where the adaptive values of the two alleles are identical in homozygotes). Alleles for which Såtenäs Hero was homozygous were expected to increase towards a frequency of 1 as relationship to him increased.

These expectations illustrate the use of the coefficient of inbreeding to correct the coefficient of relationship for the case of inbred animals with a common ancestor (p. 261).

For three simple blood group systems for which Såtenäs Hero was homozygous (F^V, j and Z), the regression of gene frequency on the coefficient of relationship was statistically significant (Rendel, 1963). In the L blood system no significant change occurred — but Såtenäs Hero was homozygous for the *l* allele, which had a frequency of over 0.9 in the population as a whole.

For the three systems for which Såtenäs Hero was heterozygous, one (*Aa*) already had a frequency close to 0.5 in the whole population and thus showed little change. The other two blood group systems for which Såtenäs Hero was heterozygous showed irregularities. Rendel (1963) explained that these irregularities could have arisen because much of Såtenäs Hero's influence was through sons and grandsons, some of which had been used more than others.

As the possible loss of heterozygosity by inbreeding is of concern to breeders and geneticists, it is surprising that there are not many publications where calculated coefficients of inbreeding are compared with actual genotype frequencies.

Finally, in due respect to Såtenäs Hero's potency, one wonders why he and his sons were so favoured. Rendel (1963, p. 231) explains the great popularity of bull 134 Såtenäs Hero as arising from 'his good body conformation and vitality, characters which were transmitted to his progeny.' However, in a breed where milk production was important the 1947 Official Progeny Test report on 168 of his dam–daughter pairs revealed that, although the butterfat levels were 'satisfactory', '. . . Såtenäs Hero seems to have carried less satisfying genes for milk yield . . .'

Rendel's finding that inbreeding was not all concentrated within a single line is one means by which inbreeding can be reconciled with the maintenance of a population with small effective numbers over a long period. The other means is the retention of heterozygosity, even within a single line, and with the possibility of forming sublines which could also be used to reduce inbreeding.

Inbreeding may improve a breed, as by the transmission of 'conformation and vitality'. It is also possible for undesirable genes to become concentrated, sometimes with more drastic consequences than 'less satisfying milk yield', thus giving rise to Wriedt's paradox.

Close (1984) noted that '. . . with a rare breed . . . there tends to be more variation of both type and quality. However, rare breeds are relatively inbred and this means that individuals are more likely to breed true to type. This fact, taken with the inherent variation, allows rapid progress'. The case of Såtenäs Hero suggests that this seeming paradox can be explained by line formation within a breed. The phenomenon observed by Close is not necessarily a characteristic of rare breeds *per se*. It seems to be associated with breeds that have a democratic structure of independently minded breeders, which prevents undue emphasis on a few fashionable élite herds (Baker, 1983, p. 10).

8.3. The South Devon

So far, most of the emphasis has been on the benefits of applying biochemical techniques to breed management. The present case history demonstrates that it is possible for biochemical techniques to be misused. It is hoped that an examination of the factors involved will prevent further incidents of this kind. The matter is far from trivial. It concerns the future of a breed and the livelihood of many breeders. Unless corrected, such incidents also raise doubts about the credibility of advice from scientists.

The South Devon is an ancient British landrace. The historical evidence is that it diverged from the same common stock as the North Devon, and that after divergence there was some gene flow from the latter. The other main contribution to the South Devon was from the Channel Island breeds, especially the Guernsey, early in the 19th century. Minor contributions may have been made by other adjacent related breeds, by the Shorthorn and, possibly, from

---

Chapter 10 references, p. 289

B. indicus (Baker, 1983, 1984).

Recently a claim has been made that the '. . . Gelbvieh and South Devon had a common ancestry on the Continent and are distinct from other British breeds such as Hereford, Angus and Jersey' (Kidd et al., 1974). This arose because a group of South African breeders of South Devon cattle wanted to cross their stock with Gelbvieh bulls and have the progeny accepted in the herd book as purebred.

The biochemical data upon which the claim rests were not published and despite a statement by Kidd et al (1974, p. 24) that 'the exact allele frequencies used are available from the authors', repeated requests for this information have been ignored. However, it was possible to assemble and analyse data from other reports. One analysis confirmed that the South Devon belongs in the English Lowland breed group and the Gelbvieh in the Yellow Mountain section of the Upland *brachyceros* breed group (Baker and Manwell, 1980). The second study, made at the level of individual breeds, placed the South Devon closer to the North Devon, Hereford and Guernsey than to the Gelbvieh. History provided no evidence that the South Devon had any 'common ancestry on the Continent' with the Gelbvieh (Baker, 1982).

Individual reasons for the discrepancies have been discussed elsewhere (Baker, 1982, 1984). For the present consideration, in relation to conservation, three aspects are important.

(1) The study of Kidd et al. (1984) did not incorporate enough internal scientific safeguards, such as: a large number of unequivocally typed systems; screening several subpopulations of South Devons (only South African South Devons were used); inclusion of close relatives of the South Devon to establish the relative values of calculated distances; and analysis of data by more than one method.

(2) Kidd et al. (1974) based their conclusions on the analysis of biochemical data. The history of the South Devon was dismissed as 'unknown'. Tracing the evolution of breeds and the relationships between them is not the function of any one discipline to the exclusion of all others, but the synthesis of information from a variety of sources.

(3) The social pressures were important. There were exporters and importers who could benefit financially from the 'right' solution. One of the scientists was based in a country which would benefit from exports. All scientists have to consider how their work will appear in competitive situations for jobs, promotions and grants. A positive result (in this case that technical skill has proved an unlikely relationship) is more attractive than a negative result.

The South Devon also demonstrates another point important for conservation. This breed did not differ significantly from the North Devon at any of the three individual loci which were available for comparison (Baker, 1982). *This does not mean that other differences do not exist.* The present North and South Devon breeds are distinct and separate by a number of traits, including the easily measured larger size, different conformation and higher average milk yields of the latter.

8.4. Beefalo and Cattalo

The case history of the Beefalo has been reviewed twice as an example of the utility of molecular markers in breed history (Baker and Manwell, 1983a,b; Stormont, 1984). It also illustrates three other topics: how breeders will persevere to create a new breed for a difficult environment; how, with a negligible contribution to that breed, agribusiness interests will try to reap the profits by manipulating reports in the media and by advertising; and how molecular markers revealed the absence of substance to agribusiness claims and vindicated the claims of the legitimate breeders.

The Beefalo is a breed based on hybridization of taurine cattle and American bison and is supposed to have, on average, three-eighths of its genes from the latter species. The idea of such hybrids can be traced to 1598, and there are isolated records of their existence in the 18th and 19th centuries (McHugh and Hobson, 1972, p. 307; Roe, 1972, p. 707). Larger experiments with such a hybrid breed were made by private breeders in Canada and the U.S.A. in the late 19th and early 20th century (Boyd, 1914; Goodknight, 1914); and Agriculture Canada investigated the hybrids from 1916 to 1964 (Peters, 1984). Formation of the hybrid breed was not easy: behavioural barriers to interspecific mating existed; there was an apparent immune response of taurine cows carrying hybrid calves which resulted in high mortality; and F_1 males from reciprocal crosses were sterile, which meant that F_1 females had to be back-crossed to the parental species (Peters, 1984). One of the early breeders named the new breed 'Cattalo', defined as the '. . . produce of the third stage in which both parents are of mixed blood' (Boyd, 1914).

Many of the traits valued by early breeders were intangibles. In Texas, Cattalo were said to be less likely to be cast (unable to get up) because they got up forelegs first, like a bison; to eat less and to go without water longer than taurine cattle; and, depending on the amount of bison, to have higher resistance to diseases such as Texas fever (Goodknight, 1914). In Canada, Cattalo survived better in heavy snow and extreme cold than taurine cattle (Smoliak and Peters, 1955). Most writers commented favourably on the yield and quality of the meat, but experimental comparisons were made against Herefords under feedlot conditions. Not surprisingly, the average performance of the Herefords was the better, although individual Cattalo and bison performed well, indicating the possibility of selection (Peters, 1958). The 'lack of finish' (i.e., less fat) which then resulted in the lower grading of bison and hybrids is now regarded as a positive attribute.

The hybrid breed remained relatively unknown until the early 1970's, when a Mr D.C. Basalo of Stockton, California, gave it considerable publicity under the name of Beefalo. Mr Basalo claimed that the Beefalo was '. . . based on the first successful crosses after more than a hundred years of experiment between a cow and a North American Buffalo' (Anon., 1973; Clayton, 1975). Other claims (without any supporting data) included: disease resistance; fattening faster on 'the poorest and scrubbiest of feeds'; high quality lean meat with '10 or 12 per cent higher protein than cattle' which was quicker to cook; production costs from 25% to 75% less than cattle; and 'It also produced fur coats' (Anon., 1973; Clayton, 1975). However, one reporter remarked sarcastically that the Beefalo '. . . was promoted as the ninth wonder of the agri-world' (Milner, 1977).

Subsequent events in the marketing of Beefalo semen (at £12.50 a dose) have been described by Milner (1977). An agreement was made with a company called EuroPacific, headed by a Mr O. Hemphill. EuroPacific became involved in a number of business manipulations to attract investors, and 'at least one' parted with $50 000. Eventually the scheme crashed, and '. . . EuroPacific filed for a Chapter XI bankruptcy with debts of more than $800 000'. At this stage the Basalos dissociated themselves from Mr Hemphill, Mrs Basalo saying: 'He was just a promoter trying to capitalise on the word Beefalo.'

Such events are damaging. Even if EuroPacific had sold large quantities of semen, there would have been many disappointed buyers. Established breeders were sceptical of many of the advertising claims, and not least in the claim that the Basalo-bred Beefalo was a hybrid of American bison. However, the bison contribution is not easy to determine from conformation. Once the stage of crossing Cattalo *inter se* was reached, 'the proportion of bison blood no longer determines the likeness to the bison' (Boyd, 1914).

Chapter 10 references, p. 289

Stormont and his colleagues have established that there are several American bison-specific markers. Using four marker loci, it has been calculated that at least one marker should be found in 99.4% of Beefalo (advertised as three-eighths bison) and in 83.3% of half-bred Beefalo (three-sixteenths bison) (Stormont, 1984). The first studies revealed *no* bison markers in seven full-blood Beefalo, and *only one* marker in *one* of 141 half-bred Beefalo; yet other cattle × bison hybrids back-crossed to cattle revealed bison markers in 9 out of 12 animals, compared with an expected 11 out of 12. Further screening of full- and half-bred Basalo Beefalo has failed to reveal *any* bison markers; but, animals described as three-eighths, one-quarter, one-eighth and one-sixteenth bison, and not of Basalo origin had frequencies of bison markers which did not differ significantly from those expected (Stormont, 1984).

8.5. Taurindicus

Although the term 'taurindicus' has no taxonomic validity, it is very useful for describing the many breeds and types of cattle derived from crosses of *Bos taurus* and *B. indicus*. At one end of the range is the Brahman, usually regarded as zebu, but with exaggerated expression of some *indicus* characteristics, such as large ears, dewlap and penis sheath; and, at the other extreme there is the Illawarra, usually regarded as taurine (pp. 238 and 275). The evolution of taurindicus has been regarded as sufficiently important for government participation in some projects, as by USDA in grading up to Brahman, and CSIRO in the formation of new breeds in Australia. These projects have led to the accumulation of a vast literature describing many production traits. But there seems to have been very little attempt to follow the process of breed formation, although information about this process would be useful for an understanding of breed evolution in general and as a yardstick for the formation of yet other breeds in the future.

An exception to this lack of synthetic studies is the series of investigations, by P.N. Bhat, Harpreet Singh and their colleagues, of the use of Friesian cattle to increase milk production in India. These investigations are of interest both because of the results obtained and because they form a model for future work.

One set of investigations concerned the records for nine production traits collected for 30 years on each of eight Holstein × Sahiwal herds (Taneja et al., 1979). The cattle were assigned on the basis of pedigree records to 40 grades, ranging from pure Sahiwal to 63/64 Holstein. The lowest performers were 'cluster I', which consisted of Sahiwal and high Sahiwal grades. The highest performers were 'cluster XI', the 63/64 Holstein grades. The next highest were the clusters with around 50% Holstein: *there was no linear increase in production above this level*, suggesting that grading up need not lead to higher production. Taneja et al. (1979) pointed out that the average expected proportion of exotic inheritance might not be achieved. They suggested that the two extremes could be absorbed into their respective pure breeds, but that the remaining cattle should be used as the basis of a stable breed, formed by the use of crossbred bulls mating *inter se* and with intensive selection.

Singh and Bhat (1980) noted the desirability of further information concerning the situation just described. A check was made on the relative contributions from the parental species and breeds, using eight electrophoretically identified loci (Singh and Bhat, 1980, 1981; Singh et al., 1981, 1983). The papers resulting from these investigations provide one of the best series of coordinated studies of biochemical polymorphism in cattle.

Gene frequencies at each locus were established for each of several indigenous breeds, for Indian-bred Friesians and for hybrids. The extreme differences found in the frequencies of some alleles between the *B. indicus* breeds and the Friesian provided several markers. For the Friesian and for each of several *B. indicus* breeds data were available for more than one herd and estimates of gene diversity were calculated. In both the *B. indicus* breeds and the Friesian the genetic structure of individual breeds was similar. Most of the total diversity was carried within herds. There were only small differences between the total population of each breed and the herds comprising the breed, and only small differences among individual herds within a breed. However, the level of heterozygosity in individual herds was not always due to similar frequencies of the same alleles.

Gene flow into the hybrid populations was followed by their gene diversities and by the migration of marker alleles, using the values of the parental populations as standards. Although the overall results were in good agreement with expectation, some interesting differences were found between different breed crosses and different herds of the same breed cross. One difference arose from the genetic distances between parental breeds: The Sahiwal was closer than the Hariana to the Friesian, and the Friesian × Sahiwal F_1 were closer than the Friesian × Hariana F_1 to the Friesian. In the back-crosses to Friesian, the overall situation was reversed, with the Hariana-based three-quarters Friesians being the closer to the Friesian. The greater overall distance of the Sahiwal-based three-quarters Friesians was due to certain herds and ascribed to the bulls which had been used. It was noted that the Hariana-based back-crosses were by bulls from local Friesian herds of long-standing which had from time to time incorporated graded up animals of 31/32 and 63/64 Friesian ancestry.

Frankel and Soulé (1981, p. 255) have asked: '. . . do we need *all* the breeds of Zebu cattle?' These authors then proceed to devise a '. . . conservation strategy . . . for *Zebu cattle in India*' which would entail the amalgamation of the existing breeds into a maximum of nine categories: milk, draught and dual-purpose × humid tropics, dry tropics and mountains (Frankel and Soulé, 1981, pp. 270–274). This scheme ignores the great diversity of geographic and socio-economic environments of the Indian subcontinent and that there are many attributes which are not covered by the nine categories. For example, when CSIRO (Sir Otto Frankel's institution) decided to import *B. indicus*, the generally low level of Australian stockmanship in northern Australia meant '. . . the search was for a quiet Zebu . . . docility being a prime requirement' (Kelley, 1959, p. ix). The 'conservation strategy' of Frankel and Soulé can only be considered destructive in view of the rich genetic diversity of Indian breeds of cattle, measured by the traditional means of morphology and adaptedness and confirmed by molecular markers.

9. APPLICATION TO PRACTICAL CONSERVATION: RECOMMENDATIONS

We believe that recommendations should be realistic. In breed conservation this means recognizing that relatively little money is available, and that the breeds which are the object of our concern are heterogeneous and widely scattered. The fundamental recommendation is to identify the causes of genetic erosion and to suggest how the loss of genetic diversity can be reduced.

Our survey reveals that much of the decline of breeds can be traced to the loss of the confidence of the breeders because of social factors which become important through the attitudes of others. One of the most important is fashion, frequently manipulated to benefit one section of the community. Another major factor is the strident emphasis of agribusiness interests on 'progress', 'efficiency' and 'production', often made with emotional reference to human needs, and especially needs arising from the human population explo-

Chapter 10 references, p. 289

sion. A more insidious but very dangerous factor is the cult of the expert. The expert can advocate or support policies injurious to independent breeders under the guise of academic conclusions: e.g., the technically worded genetic argument of Donald and El Itriby (1945) that small herds are inefficient, presented without any reference to the opposite genetic theory that evolution is fastest in small demes. Probably the most damaging personal experience of breeders trying to maintain a breed, is that when they seek help, some expert pronounces that the breeds in question are '... varieties ... not sufficiently distinct to be given separate breed status,' or '... no longer true breeds because of crossbreeding' (Alderson, 1981, p. 55). Yet, such pronouncements are made without any attempt to obtain accurate measures of genetic uniqueness, utilizing molecular and other markers, research techniques that have been available for years.

All counter-measures to genetic erosion ultimately rest on knowledge. But social factors are important in making sure that knowledge is applied. First we must mention a social topic which we have not discussed as it has been dealt with adequately by others: the stabilization and reduction of human populations, which is basic to all conservation (Hawkes, 1978, p. 156; Ehrlich and Ehrlich, 1982). It is only by the conservation of the whole environment that the peace, privacy and beauty necessary for the uniquely human properties of aesthetic and cultural development will be available to all and not just a privileged few.

As pointed out by Rognoni and Finzi (1984) breed conservation is a political process and, for success, requires participation from all sections of the community. In France and Italy the breed conservation movement was led by groups of scientists (Laurans, 1974; Rognoni and Finzi, 1984). In the U.K. the academic community was in default and the initiative came from breeders (Ryder, 1976). Fortunately the latter included several who had high social rank. This meant that they were able to place information before the public, and that they were not vulnerable to victimization. They could not be dismissed as cranks as many had important personal attributes and achievements in addition to inherited status. For example, one of the founders of the Rare Breeds Survival Trust, Sir Dudley Forwood, Bt., is '... a one-time soldier, also a diplomat and farmer' (Paris, 1983).

The right to express dissent without fear of subsequent victimization is important. As pointed out by Maijala (1974; see also p. 228) it is easy to dismiss a dissident as 'unrealistic' — and worse can follow (Martin et al., 1986). A major aspect of suppression is the cult of the expert. This is manifest when one or a few people try to monopolize 'their' field to the exclusion of other workers. Another sign is the assumption that, from an expert, a mere statement without supporting evidence is adequate. As no one person or group can possess complete knowledge of even a single discipline, the cult of the expert impedes the development of new insights. The problem can be overcome if both professionals and laymen uphold the right to express a variety of viewpoints, encouraging everyone to examine the evidence critically and dispassionately, but without insensitivity to cultural factors.

Of particular importance is the necessity to reform the peer review procedures used in judging the 'quality' of research and the access to funds and to jobs. It is not generally realized by many scientists that a number of recent studies on the peer review process have shown serious bias, with personal and political factors often determining how public money is spent on science (reviewed: Manwell and Baker, 1986). Among many examples of the suppression of agriculturally relevant research have been studies on marker genes in both rare and economically important livestock in Australia (Manwell, 1979). Organizations concerned with gene conservation and rare breeds should take a more active role in supporting research and use their influence to counter the abuses that occur within government and academe.

The influence of education is almost limitless. Schools of Agriculture (at all levels) should be expected to keep local breeds for use in teaching and research. The latter should include reasonable access by any bona fide workers whether or not they are employed by the institution. In this way, information about a variety of breeds would spread by two routes: by former students to the community at large; and by research publications. Many agricultural institutions do not keep less popular breeds on the grounds that these are 'uneconomic'. As most educational institutions receive support from public funds, such excuses should not be tolerated. Furthermore, rare and lesser-known breeds should not be presented to students from the economic standpoint alone — quite apart from the evidence reviewed by us earlier, that a number of rare breeds show real economic value in the right situation.

Most discussions of breed conservation point to the need for further information and bewail the lack of research funding. We agree with these statements. However, there are a number of projects which could be carried out by individual independent workers at very little cost:

(1) Studies of breed history, preferably on a multi-disciplinary basis.

(2) Analysis of breed structure using herd book data, protein polymorphisms or both, and integrating the findings with breed history.

(3) Methodical recording of the occurrence and frequency of phenotypic variation such as colour and body measurements.

(4) The collection of more gene frequency data for biochemical polymorphisms. Emphasis should be on electrophoretically identified markers. Immunologically detected markers are complicated by the breed- or species-specifities of reagents; and some systems require pedigree information from large families before the reactions can be interpreted. Gene frequency data could be assembled in several ways. It would cost very little extra for organizations which do parentage testing to include more proteins. Another source of information would be to use electrophoretic markers to follow the progress of government-financed breeding schemes. The additional cost would be very small in relation to the total costs. Finally, a number of small grants to individual workers could be used to extend studies to many of the less common breeds. It is particularly desirable to type every individual in a small breed for a large number of loci. Many rare breeds are important as missing links in history and evolution (Ryder, 1976).

(5) The synthesis of information from published sources.

These suggestions lead to the problem of accessibility. For example, Alderson (1981) has claimed that the structure of several British rare breeds has been analysed. Such information could be useful to workers concerned with other rare breeds. But the only definitive publication is that on the Dexter (Young, 1953). This not only demonstrated that inbreeding need not rise, but showed that even in a numerically small breed selection was possible.

Some editors take the attitude '. . . what is the point of recording more and more variants in further species? This activity unless taken to answer specific questions in a precise and quantitative fashion seems to me to have the same intellectual content as stamp collecting' (F.W. Robertson, 1972, p. 50). First, such research should only be rejected for publication if there is evidence for unreliability, or fundamental errors in experimental design — and we all know of published papers which have those drawbacks. Secondly, it is only by 'recording more and more variants' that we will attain more accurate measures of genetic diversity; even the most casual acquaintance with the recent literature on population genetics reveals the number of important papers which used the data published by others on 'more and more variants in further species.' A number of fundamental problems relating to the role of selection versus the theory of neutral alleles may only become decidable with the

Chapter 10 references, p. 289

analysis of very large data bases. Especially in research on livestock, each new marker gene locus provides the potential for more accurate assessment of pedigrees, relationships and population structure — quite apart from the fact that the marker genes may have direct or indirect relevance to traits of economic importance. Each new set of gene frequency data helps to provide a better understanding of population stratification and breed organization.

Suggestions have been made that herd books should be replaced by computer storage (e.g., Barton, 1984). We regard any suggestion to impose secrecy as a retrograde step. Making the pedigrees of livestock public knowledge was a major conceptual advance. We would prefer to see computers used to improve herd books. Computerization could have enormous benefits, but it must not be allowed to fall into the hands of a few scientists and information entrepreneurs. The final print-out could include information on coefficients of relationship to particular sires or dams, coefficients of inbreeding, and data on biochemical or other markers. Computerization, if integrated with other scientific advances, could produce herd books which are more informative and more useful.

We have not given recommendations for minimum numbers, mating systems or other aspects of breeding schemes. There is always a danger that such estimates become criteria for rejection or acceptance. With care and luck, a species can be saved even when the numbers drop as low as 12 (p. 271). The fact that for a number of species of ungulates, including both wild species and domesticates, large and flourishing populations have arisen from introductions as small as 2–18 individuals, reveals that, in a satisfactory environment, narrow bottlenecks do not necessarily lead to extinction (Baker and Manwell, 1981).

Set systems of breeding are often counter-productive. Each breed — indeed, each herd — has idiosyncrasies which should not be ignored.

For the same reasons we do not propose any rules for acceptance, rejection or amalgamation of a breed. But the bases of some decisions are to be deplored. The Ad Hoc Committee (NRC, 1983, p. 20) state that in Madura cattle '. . . genetic variation has been largely removed during 1500 years of continuous breeding.' In fact, Namikawa et al. (1982) found the Madura had the highest heterozygosity of several breeds of Indonesian cattle ($H = 0.2194$). Alderson (1981, p. 55) may be premature to dismiss the White Galloway as merely a colour variant. Apart from the technicality that it has its own herd book, the same could be said of the Belted Galloway. Yet this differs markedly from the Galloway in the frequencies of transferrin variants (Jamieson, 1966) and in skin structure (Jenkinson and Nay, 1972). The biochemical genetics of variants such as the Bolian Gwynion and White Galloway and their parental breeds (the Welsh Black and the Galloway) should be investigated with care. If the variants differ from the parental breeds, separate status should be recognized. If there are no significant differences, the parental breeds should be asked to drop the requirements of colour. It is no longer essential as a trademark now that breed purity can be guaranteed by parentage tests.

When acceptance or rejection of individual breeds is considered, it should always be remembered that failure to find differences only means that differences were not demonstrated by use of the techniques available. Other differences may exist.

The 20th century trend to breed extinction has reached the point where, for milk production, a single breed dominates 80–90% of the numbers in several First World countries. It is instructive to compare the situation of breeds with that for species. In stable environments the number of species is much greater than in unstable or polluted environments. Competition encourages specialization, with each of the many species in stable environments adapted best for some specialized niche. In unstable environments, the boom-or-bust economy of nutrients prevents such species diversity; instead, selection favours those few species which have general tolerance to the degraded environment and the ability to reproduce rapidly (*r*-selection).

Thus, if man is to come to terms with his environment he will need more breeds, not less. Each breed is adapted to a specialized niche, a niche defined by the type of animal husbandry and the economic utilization. For greatest efficiency in the overall system, each breed will be *optimally* specialized (which will include some dual-purpose and triple-purpose generalists as well). As competition for resources increases, in particular as the cost of energy and food concentrates increases faster than the general rate of inflation, man will be less able to afford the luxury of creating uniform environments for his domesticates. It will be necessary to reach a balance with the immediate environment, choosing breeds best able to produce on the immediately available inputs in each of the diverse habitats where man and his domesticates live.

The decline in breed numbers, the loss of genetic diversity, is a consequence of our environmental degradation, a degradation brought on by agribusiness. While this situation is in the best short-term interests of a few, measured in terms of profits of agribusiness and prestige of compliant scientists, it is basically unnatural. The long-term interests will be best served by conforming to the model of species specialization in a stable environment, maintaining, indeed encouraging, a diversity of breeds to fill most efficiently the complex requirements of man and his domesticates.

Genetic markers offer new opportunities to understand the evolution, relationships and structure of cattle breeds. The present accumulation of knowledge is only a beginning but it emphasizes the urgency of conservation. Our domesticated bovines are one of the most precious legacies of many thousand years of coevolution of man and beast.

10. ACKNOWLEDGEMENTS

We thank the many people who have provided us with reprints and other information, especially Dr T. Amano for the publications of the Society for Research on Native Livestock; Miss C.J. Baker for the article by Dent (1983); Miss E.L. Henson for the manuscript based on her research on the Gloucester breed; Dr A. Jamieson for discussions on exclusion probabilities; Dr E.P. Kelly for the data on the Kerry breed; Dr K. Maijala for the unpublished data from Maijala et al. (1984); and Dr H.F. Peters for information on the Cattalo. We also thank the librarians who helped us to obtain a number of references at short notice: the staff in the Reading Room of the National Library, Boston Spa, Yorkshire, especially S. Bygott, M. Marcus and P. Whitehead; and the staff of the Inter-Library Loan service of the University of Adelaide, especially M. van der Wilk, M. Furlan, L.-A. Harris and Marjolijn Jones.

11. REFERENCES

Accredited Poultry Breeders' Federation of England and Wales, 1963. British poultry supremacy must be maintained. Poultry Industry, October, p. 373.

Adams, J. and Ward, J.H., 1973. Admixture studies and the detection of selection. Science, 180: 1137–1143.

Adams, M.B., 1979. From 'Gene Fund' to 'Gene Pool': on the evolution of evolutionary language. Studies History Biol., 3: 241–285.

Alderson, G.L.H., 1981. The conservation of animal genetic resources in the United Kingdom. In: Animal Genetic Resources Conservation Management. Animal Production and Health Paper 24, Food and Agriculture Organization, Rome, pp. 53–76.

Alderson, L., 1978. The Chance to Survive. Rare Breeds in a Changing World. Cameron and Tayleur in association with David and Charles, Newton Abbot.

Amano, T., 1974. Blood groups and serum protein polymorphisms in Thai Water buffalo. Report No. 6, Society for Researches on Native Livestock, pp. 87–91, 163–164, 179–180. (Japanese with English figure and table legends and summary.)
Amano, T., 1978. Coat colour variation and blood protein polymorphisms of the Water buffaloes in the Philippines. Report No. 8, Society for Researches on Native Livestock, pp. 40–48. (Japanese with English figure and table legends and summary.)
Amano, T., 1983. Genetic differences between swamp and river buffaloes in biochemical and immunological characteristics. In: H. Shimizu (Editor), Current Development and Problems in Swamp Buffalo Production, Proc. Preconference Symposium of the 5th World Conference on Animal Production, Tsukaba, Japan, 1983, pp. 131–135.
Amano, T. and Martojo, H., 1983. Karyotypes of water buffaloes and anoas. Report No. 10, Society for Researches on Native Livestock, pp. 98–110, 239, 253. (Japanese with English figure and table legends and summary.) N.B. Swamp and River autosomes also morphological diffs.
Amano, T., Suzuki, S. and Masangkay, J., 1980 Body conformation of water buffaloes on Luzon Island of the Philippines. J. Agric. Sci., Tokyo University Agric., 25: 18–26. (Japanese with English summary and figure and table legends.)
Amano, T., Katsumata, M., Suzuki, S., Nozawa, K., Kawamoto, Y., Namikawa, T., Martojo, H., Abdulgani, I.K. and Nadjib, H., 1981. Morphological and genetical survey of Water buffaloes in Indonesia. In: The Origin and Phylogeny of Indonesian Native Livestock, Vol. II, Investigation on the Goats, Horses and Water Buffaloes. The Research Group of Overseas Scientific Survey, 1981. Grant-in-Aid for Overseas Scientific Survey, Japan, pp. 31–54.
Amano, T., Namikawa, T. and Martojo, H., 1982a. Blood groups of the Banteng (*Bos banteng*) and Indonesian cattle.In: The Origin and Phylogeny of Indonesian Native Livestock, Vol. III, Morphological and Genetical Investigations on the Interrelationship between Domestic Animals and Their Wild forms in Indonesia. The Research Group of Overseas Scientific Survey, 1982, Grant-in-Aid for Overseas Scientific Survey, Japan, pp. 49–52.
Amano, T., Namikawa, T. and Natasamita, S., 1982b. Blood protein polymorphisms of water buffaloes and anoas in Indonesia. In: The Origin and Phylogeny of Indonesian Native Livestock, Vol. III, Morphological and Genetical Investigations on the Interrelationships between Domestic Animals and Their Wild forms in Indonesia. The Research Group of Overseas Scientific Survey, 1982, Grant-in-Aid for Overseas Scientific Survey, Japan, pp. 57–65.
Amano, T., Namikawa, T. and Martojo, H., 1983. Body measurements, blood groups and buffaloes and Anoas in Indonesia. Report No. 10, Society for Researches on Native Livestock, pp. 82–97, 238–239, 252–253. (Japanese with English figure and table legends and summary.)
Anderson, E., 1949. Introgressive Hybridization. Wiley, New York.
Anon., 1973. Have a slice of roast Beefalo. Time, 9 July, p. 41.
Anon., 1974a. Los Toros: Bullfighting. Magallanes, Madrid.
Anon., 1974b. Snow problem. Advertiser (Adelaide), 30 July, p. 2.
Anon., 1982. Proc. Second International Bovine Lymphocyte Antigen (BoLA) Workshop. Anim. Blood Groups Biochem. Genet., 13: 33–53.
Anon., 1984. Triumph for White cattle breeds. Ark, 11 (August): 228.
Ansay, M. and Hanset, R., 1979. Anatomical, physiological and biochemical differences between conventional and double-muscled cattle in the Belgian Blue and White breed. Livestock Prod. Sci. 6: 5–13.
Archibald, A.L., 1981. Bovine serum amylase polymorphism. PhD thesis, University of Edinburgh.
Archibald, J.D.H., 1963. On the banks of a gene pool. Poultry Farmer and Packer, 20 November, p. 11.
Ashton, G.C., 1958. Genetics of beta-globulin polymorphism in British Cattle. Nature, 182: 370–372.
Astolfi, P., Pagnacco, G. and Guglielmino-Matessi, C.R., 1983. Phylogenetic analysis of native Italian cattle breeds. Z. Tierz. Züchtungsbiol., 100: 870–100.
Aupetit, R.Y., 1985. Analyse des relations phylogénétique entre les races bovines françaises par le polymorphisme biochimique. Doctoral Thesis, University of Paris.
Austin, H.B., 1943. The Merino. Past, Present and Probable. Grahame Book Co., Sydney.
Austin, N., 1984a. Where $2000 buys a rare kill. The Australian, 18 September, p. 9.
Austin, N., 1984b. N.T. buffalo to be wiped out in mass slaughter. Weekend Australian, 6–7 October, pp. 1–2.
Bachman, K.L. and Christensen, R.P., 1967. The economics of farm size. In: H.M. Southworth and B.F. Johnston (Editor), Agricultural Development and Economic Growth. Cornell University Press, Ithaca, NY, pp. 234–257.
Bailey, L.F., 1968. Inherited biochemical polymorphisms and their association with production in dairy cattle. PhD thesis, University of Adelaide.
Baker, C.M.A., 1963. Depths of a gene pool. Poultry Farmer and Packer, 25 December, p. 6.
Baker, C.M.A, 1965. Molecular genetics of avian proteins. IV. The egg white proteins of the Golden Pheasant, *Chrysolophus pictus* L., and Lady Amherst's Pheasant, *C. amherstiae* Leadbeater and their possible evolutionary significance. Comp. Biochem. Physiol. 16: 93–101.
Baker, C.M.A., 1982. The use of genetic relationships among cattle breeds in the formulation of

rational breeding policies: a re-examination of the example of the South Devon and the Gelbvieh. Anim. Blood Groups Biochem. Genet., 13: 199–212.
Baker, C.M.A., 1983. A history of South Devon cattle. Aust. South Devon Cattle Breeders' Assoc. Newsl., No. 19, pp. 2–9; No. 20, pp. 2–6; No. 21, pp. 3–7, 10.
Baker, C.M.A., 1984. The origin of South Devon cattle. Agric. History Rev., 32: 145–158.
Baker, C.M.A. and Manwell, C., 1976. Contribution to the study of the evolution of animals at the molecular level with particular reference to the domestic fowl. Philosophical Transactions of the Royal Society of London, B275: 109–113.
Baker, C.M.A. and Manwell, C., 1980. Chemical classification of cattle. I. Breed groups. Anim. Blood Groups Biochem. Genet. 11: 127–150.
Baker, C.M.A. and Manwell, C., 1981. 'Fiercely feral': on the survival of domesticates without care from man. Z. Tierz. Züchtungsbiol., 98: 241–257.
Baker, C.M.A. and Manwell, C., 1983a. Electrophoretic variation of erythrocyte enzymes of domesticated mammals: paradigm shifts, practical problems and phylogenetic speculations. In: N.S. Agar and P.G. Board (Editor), Red Blood Cells of Domestic Mammals. Elsevier, Amsterdam, pp. 367–412.
Baker, C.M.A. and Manwell, C., 1983b. Man and Elephant: The 'dare theory' of domestication and the origin of breeds. Z. Tierz. Züchtungsbiol., 100: 55–75.
Baker, C.M.A. and Manwell, C., 1984. Biochemical markers and the genetic structure of the Jersey breed of cattle. XIXth Conference of the International Society for Animal Blood Group Research, Göttingen, 1984, p. 45.
Baker, R.D., Large, R.V. and Spedding, C.R.W., 1973. Size of animal in relation to productivity with special reference to ruminant-economic aspects. Proc. Br. Soc. Anim. Prod., 2: 35–42.
Balakrishnan, V. and Sanghvi, L.D., 1968. Distance between populations on the basis of attribute data. Biometrics, 24: 859–865.
Barlow, R., 1984. Selection for growth and size in ruminants: is it time to call a moratorium. In: Proc. Second World Congress on Sheep and Beef Cattle Breeding, Pretoria, Vol. 1, Paper No. 39, pp. 1–12.
Barrett, M.A. and Larkin, P.J., 1974. Milk and Beef Production in the Tropics. Oxford University Press, Oxford.
Barton, R.A., 1984. The role of breed societies: past, present and probable. In: Proc. Second World Congress on Sheep and Beef Cattle Breeding, Pretoria, Vol. 1, Paper No. 15, pp. 1–9.
Basrur, P.K., 1969. Hybrid sterility. In: K. Benirschke (Editor), Comparative Mammalian Cytogenetics. Springer-Verlag, New York, pp. 107–131.
Beevor, T., 1788. On the Suffolk breed of cows; raising potatoes, etc. Bath and West and Southern Counties Letters and Papers, 3: 280–285.
Bell, K., 1983. The blood groups of domestic mammals. In: N.S. Agar and P.G. Board (Editor), Red Blood Cells of Domestic Mammals. Elsevier, Amsterdam, pp. 133–164.
Bell, K., Hopper, K.R. and McKenzie, H.A., 1981a. Bovine α-lactalbumin C and α_{SI}-, β- and $\varkappa$-caseins of Bali (Banteng) cattle, *Bos (Bibos) javanicus*. Aust. J. Biol. Sci. 34: 149–159.
Bell, K., McKenzie, H.A. and Shaw, D.C., 1981b. Bovine β-lactoglobulin E,F. and G of Bali (Banteng) cattle, *Bos (Bibos) javanicus*. Aust. J. Biol. Sci., 34: 133–147.
Bernoco, D., Lewin, H.A. and Howland, J., 1984. Role of the bovine major histocompatibility complex in infection and transformation by bovine leukemia virus. XIXth Conference of the International Society for Animal Blood Group Research, Göttingen, p. 53.
Betancourt, A., Gutierrex, C. and Sanchez, A., 1974. Los cromosomas del '*Bos taurus*', '*Bos indicus*', '*Bison bonasus*' y sus hibridos. First World Congress on Genetics Applied to Livestock Production. Vol. 3, pp. 173–176.
Bettini, T.M. and Masina, P., 1972. Proteine e polimorfismo proteico del latte vaccino. Produzione Anim., 11: 107–126.
Bhat, P.N., 1981a. In: S. Sachdeva (Editor), Animal Genetic Resources in India. Indian Veterinary Research Institute, Izatnagar, pp. 4–30.
Bhat, P.N., 1981b. Conservation of animal genetic resources in India. In: Animal Genetic Resources Conservation Management. Animal Production and Health Paper 24, Food and Agriculture Organization, Rome, pp. 86–95.
Blokhuis, H.J. and Buis, R.C., 1979. Genetic relationships between breeds of horses and ponies in the Netherlands. Anim. Blood Groups Biochem. Genet., 10: 27–38.
Bohlken, H., 1961. Der Kouprey, *Bos (Bibos) sauveli* Urbain 1937. Z. Säugetierkunde, 26: 193–256.
Bojanus, L.H., 1827. De uro nostrate eiusque sceleto commentatio. Verhandlingen Kaiserlichen Leopoldinisch – Carolinischen Akadademie Naturforscher, 13(2): 413–478.
Bongso, T.A. and Hilmi, M., 1982. Chromosome banding homologies of a tandem fusion in river, swamp and crossbred buffaloes (*Bubalus bubalis*). Can. J. Genet. Cytol., 24: 667–673.
Bonsma, J.C., 1955. The improvement of indigenous breeds in subtropical environments. In: A.O. Rhoad (Editor), Breeding Beef Cattle for Unfavourable Environments. University of Texas Press, Austin, pp. 170–186.
Bowen, J., 1983. Cattle Baron truly a breed apart. Weekend Australian Mag., 2–3 April, p. 14.
Bowly, E., 1868. Report on the exhibition of live stock at Leicester. J. Royal Agric. Soc. England,

2nd Series, 4: 435–448.
Boyd, M.M., 1914. Crossing bison and cattle. J. Heredity, 5: 189–197.
Boyer, J.P., 1965. De la creation d'un conservatoire national des races Françaises. In: Proc. Second European Poultry Conference, Bologna, 1964 pp.
Braend, M., 1975. Blood group structure of Norwegian Red cattle (NRF). Acta Agric. Scand., 25: 103–108.
Braend, M., 1979. Blood groups of Nigerian cattle. Comparative aspects. Anim. Blood Groups Biochem. Genet., 10: 49–56.
Braend, M., 1981. Measures of genetic variability and aids to selection using blood types. In: Animal Genetic Resources Conservation Management. Animal Production and Health Paper 24, Food and Agriculture Organization, Rome, pp. 243–267.
Braend, M. and Stormont, C., 1963. Haemoglobin and transferrin types in the American buffalo. Nature, 197: 910–911.
Braend, M., Berg, I.H. and Lie, H., 1964. Blood groups of Norwegian cattle. Studies on South and West Norway cattle (SV) and Coloursided Trønder cattle (ST). Acta Agric. Scand. 14: 150–164.
Briggs, H.M. and Briggs, D.M., 1980. Modern Breeds of Livestock, (4th Edition). Macmillan, London.
Brothwell, D., 1978. On the complex nature of man–animal relationships from the Pleistocene to early agricultural societies. In: J.G. Hawkes (Editor), Conservation and Agriculture. Duckworth, London, pp. 45–59.
Brown, A.H.D., 1978. Isozymes, plant population genetic structure and genetic conservation. Theor. Appl. Genet., 52: 145–157.
Brown, H., 1984. Cattlemen fear for their future as the bureaucrats ride in. Weekend Australian Mag., 21–22 July, p. 9.
Brownlee, J.W.I., 1977. The Nkone cattle of Rhodesia. Part I. Rhodesian Agric. J. 74: 1–9.
Buck, C.D., 1949. A Dictionary of Selected Synonyms in the Principal Indo-European Languages. A Contribution to the History of Ideas. University of Chicago Press, Chicago.
Caldwell, H.S. (Editor), 1977. The Water Buffalo. Animal Production and Health Series 4. Food and Agriculture Organization, Rome.
Caldwell, J., Cumberland, P.A., Weseli, D.F. and Williams, J.D., 1979. Breed differences in frequency of BoLA specificities. Anim. Blood Groups Biochem. Genet., 10: 93–98.
Chandler, R.L., 1958. Studies on the tolerance of N'Dama cattle to trypanosomiasis. J. Comp. Pathol., 68: 253–266.
Chapman, A.B., 1974. Significance of breeds. In: H.H. Cole and M. Ronning (Editor), Animal Agriculture. W.H. Freeman and Co., San Francisco, pp. 270–279.
Chatterjee, N., 1926. The Condition of Cattle in India. All India Cow Conference Association. Cited by Simoons, F.J. and Simoons, E.S., 1968. A Ceremonial Ox of India. University of Madison Press, Wisconsin, p. 26.
Chesser, R.K., 1983. Isolation by distance: relationship to the management of genetic resources. In: C.M. Schonewald-Cox, S.M. Chambers, B. MacBryde and W.L. Thomas (Editor), Genetics and Conservation. Benjamin/Cummings, Menlo Park, CA, pp. 66–77.
Chevallier, J.B., 1910. Red Poll cattle. J. Royal Agric. Soc. England, 71: 46–56.
Clayton, H., 1975. Red tape holds up new breed. The Times, 20 October, p. 1.
Clegg, M.T., Brown, A.H.D. and Whitfeld, P.R., 1984. Chloroplast DNA diversity in wild and cultivated barley: implications for genetic conservation. Genet. Res., 43: 339–343.
Close, P., 1984. Rare breed cattle in commercial farming today. Ark, 11: 97–99.
Clutton-Brock, J., 1981. Domesticated Animals from Early Times. Heinemann and The British Museum (Natural History), London.
Cockrill, W.R. (Editor), 1974. The Husbandry and Health of the Domestic Buffalo. Food and Agriculture Organization, Rome.
Cockrill, W.R. 1975. The domestic buffalo. The Blue Book, 25: 121–131.
Cockrill, W.R. 1976. The Buffaloes of China. Food and Agriculture Organization, Rome.
Coles, J., 1973. Archaeology by Experiment. Hutchinson, London.
Coolidge, H.J., 1940. The Indo-Chinese Forest Ox or Kouprey. Memoirs Museum Comp. Zool. Harvard, 54: 421–431.
Coolidge, H.J., 1955. The Forest Ox or Kouprey of South East Asia. In: A.O. Rhoad (Editor), Breeding Beef Cattle for Unfavourable Environments. University of Texas Press, Austin, pp. 109–112.
Crawford, M.A., 1968. Fatty-acid ratios in free living and domestic animals. The Lancet, 1: 1329–1332.
Darwin, C., 1875. The Variation of Animals and Plants Under Domestication, 2 vols. John Murray, London.
Davidson, B.R., 1966. The Northern Myth. University of Melbourne Press, Melbourne.
Deaton, O.W., 1981. The disappearance of local breeds. In: Animal Genetic Resources Conservation Management. Animal Production and Health Paper 24, Food and Agriculture Organization, Rome, pp. 212–229.
Denniston, C., 1976. A note on serological interpretations. Anim. Blood Groups Biochem. Genet., 7: 101–108.

Dent, A.A., 1983. Wild cattle of the Basque country. Country Life, 30 June, p. 1755.
Dent, J.D.D., 1864. Report to the Council on the cattle exhibited at Newcastle. J. Royal Agric. Soc. England, 25: 425–448.
Devillard, J.M., 1981. La politique Française de conservation des races domestiques en peril. In: Animal Genetic Resources Conservation Management. Animal Production and Health Paper 24, Food and Agriculture Organization, Rome, pp. 96–120.
De Young, H.G., 1973. The bison is beleaguered again. Natural History, 82: 48–55.
Dickerson, G., 1969. Experimental approaches in utilising breed resources. Anim. Breeding Abstr., 37: 191–202.
Dickerson, G.E., 1978. Animal size and efficiency: basic concepts. Anim. Prod., 27: 367–379.
Dickinson, W., 1852. On the farming of Cumberland. J. Royal Agric. Soc. England, 13: 207–300.
Dixon, H.H., 1865a. Rise and progress of Shorthorns. J. Royal Agric. Soc. England, 2nd Series, 1: 317–329.
Dixon, H.H., 1865b. Field and Fern, 2 vols. Rogerson and Tuxford, Strand.
Dobie, J.F., 1941. The Longhorns. Bramhall House, New York.
Donald, H.P., 1944. Pedigree bull production in relation to bull licensing. Vet. Rec., 56 (23 September): 352–353.
Donald, H.P. and El Itriby, A.A., 1945. Herd size and its genetical significance in pedigree cattle breeding. J. Agric. Sci., 35: 84–94.
Dove, W.F., 1935. Physiology of horn growth. J. Exp. Zool., 69: 347–405.
Downs, J.F. and Ekvall, R.B., 1965. Animals and social types in the exploitation of the Tibetan Plateau. In: A. Leeds and A.P. Vayda (Editor), Man, Culture and Animals. Publication 78, American Association for the Advancement of Science, Washington, DC, pp. 169–184.
Duke, J.B., 1979. Animal Physiology: Adaptation and Environment. Cambridge University Press, Cambridge.
Dziurdzik, B., 1975. Key to the identification of hairs of mammals from Poland. Acta Zool. (Cracow), 18: 73–109.
Dziurdzik, B., 1978. Histological structure of the hair in hybrids of European bison and domestic cattle. Acta Theriologia, 23: 277–284.
Edwards, J. (Editor), 1959. Genetic Considerations in Breeding Two Million Cattle to Two Hundred Sires. Milk Marketing Board, Thames Ditton, Surrey, U.K.
Edwards, K., 1983. A Town Like Alice. A breed like South Devon? Aust. South Devon Cattle Breeders' Assoc. Newsl., No. 21 (September), p. 15.
Ehrlich, P., 1983. Genetics and the extinction of butterfly populations. In: C.M. Schonewald-Cox, S.M. Chambers, B. MacBryde and W.L. Thomas (Editor), Genetics and Conservation. Benjamin/Cummings, Menlo Park, CA, pp. 152–163.
Ehrlich, P. and Ehrlich, A., 1982. Extinction: the Causes and Consequences of the Disappearance of Species. Victor Gollancz, London.
Eldridge, F. and Blazak, W.F., 1977. Comparison between the Y chromosomes of Chianina and Braham cross bred steers. Cytogenet. Cell Genet., 18: 57–60.
Epstein, H., 1971. The Origin of the Domestic Animals of Africa, Vols I and II. Africana, New York.
Epstein, H. and Mason, I.L., 1984. Cattle. In: I.L. Mason (Editor), Evolution of Domesticated Animals. Longman, London, pp. 6–27.
Evans-Pritchard, E.E., 1940. The Nuer. Oxford University Press, Oxford.
Faber, H.E. and Stone, W.H., 1976. Cattle allotypes: a review and suggested nomenclature. Anim. Blood Groups Biochem. Genet., 7: 39–50.
Fahimuddin, M., 1975. Domestic Water Buffalo. Oxford and IBH Publishing, New Delhi.
Ferguson, A., 1980. Biochemical Systematics and Evolution. Blackie, Glasgow.
Finch, V.A. and Western, D., 1977. Cattle colors in pastoral herds: natural selection or social preference? Ecology, 58: 1384–1392.
Fiorentini, A., Braend, M. and Mzee, R.M., 1980. Red blood cell groups of East African Zebu cattle. Anim. Blood Groups Biochem. Genet., 11: 43–47.
Fischer, H., 1969. Die chromosomensätze des Bali-rindes (*Bibos banteng*) und des Gayal (*Bibos frontalis*). Z. Tierz. Züchtungsbiol., 86: 52–57.
Fischer, H. and Hohn, H., 1976. Der Karotyp eines weiblichen Tamarau (*Anoa mindorensis*). Giessnener Beitr. Erbpathol. Züchthyg., 6: 173–177.
Fisher, R.A., 1930. The Genetical Theory of Natural Selection. Clarendon Press, Oxford.
Fisher, R.A., 1931. The evolution of dominance. Biol. Rev., 6: 345–368.
Fisher, R.A., 1934. Some results of an experiment on dominance in poultry, with special reference to polydactyly. Proc. Linnean Soc. Lond., 147: 71–81.
Fisher, R.A., 1935. Dominance in poultry. Phil. Trans. Royal Soc. Lond., B, 225: 197–226.
Ford, J., 1982. Cool cows to break the Top End milk drought. The Australian, 6 August, p. 7.
Francis, J., 1970. Breeding cattle for the tropics. Nature, 227: 557–560.
Frankel, O.H. and Soulé, M.E., 1981. Conservation and Evolution. Cambridge University Press, Cambridge.
Fredeen, H.T., 1977. Animal breeding today — its dimensions and accomplishments. Can. J. Genet. Cytol., 19: 193–210.

Gahne, B., 1980. Immunogenetics: a review and future prospects. Livestock Prod. Sci., 7: 1–12.

Gardiner, M.R., Anderson, J.L. and Robertson, D.E., 1972. Cancer eye of cattle. J. Agric., West Australia, 13: 53–56.

Gasparski, J.M., 1965. Investigations on the blood groups of wisents (*Bison bonasus*) and hybrids in comparison with the blood groups of cattle. In: Proc. IXth European Blood Group Conference, Prague, 1965, pp. 93–97.

Gasparski, J.M., 1972. Serum amylase isozymes in Wisents and cattle–wisent hybrids. XIIth European Conference on Animal Blood Groups and Biochemical Polymorphism, Budapest, 1970, pp. 181–182.

Gates, G.M., 1952. Breeds of cattle found in Nigeria. Farm and Forest, 1952: 19–29.

Gaunt, D.S., 1984. Beef breed societies — the way ahead. In: Proc. Second World Congress on Sheep and Beef Cattle Breeding, Pretoria, Vol. I, Paper No. 17, pp. 1–11.

Goodknight, C., 1914. My experience with bison hybrids. J. Heredity, 5: 197–199.

Gowen, J.W., 1927. A resumé of cattle inheritance. Bibliograph. Genetica, 3: 87–140.

Gowen, J.W., 1933. On the genetic constitution of Jersey cattle as influenced by inheritance and environment. Genetics, 18: 415–440.

Graml, R., 1984. Importance of correct pedigrees to genetic progress. XIXth Conference of the International Society for Animal Blood Group Research, Göttingen, 1984, p. 106.

Gray, A.P., 1972. Mammalian Hybrids. A Check-List with Bibliography. Commonwealth Agricultural Bureaux, Farnham Royal, U.K.

Grigson, C., 1980, The craniology and relationships of four species of *Bos*. 5. *Bos indicus* L. J. Archaeol. Sci., 7: 3–32.

Grigson, C., 1984. Bifid dorsal spines and *Bos indicus* — a reply to Stallibrass. J. Archaeol. Sci., 11: 117.

Grosclaude, F., Mahé, M-F., Mercier, J.C., Bonnemaire, J. and Teissier, J.H., 1976. Polymorphisme des lactoprotéines de bovinés népalais. 1. Mise en evidence chez le Yak, et caractérisation biochemique de deux nouveaux variants: β-lactoglobulin D_{Yak} et caséine α_{s1}E. Ann. Génét. Sélection Anim., 8: 461–479.

Grosclaude, F., Mahé, M-F. and Accolas, J.P., 1982. Note sur le polymorphisme génétique des lactoprotéines de bovins et de yaks Mongols. Ann. Génét. Sélection Anim., 14: 545–550.

Groves, C.P., 1969. Systematics of the anoa (Mammalia, Bovidae). Beaufortia, 17: 1–12.

Gupta, P., Singh, L. and Ray-Chaudhuri, S.P., 1974. Chromosomes of India breeds of cattle. Nucleus, 17: 129–132.

Gustavsson, I., 1969. Cytogenetics, distribution and phenotype effects of a translocation in Swedish cattle. Hereditas, 63: 68–169.

Gustavsson, I., 1980. Banding techniques in chromosome analysis of domestic animals. Adv. Vet. Sci. Comp. Med., 24: 245–289.

Gustavsson, I. and Rockborn, G., 1964. Chromosome abnormality in three cases of lymphatic leukaemia in cattle. Nature, 203: 990.

Hadorn, E., 1961. Developmental Genetics and Lethal Factors. Methuen, London. (Translated by Ursula Mittwoch.)

Hadžiselimovic, F., 1971. Über das chromosomenbild und das geschlechtoschromatin der Zwergform des Indischen Zebu (*Bos indicus nanus*) Ceylon. Acta Anatom., 80: 418–425.

Haldane, J.B.S., 1962. The argument from animals to man: an examination of its validity for anthropology. In: M.F.A. Montagu (Editor), Culture and Evolution of Man. Oxford University Press, Oxford, pp. 65–83.

Halder, U., 1976. Ökologie und Verhalten des Banteng (*Bos javanicus*) in Java. Paul Parey, Hamburg.

Halnan, C.R.E. and Francis, J., 1976. *Bos taurus* Y chromosome of Africander cattle and the development of improved breeds for the Tropics. Veterinary Record, 96: 88–90.

Halnan, C.R.E., Watson, J.I. and McKee, J.J., 1981. G-Band patterns of the karyotype of *Bos indicus*. Vet. Rec., 11 July, pp. 34–37.

Hamburger, H. and Ramsay, K.A., 1984. The current status and future of animal production and breeding in developing countries: the southern African region. Proc. Second World Congress on Sheep and Beef Cattle Breeding, Pretoria, Vol. I, Paper No. 13, pp. 1–31.

Harris, E.J., Weiermans, J.E., Nel, N.D. and Meyer, E.H.H., 1984. An investigation of chromosomal abnormalities in certain southern African cattle breeds. Proc. Second World Congress on Sheep and Beef Cattle Breeding, Pretoria, Vol. II, Paper No. P12, pp. 1–5.

Harris, H., 1983. Applications of monoclonal antibodies in enzyme genetics. Ann. Rev. Genet., 17: 279–314.

Harris, H. and Hopkinson, D.A., 1976. Handbook of Enzyme Electrophoresis in Human Genetics. North-Holland, Amsterdam.

Harris, M., 1966. The cultural ecology of India's sacred cattle. Current Anthropol., 7: 51–60.

Harris, M.J., Wilson, J.B. and Huisman, T.H.J., 1973. Two hemoglobin phenotypes in the American Bison (*Bison bison*): a possible genetic explanation based on structural studies. Biochem. Genet., 9: 1–11.

Hashiguchi, T., Nishida, T., Hayashi, Y. and Mansjoer, S.S., 1982. Blood protein variations of the native and the Jungle fowls in Indonesia. In: The Origin and Phylogeny of Indonesian Native

Livestock, Vol. III, Morphological and Genetical Investigations on the Interrelationship between Domestic Animals and Their Wild Forms in Indonesia. The Research Group of Overseas Scientific Survey, 1982, Grant-in-Aid for Overseas Scientific Survey, Japan, pp. 97–109.

Hauswirth, W.W. and Laipis, P.J., 1982. Mitochondrial DNA polymorphism in a maternal lineage of Holstein cows. Proc. Nat. Acad. Sci., U.S.A., 79: 4686–4690.

Hawkes, J.G. (Editor), 1978. Conservation and Agriculture. Duckworth, London.

Hayashi, Y., Otsuka, J., Nishida, T. and Martojo, H., 1982. Multivariate cranimetrics of wild banteng, *Bos banteng* and five types of native cattle in Eastern Asia. In: The Origin and Phylogeny of Indonesian Native Livestock, Vol. III, Morphological and Genetical Investigations on the Interrelationship Between Domestic Animals and Their Wild Forms in Indonesia. The Research Group of Overseas Scientific Survey, 1982, Grant-in-Aid for Overseas Scientific Survey, Japan, pp. 19–30.

Hayman, R.H., 1965. Hair growth in cattle. In: A.G. Lyne and B.F. Short (Editor), Biology of the Skin and Hair Growth. Angus and Robertson, Sydney, pp. 575–590.

Hazel, L.N., 1943. The genetic basis for constructing selection indexes. Genetics, 28: 476–490.

Heath-Agnew, E., 1983. A History of Hereford Cattle and Their Breeders. Duckworth, London.

Henson, E.L., 1981. An examination of the breed relationship of the Gloucester cattle breed using immunological and electrophoretic techniques. MSc thesis, University of Edinburgh.

Henson, E.L., Archibald, A.L., Oliver, R.A. and Ross, D.S., 1983. Red blood cell antigens, lymphocyte antigens and biochemical polymorphisms in Gloucester cattle, unpublished manuscript.

Henson, J.L., 1978. Preserving Britain's historic farm animals. In: J.G. Hawkes (Editor), Conservation and Agriculture. Duckworth, London, pp. 151–154.

Hermanns, M., 1949. Die Nomaden von Tibet. Verlag Herold, Wien.

Heslop-Harrison, J., 1976. Introduction. In: J.B. Simmons, R.I. Beyer, P.E. Brandham, G.Ll. Lucas and V.T.H. Parry (Editors), Conservation of Threatened Plants. Plenum Press, New York, pp. 3–7.

Heston, A., 1971. An approach to the sacred cow of India. Curr. Anthropol., 12: 191–209.

Heuch, I., 1975. The relationship between separation time and genetic distance based on angular transformation of gene frequencies. Biometrics, 31: 685–700.

Hickman, C.G., 1981. Breeding programmes for indigenous breeds. In: Animal Genetic Resources Conservation Management. Animal Production and Health Paper 24. Food and Agriculture Organization, Rome, pp. 299–317.

Hickman, C.G., 1982. Cattle breeding in Bhutan, Ceres, FAO, March–April.

Hickman, C.G., 1984. Management aspects of animal genetic resources. Proc. Second World Congress on Sheep and Beef Cattle Breeding, Pretoria, 1984. Vol. I, Paper No. 10, pp. 1–21.

Hines, H.C., 1977. Blood group examination of cattle breed purity. Anim. Blood Groups Biochem. Genet., 8 (Suppl. 1): 31–32.

Hodgson, R.E. (Editor) 1961. Germ Plasm Resources. Publication 66, American Association for the Advancement of Science, Washington, DC.

Hoffpauir, R., 1982. The water buffalo: India's other bovine. Anthropos, 77: 215–238.

Holmberg, S.D., Osterholm, M.T., Senger, K.A. and Cohen, M.L., 1984a. Drug-resistant Salmonella from animals fed antimicrobials. New Engl. J. Med., 311: 617–622.

Holmberg, S.D., Wells, J.G. and Cohen, M.L., 1984b. Animal-to-man transmission of antimicrobial-resistant Salmonella: investigations of U.S. outbreaks, 1971–1983. Science, 225: 833–835.

Hooijer, D.A., 1956. The valid name of the banteng *Bibos javanicus* d'Alton. Zoöl. Mededeling. Rijksmuseum Natuurlijke Historie Leiden, 34: 223–226.

Hopkins, G.M., 1967. Pied beauty. In: W.H. Gardiner and N.H. Mackenzie (Editors), The Poems of Gerard Manley Hopkins. Oxford University Press, London, pp. 69–70 and Io (p. 141).

Hopper, P., 1984. The role of rare breed cattle on a small diary farm. Ark, 11 (August): 240–241, 244–245.

Hsu, T.C., 1979. Human and Mammalian Cytogenetics. An Historical Perspective. Springer-Verlag, New York.

Hsu, T.C. and Benirschke, K., 1967–1977. An Atlas of Mammalian Chromosomes. Springer-Verlag, New York.

Hunter, G., 1970. The administration of Agricultural Development. Oxford University Press, Oxford.

Hutchison, C.A., Newbold, J.E., Potter, E.S. and Edgell, M.H., 1974. Maternal inheritance of mammalian mitochondrial DNA. Nature, 251: 536–538.

Ianelli, D., 1978. Water buffalo (*Bubalus bubalus arnee*) allotypes: identification of a multiple allelic system. Anim. Blood Groups Biochem. Genet., 9: 105–113.

Ibsen, H.L., 1933. Cattle inheritance. I. Color. Genetics, 18: 441–480.

Jaap, R.G., 1965. Minimum population size and source of stock. In: Proc. Second European Poultry Conference, Bologna, 1964, pp. 429–431.

James, P.G., 1971. Agricultural Policy in Wealthy Countries. Angus and Robertson, Sydney.

Jamieson, A., 1965. The genetics of transferrins in cattle. Heredity, 20: 419–441.

Jamieson, A., 1966. The distribution of transferrin genes in cattle. Heredity, 21: 191–218.

Jamieson, A., 1967. The application of a blood group formula. Xth European Conference on Animal Blood Groups and Biochemical Polymorphisms, Paris, 1966, pp. 461–464.

Jamieson, A., 1978. Electromorphs and erroneous pedigrees. XVIth International Conference on Animal Blood Groups and Biochemical Polymorphism, Leningrad, Abstracts, p. 27.

Jenkinson, D.M. and Nay, T., 1972. The sweat glands and hair follicles of European cattle. Aust. J. Biol. Sci., 25: 585–595.

Jenkinson, D.M. and Nay, T., 1973. The sweat glands and hair follicles of Asian, African and South American cattle. Aust. J. Biol. Sci., 26: 259–275.

Jenkinson, D.M. and Nay, T., 1975. The sweat glands and hair follicles of different species of Bovidae. Aust. J. Biol. Sci., 28: 55–68.

Jewell, P.A., 1971. The case for the preservation of rare breeds of domestic livestock. Vet. Rec., 13 November, pp. 524–527.

Jewell, P.A. and Alderson, G.L.H., 1977. Genetic conservation in domestic animals: purposes and actions to preserve rare breeds. J. Royal Soc. Arts, 125: 693–710.

Johansson, I. and Rendel, J., 1968. Genetics and Animal Breeding. Oliver and Boyd, Edinburgh. (Translated from the Swedish by Michael Taylor).

Johnston, T.H. and Bancroft, M.J., 1918. A tick-resistant condition in cattle. Proc. Royal Soc. Queensland, 30: 219–317.

Jope, E.M., 1976. The evolution of plants and animals under domestication: the contribution of studies at the molecular level. Phil. Trans. Royal Soc. Lond., B, 275: 99–109.

Joubert, D.M. and Hammond, J., 1958. A crossbreeding experiment with cattle, with special reference to the maternal effect in South Devon–Dexter crosses. J. Agric. Sci., 51: 325–341.

Kaczmarek, A. and Dorynek, Z., 1979. Influence of the selection criteria on the blood group structure in breeding bulls of Lowland Black and White breed in Poland. In: Proc. XVIth International Conference on Animal Blood Groups and Biochemical Polymorphism, Leningrad, 1978, Vol. 2, pp. 142–152.

Kalia, H.R., 1974. Appraisal of the cow (*Bos indicus*) × yak (*Bos grunniens*) crossbreeding work in cold and elevated regions of Himachal Pradash (India). First World Congress on Genetics Applied to Livestock Production, Vol. 3, pp. 723–730.

Karlikov, D.V., Sorokovoj, P.F., Yakushenkov, A.M. and Grinberg, R.O., 1979. Analysis of association between blood group marker genes and bovine leukosis incidence. In: Proc. XVIth International Conference on Animal Blood Groups and Biochemical Polymorphism, Leningrad, 1978, Vol. II, pp. 219–224.

Kästli, F., 1979. Blood groups and biochemical polymorphisms in the Hérens cattle breed in Switzerland. In: Proc. XVIth International Conference on Animal Blood Groups and Biochemical Polymorphism, Leningrad, 1978, Vol. 2, pp. 101–108.

Kelley, R.B., 1959. Native and Adapted Cattle. Angus and Robertson, Sydney.

Kelly, J.H., 1971. Beef in Northern Australia. Australian National University Press, Canberra.

Kidd, K.K., 1969. Phylogenetic Analysis of Cattle Breeds. PhD thesis, University of Wisconsin. (University Microfilms, Ann Arbor, Michigan, No. 70–3581.)

Kidd, K.K. and Pirchner, F., 1971. Genetic relationships of Austrian cattle breeds. Anim. Blood Groups Biochem. Genet., 2: 145–148.

Kidd, K.K., Osterhoff, D., Erhard, L. and Stone, W.H., 1974. The use of genetic relationships among cattle breeds in the formulation of rational breeding policies: an example with South Devon (South Africa) and Gelbvieh (Germany). Anim. Blood Groups Biochem. Genet., 2: 145–158.

Kidd, K.K., Stone, W.H., Crimella, C., Carenzi, C., Casati, M. and Rognoni, G., 1980. Immunogenetic and population genetic analyses of Iberian cattle. Anim. Blood Groups Biochem. Genet., 11: 21–28.

Kimura, M. and Crow, J.F., 1964. The number of alleles that can be maintained in a finite population. Genetics, 49: 725–738.

Kimura, M. and Ohta, T., 1971. Theoretical Aspects of Population Genetics. Princeton University Press, New Jersey.

Kimura, M., Oniwa, K., Ito, S. and Isogai, I., 1983. Protein polymorphism in two populations of the wild quail *Coturnix coturnix japonica*. Anim. Blood Groups Biochem. Genet., 15: 13–22.

King, J.W.B., 1981. Genetic exhaustion in single purpose breeds. In: Animal Genetic Resources Conservation Management. Animal Production and Health Paper 24. Food and Agriculture Organization, Rome, pp. 230–242.

King, J.W.B. and Ménissier, F. (Editors), 1982. Muscular Hypertrophy of Genetic Origin and Its Use to Improve Beef Production. Martinus Nijhoff, The Hague.

Kirby, G.W.M., 1979. Bali cattle in Australia. World Anim. Rev., 31: 24–29.

Kraay, G.J., Giebelhaus, E.D. and Colling, D.T., 1978. A case of unrelated twins in cattle. Can. Vet. J., 19: 279–283.

Krumbiegal, I., 1980. Die unterartliche Trennung des Bisons, *Bison bison* (Linné, 1788), und seine Rückzüchtung, Säugetierkund. Mitteil., 28: 148–160.

Lalthantluanga, R. and Barnabas, J., 1974. Hemoglobin alpha chain allelic variants in Gayal (*Bos gaurus frontalis*). Folia Biochemica et Biologica Graeca, 11: 65–69.

Lalthantluanga, R. and Braunitzer, G., 1981. The primary structure of the β^{I}- and β^{II}-chains of yak hemoglobins (Bovidae). Hoppe-Seyler's Z. Physiol. Chem., 362: 1405–1409.

Lalthantluanga, R., Gulati, J.M. and Barnabas, J., 1975. Hemoglobin genetics in bovines and equines. Ind. J. Biochem. Biophys., 12: 51–57.

Landauer, W., 1945. Shall we lose or keep our plant and animal stocks? Science, 101: 497–499.

Lasley, J.F., 1963. Genetics of Livestock Improvement. Prentice-Hall, Englewood Cliffs, NJ.

Latimer, F.G., Wilson, L.L., Cain, M.F. and Stricklin, W.R., 1982. Scrotal measurements in beef bulls: heritability estimates, breed and test station effects. J. Anim. Sci., 54: 473–479.

Laurans, R., 1974. Le probleme de la conservation du materiel génétique en France. First World Congress on Genetics Applied to Livestock Production, Vol. 2, pp. 75–84.

Lauvergne, J.J., 1966. Génétique de la couleur du pelage des bovins domestiques (*Bos taurus* Linné). Bibliograph. Genet., 20: 1–68.

Lauvergne, J.J., 1977. The current status of cattle breeds in Europe. World Anim. Rev., 21: 42–47.

Lauvergne, J.J., 1979. France. In: I.L. Mason (Editor), Inventory of Special Herds. FAO/UNEP Project No. FP/1108-76-02 (833), Conservation of Animal Genetic Resources, Food and Agriculture Organization, Rome, pp. 29–39.

Lauvergne, J.J., 1981. Organization of the conservation and management of genetic stocks of large farm animals. In: Animal Genetic Resources Conservation Management. Animal Production and Health Paper 24, Food and Agriculture Organization, Rome, pp. 318–331.

Lauvergne, J.J. and Laurans, R., 1979. Inventaire et conservation du matériel génétique animal de ferme en France et écodévelopment: une bibliographie signalétique, 1961–1979. Ann. Génét. Sélection Anim., 11: 165–185.

Lauvergne, J.J., Boyazoglu, J.G. and Hubert, D., 1968. Le phénoméne culard chez les bovins: bibliographie annotée. Institut Nationale Recherches Agronomiques, Paris.

Leeds, A. and Vayda, A.P. (Editors), 1965. Man, Culture and Animals. Publication 78, American Association for the Advancement of Science, Washington, DC.

Lehrer, A.R., Brown, M.B., Schindler, H., Holzer, Z. and Larsen, B., 1977. Paternity tests in multisired beef herds by blood grouping. Acta Vet. Scand., 18: 433–441.

Leipold, H.W., Dennis, S.M. and Huston, K., 1972. Congenital defects of cattle: nature, cause and effect. Adv. Vet. Sci., 16: 103–150.

Lerner, I.M. and Donald, H.P., 1966. Modern Developments in Animal Breeding. Academic Press, London.

Longenecker, B.M., 1982. Preparation and properties of monoclonal antibodies against cell surface polymorphic or allelic determinants: their use in blood typing and the study of cell differentiation. Anim. Blood Groups Biochem. Genet. 13: 225–238.

Longsworth, J.W., 1983. Beef in Japan. Politics, Production, Marketing and Trade. University of Queensland Press, St Lucia.

Lush, J.L., 1945. Animal Breeding Plans. Iowa State College Press, Ames, Iowa.

Lydekker, R., 1894. The Royal Natural History, Vol. 2. Frederick Warne, London.

Lydekker, R., 1898. Wild Oxen Sheep and Goats of All Lands, Living and Extinct. Rowland Ward, London.

McCaffrey, F., 1909. First Century of Dairying in New South Wales. Sydney and Melbourne Publishing, Sydney.

McCormick, J.M. and Mascareñas, M.S., 1967. The Complete Aficionado. World Publishing, Cleveland and New York.

McCoubrey, C.M., Sales, D.I. and Archibald, A.L., 1983. Testing genetic models in populations which contain pedigree errors. Anim. Blood Groups Biochem. Genet., 14: 257–268.

McDermid, E.M., Agar, N.S. and Chai, C.K., 1975. Electrophoretic variation of red cell enzyme systems in farm animals. Anim. Blood Groups Biochem. Genet., 6, 127–174.

Machado, M.A., 1981. The North Mexican Cattle Industry 1910–1975. Texas A. & M. University Press, College Station, Texas.

McHugh, T. and Hobson, V., 1972. The Time of the Buffalo. Alfred A. Knopf, New York.

McKenzie, H.A. (Editor), 1971. Milk Proteins, 2 vols. Academic Press, New York.

McKnight, T., 1976. Friendly Vermin: Feral Livestock in Australia. University of California Press, Berkeley.

Mahé, M.F. and Grosclaude, M., 1982. Polymorphisme de la caséine α_{S2} des Bovinés: caractérisation du variant C du Yak (*Bos grunniens*). Ann. Génét. Sélection Anim., 14: 401–406.

Maijala, K., 1974. Conservation of animal breeds in general. First World Congress on Genetics Applied to Livestock Production, Vol. 2, pp. 37–46.

Maijala, K. and Lindström, G., 1966. Frequencies of blood group genes and factors in the Finnish cattle breeds with special regard to breed comparisons. Ann. Agric. Fenniae, 5: 76–93.

Maijala, K., Cherekaev, A.V., Devillard, H-M., Reklewski, Z., Rognoni, G., Simon, D.L. and Steane, D.E., 1984. Conservation of animal genetic resources in Europe. Final Report of an EEAP Working Party. Livestock Prod. Sci., 11: 3–22.

MacKellar, J.C., 1960. The occurrence of muscular hypertrophy in South Devon cattle. Vet. Rec., 72: 507–510.

Makaveev, T., 1970. Albumins, transferrins, serum amylase and blood groups in Bulgarian Water Buffalo. XIth European Conference on Animal Blood Groups and Biochemical Polymorphism, Warsaw, 1968, pp. 235–238.

Makaveev, T., 1984. Biochemical polymorphisms and breeding water buffaloes in Bulgaria. XIXth Conference of the International Society for Animal Blood Group Research, Göttingen, p. 83.
Makino, S., 1944. Karyotypes of domestic cattle, zebu and domestic water buffalo. Cytologia, 13: 247–264.
Manwell, C., 1979. Peer review: a case history from the Australian Research Grants Committee. Search (ANZAAS), 10: 81–86.
Manwell, C. and Baker, C.M.A., 1970. Molecular Biology and the Origin of Species: Heterosis, Protein Polymorphism and Animal Breeding. Sidgwick and Jackson, London.
Manwell, C. and Baker, C.M.A., 1976. Protein polymorphisms in domesticated species: evidence for hybrid origin? In: S. Karlin and E. Nevo (Editors), Population Genetics and Ecology. Academic Press, New York, pp. 105–139.
Manwell, C. and Baker, C.M.A., 1980. Chemical classification of cattle. 2. Phylogenetic tree and specific status of the Zebu. Anim. Blood Groups Biochem. Genet., 11: 151–162.
Manwell, C. and Baker, C.M.A., 1982. Heterozygosity versus population structure in cattle, evidence for different patterns of selection for β-lactoglobulin and for transferrin. XVIIIth International Conference on Animal Blood Groups and Biochemical Polymorphisms, Ottawa, p. 95.
Manwell, C. and C.M.A. Baker, 1986. Evaluation of performance in academic and scientific institutions. In: B. Martin, C.M.A. Baker, C. Manwell and C. Pugh (Editors), Intellectual Suppression. Angus and Robertson, Sydney, pp. 264–300.
Manwell, C., Baker, C.M.A. and Childers, W., 1963. The genetics of hemoglobin in hybrids. I. A molecular basis for hybrid vigor. Comp. Biochem. Physiol., 10: 103–120.
Markham, G., 1615. Countrey Contentments. R. Jackson, London.
Marshall, W., 1796. The Rural Economy of Gloucestershire. G. Nicol, Pall-Mall. (Reprinted 1979 by Allan Sutton, Gloucester).
Marshall, W., 1818. The Review and Abstract of the County Reports to the Board of Agriculture. 5 vols. T. Wilson and Sons, York. (First edition, 1808. 1818 edition reprinted 1968 by Augustus M. Kelley, New York.)
Martin, B., Baker, C.M.A., Manwell, C. and Pugh, C. (Editors), 1985. Intellectual Suppression. Angus and Robertson, Sydney.
Mason, I.L., 1969. A Dictionary of Livestock Breeds. Commonwealth Agricultural Bureaux, Farnham Royal, U.K.
Mason, I.L., 1971. Comparative beef performance of the large cattle breeds of Western Europe. Anim. Breeding Abstr., 39: 1–29.
Mason, I.L., 1973. The role of natural and artificial selection in the origin of breeds of farm animals. Z. Tierz. Züchtungsbiol., 90: 229–244.
Mason, I.L., 1974. Introduction to the Round Table on the Conservation of Animal Genetic Resources. First World Congress on Genetics Applied to Livestock Production, Vol. 2, pp. 13–21.
Mason, I.L. (Editor), 1979. Inventory of Special Herds. FAO/UNEP Project No. FP/1108-76-02(833), Conservation of Animal Genetic Resources, Food and Agriculture Organization, Rome.
Matsuda, Y., Namikawa, T., Kondo, K. and Martojo, H., 1980. A study on karyotypes of the Bali cattle. In: The Origin and Phylogeny of Indonesian Native Livestock. Investigation on Cattle, Fowl and Their Wild Forms. The Research Group of Overseas Scientific Survey, 1980. Grant-in-Aid for Overseas Scientific Survey (Synthesis), Japan, pp. 29–33.
Medawar, P.B., 1960. The Future of Man. Methuen, London.
Meijer, W.C.P., 1962. Das Balirind. A. Zeimsen Verlag, Wittenberg.
Metenier, L. and Grosclaude, J., 1984. The production of monoclonal antibodies to horse and cattle red cells. XIXth International Conference on Animal Blood Groups and Biochemical Polymorphisms, Göttingen, p. 122.
Meyer, H.H., 1984. Chromosomal and biochemical genetic markers of cattle breeds in southern Africa. In: Proc. Second World Congress on Sheep and Beef Cattle Breeding, Pretoria, Vol. I, Paper No. 31, pp. 1–12.
Meyer, E.H.H., Reid, G. and du Plessis, S.J., 1984. Practical experience with blood typing for genetic counselling to breed societies on embyro transfer. XIXth Conference of the International Society for Animal Blood Group Research, Göttingen, p. 153.
Meyn, K., 1984. Requirements and constraints for cattle breeding programmes in developing countries. In: Proc. Second World Congress on Sheep and Beef Cattle Breeding, Pretoria, Vol. I, Paper No. 4, pp. 1–12.
Milburn, M.M., 1848. On the farming of the North Riding of Yorkshire. J. Royal Agric. Soc. England, 9: 496–421.
Miller, R.H., 1977. The need for and potential application of germ plasm conservation in cattle. J. Heredity, 68: 365–374.
Mills, H.D., 1953. *Bos brachyceros* in Africa. Vet. Rec., 65: 587–588.
Milner, R., 1977. Inside business. Cowboys and the incredible Beefalo. Sunday Times (London), 19 June, p. 72.
Mkrtchyan, S.A., 1975. Polimorfizm gemoglobina yakov vysokogornogo Altaya; Mongol'skoi

Naradnoi Respubliki. Trudy Altaiskogo Nauchno-Issledovatel'skogo i Proektno-Teknologicheskogo Instituta Zhivotnovodstva za 1969–1973, 1: 198–202.
Mloszewski, M.J., 1983. The Behaviour and Ecology of the African Buffalo. Cambridge University Press, Cambridge.
Mohr, E., 1949. Development of the European bison during recent years and present state. J. Soc. Preserv. Fauna Empire, N.S. 59: 29–33.
Mortelmans, J. and Kageruka, P., 1976. Trypanotolerant cattle breeds in Zaïre. World Anim. Rev., 19: 14–17.
Mourant, A.E. and Zeuner, F.E. (Editors), 1963. Man and Cattle. Occasional Paper No. 18, Royal Anthropological Institute, London.
Mumford, R.G.R., 1981. Views on the polling factor. Aust. South Devon Cattle Breeders' Assoc. News., No. 14, p. 8.
Murray, L.A., 1972. The names of the humble. In: L.A. Murray (Editor), Poems Against Economics. Angus and Robertson, Sydney, pp. 42–44.
Murray, M., Morrison, W.I., Murray, P.K., Clifford, D.J. and Trail, J.C.M., 1979. Trypanotolerance — a review. World Anim. Rev. 31: 2–12.
Myers, N., 1979. The Sinking Ark. Pergamon Press, Oxford.
Naik, S.N., 1978. Origin and domestication of zebu cattle (*Bos indicus*). J. Human Evolut., 7: 23–30.
Namikawa, T., Matsuda, Y-I., Kondo, K., Pangestu, B. and Martojo, H., 1980. Blood groups and blood protein polymorphisms of different types of the cattle in Indonesia. In: The Origin and Phylogeny of Indonesian Native Livestock. Investigation on the Cattle, Fowl and Their Wild Forms. The Research Group of Overseas Scientific Survey, 1980, Grant-in-Aid For Overseas Scientific Survey, Japan, pp. 35–45.
Namikawa, T., Orsuka, J. and Martojo, H., 1982. Coat color variations in Indonesian cattle. In: The Origin and Phylogeny of Indonesian Native Livestock, Vol. III, Morphological and Genetical Investigations on the Interrelationship Between Domestic Animals and Their Wild Forms in Indonesia. The Research Group of Overseas Scientific Survey, Grant-in-Aid for Overseas Scientific Survey (Synthesis), Japan, pp. 31–34.
Namikawa, T., Amano, T., Kondo, K. and Martojo, H., 1983a. A comparison of karyotypes of the Bali cattle and the bantengs. Report No. 10, Society for Researches on Native Livestock, pp. 59–64 and 249–250. (Japanese with English figure and table legends and summary.)
Namikawa, T., Amano, T., Takenaka, O., Martojo, H. and Widodo, W., 1983b. Studies on the blood groups and biochemical polymorphisms in the different types of cattle and the Bantengs in Indonesia. Report No. 10, Society for Researches on Native Livestock, pp. 68–81, 250–251. (Japanese with English figure and table legends and summary.)
Namikawa, T., Takenaka, O. and Takahashi, K., 1983c. Hemoglobin Bali (Bovine): β^A18(Bl) Lys → His: one of the 'missing links' between β^A and β^B of domestic cattle exists in Bali cattle (Bovinae, *Bos banteng*). Biochem. Genet., 21: 787–796.
Namikawa, T., Ito, S. and Amano, T., 1984. Genetic relationships and phylogeny of East and Southeast Asian cattle: genetic distance and principal component analyses. Z. Tierz. Züchtungsbiol., 101: 17–32.
Nei, M., 1972. Genetic distance between populations. Am. Naturalist, 106: 283–292.
Nei, M., 1973. Analysis of gene diversity in subdivided populations. Proc. Nat. Acad. Sci., U.S.A., 70: 3321–3323.
Nei, M., 1975. Molecular Population Genetics and Evolution. North Holland, Amsterdam.
Nei, M., 1976. Mathematical models of speciation and genetic distance. In: S. Karlin and E. Nevo, (Editors), Population Genetics and Ecology. Academic Press, New York, pp. 723–765.
Nei, M., 1977. F-Statistics and analysis of gene diversity in subdivided populations. Ann. Human Genet., 41: 225–233.
Nei, M., 1978. Estimation of average heterozygosity and genetic distance from a small number of individuals. Genetics, 89: 583–590.
Nei, M., 1980. Stochastic theory of population genetics and evolution. In: C. Barigozzi (Editor), Lecture Notes in Mathematics No. 39, Vito Volterra Symposium on Mathematical Models in Biology. Springer Verlag, Berlin, pp. 17–47.
Nei, M. and Koehn, R.K. (Editors), 1983. Evolution of Genes and Proteins. Sinauer Associates, Sunderland, MA.
Nei, M., Maruyama, T. and Chakraborty, R., 1975. The bottleneck effect and genetic variability in populations. Evolution, 29: 1–10.
Neimann-Sørensen, A., 1956. Blood groups and breed structure as exemplified by three Danish breeds. Acta Agric. Scand., 6: 115–137.
Nevo, E., 1978. Genetic variation in natural populations: patterns and theory. Theor. Population Biol., 13: 121–177.
Nicholls, S.E., 1957. Livestock Improvement (4th Edition). Oliver and Boyd, Edinburgh.
Nisbett, A., 1976. Konrad Lorenz, J.M. Dent, London.
Nozawa, K., 1979. Phylogenetic studies on the native domestic animals in East and Southeast Asia. In: SABRAO 1979. Animal Genetic Resources in Asia and Oceania. Tropical Agriculture Research Center, Ministry of Agriculture, Forestry and Fisheries, Yatabe, Tsukuba, Ibaraki

305, Japan, pp. 23–43.

NRC, 1983. Managing Tropical Animal Resources. Ad Hoc Panel of the Advisory Committee on Technology Innovation, National Research Council, U.S.A. National Academy Press, Washington, DC.

Odend'hal, S., 1972. Energetics of Indian cattle in their environment. Human Ecol., 1: 3–22.

OhUigin, C. and Kelly, E.P., 1984. A survey of the pedigree Kerry cattle population. XIXth Conference of the International Society for Animal Blood Group Research, Göttingen, p. 43.

Oliver, J., 1966. The origin, environment and description of the Mashona cattle of Rhodesia. Exp. Agric., 2: 81–88.

Oliver, R.A., McCoubrey, C.M., Millar, P., Morgan, A.L.G. and Spooner, R.L., 1981. A genetic study of bovine lymphocyte antigens (BoLA) and their frequency in several breeds. Immunogenetics, 13: 127–132.

Olson, T.A. and Willham, R.L., 1982. Inheritance of coat coloration and spotting patterns of cattle: a review. Research Bulletin, Agriculture and Home Economics Experiment, Iowa State University of Science and Technology, No. 595.

Osman, A.H., 1981. Genetic types for different environments. In: Animal Genetic Resources Conservation Management. Animal Production and Health Paper 24, Food and Agriculture Organization, Rome, pp. 162–177.

Osterhoff, D.R., 1966 (published 1967). Blood group gene frequencies in South African cattle breeds. Xth European Conference on Animal Blood Groups and Biochemical Polymorphisms, Paris, pp. 107–114.

Osterhoff, D.R. and Young, E., 1966 (published 1967). Blood groups in African buffalo (*Syncerus caffer*). Xth European Conference on Animal Blood Groups and Biochemical Polymorphisms, Paris, pp. 133–135.

Osterhoff, D.R., Young, E. and Ward-Cox, I.S., 1970. A study of genetic blood variants in African buffalo. J. South African Vet. Med. Assoc., 4: 33–37.

Otsuka, J., Namikawa, T., Nozawa, K. and Martojo, H., 1982. Statistical analysis on the body measurements of the East Asian native cattle and Bantengs. In: The Origin and Phylogeny of Indonesian Native Livestock, Vol. III, Morphological and Genetical Investigations on the Interrelationship Between Domestic Animals and Their Wild Forms in Indonesia. The Research Group of Overseas Scientific Survey, Grant-in-Aid for Overseas Scientific Survey, Japan, pp. 7–17.

Paris, A., 1983. Inspired instigator. Ark, 10: 431.

Payne, F.G., 1969. The Welsh Plough Team to 1600. In: G. Jenkins (Editor), Studies in Folk Life. Routledge and Kegan Paul, London, pp. 236–252.

Payne, W.J.A. and Rollinson, D.H.L., 1976. Madura cattle. Z. Tierz. Züchtungsbiol., 93: 89–100.

Perry, P.J., 1982. The Shorthorn comes of age (1822–1843): agricultural history from the herdbook. Agric. History, 56: 560–566.

Peters, G.H., 1968. Farming as a successful business. In: G.L.D. Shackle (Editor), On the Nature of Business Success. University of Liverpool Press, Liverpool, pp. 35–51.

Peters, H.F., 1958. A feedlot study of bison, cattalo and Hereford calves. Can. J. Anim. Sci., 38: 87–90.

Peters, H.F., 1984. American bison, and bison-cattle hybrids. In: I.L. Mason (Editor). Evolution of Domesticated Animals. Longman, London, pp. 46–49.

Peters, H.F. and Slen, F.B., 1964. Hair coat characteristics of bison, domestic × bison hybrids, cattalo and certain domestic breeds of beef cattle. Can. J. Anim. Sci., 44: 48–57.

Petit, J.P. and Queval, R., 1973. Le Kouri: race bovine du lac Chad. Rev. d'Elevage Méd. Vét. Pays Tropicaux, 26: 97–104.

Pfeffer, P. and Kim-San, O., 1967. Le Kouprey *Bos (Bibos) sauveli* Urbain 1937: discussion systématique et statut actuel. Hypothése sur l'origine du Zebu (*Bos indicus*). Mammalia, 31: 521–536.

Phillips R.W., Johnson, R.G. and Moyer, R.T., 1945. The Livestock of China. United States Government Printing Office. Washington D.C.

Pieper, U. and Geldermann, H., 1984. Influence of misidentified offspring on the estimation of breeding values in cattle. XIXth Conference of the International Society for Animal Blood Group Research, Göttingen, p. 47.

Pinheiro, L.E.L., Moraes, J.C.F., Mattevi, M.S., Erdtmann, B., Salzona, F.M. and Filho, A.M., 1980. Two types of Y chromosome in a Brazilian cattle breed. Caryologia, 33: 25–32.

Pirchner, F., 1984. Breeding for milk and meat in dual purpose cattle. In: Proc. Second World Congress on Sheep and Beef Cattle Breeding, Pretoria, Vol. II, Paper No. 49, pp. 1–15.

Popescu, C.P., 1969. Idiograms of yak (*Bos grunniens*), cattle (*Bos taurus*) and their hybrid. Ann. Génét. Sélection Anim., 1: 207–217.

Popescu, C.P. 1977., Les anomalies chromosomiques des bovins (*Bos taurus* L.). État actuel des connaissances. Annales de Génétique et de la Sélection Animale, 9: 463–470.

Popescu, C.P., 1981. Cytogenetics of domesticated animals: present statement and perspectives. In: Topicos Avançados en Reproducao Animal: 10 Simposio Nacional-Jaboticabal. Sociedade Brasileira de Genética. Sao Paulo, Brasil, pp. 135–152.

Popescu, C.P., Cribiu, E.P., Poivey, J.P., Seitz, J.L. and Boscher, J., 1979. Étude cytogénétique

d'une population bovine de Côte-d'Ivoire. Revue d'Élevage et de Médicine Vétérinaire des Pays Tropicaux, 32: 81–84.
Potter, S.S., Newbold, J.E., Hutchison, C.A. and Edgell, M.H., 1975. Specific cleavage analysis of mammalian mitochondrial DNA. Proc. Nat. Acad. Sci., U.S.A., 72: 4496–4500.
Powell, J.R., 1983. Molecular approaches to studying founder effects. In: C.M. Schonewald-Cox, S.M. Chambers, B. MacBryde and W.L. Thomas (Editors), Genetics and Conservation. Benjamin/Cummings, Menlo Park, CA, pp. 229–240.
Prentice, E.P., 1942. American Dairy Cattle Their Past and Future. Harper, New York.
Ram, C. and Khanna, N.D., 1961. Studies on blood groups of Indian cattle. Ind. J. Vet. Sci., 31: 257–267.
Ram, C., Khanna, N.D. and Prabhu, S.S., 1964. Studies on Indian bovine blood groups. I. Buffalo blood antigenic factors detected through cattle blood-group reagents. Ind. J. Vet. Sci., 34: 84–88.
Ranjekar, P.K. and Barnabas, J., 1969. Haemoglobin phenotypes in Water Buffalo (*Bos bubalus*) during development. Comparative biochemistry and physiology, 28: 1395–1401.
Rastogi, R., 1978. Regional livestock resources for meat production. J. Agric. Soc. Trinidad Tobago, 78: 118–120, 122.
Raven, P.H., 1976. Ethics and attitudes. In: J.B. Simmons, R.I. Boyer, P.E. Brandham, G.Ll. Lucas and V.T.H. Parry (Editors), Conservation of Threatened Plants. Plenum Press, New York, pp. 155–179.
Raynbird, H., 1847. On the farming of Suffolk. J. Royal Agric. Soc. England, 8: 261–329.
Rendel, J., 1957. Blood groups of farm animals. Anim. Breeding Abstr., 25: 223–238.
Rendel, J., 1958a. Studies of cattle blood groups. II. Parentage tests. Acta Agric. Scand., 8: 131–161.
Rendel, J., 1958b. Studies of cattle blood groups. IV. The frequency of blood group genes in Swedish cattle breeds with special reference to breed structure. Acta Agric. Scand., 8: 191–215.
Rendel, J., 1963. An example of changes in the genetic compositions of a cattle breed due to one popular bull. Acta Agric. Scand., 13: 227–238.
Rendel, J. and Gahne, B., 1961. Parentage tests in cattle using erythrocyte antigens and serum transferrins. Anim. Prod., 3: 307–314.
Rendel, J.M., 1980. Low calving rates in Brahman cross cattle. Theor. Appl. Genet., 58: 207–210.
Reynolds, P.J., 1979. Iron-Age Farm: The Butser Experiment. British Museum Publications, London.
Robertson, A., 1953. A numerical description of breed structure. J. Agric. Sci., 43: 334–336.
Robertson, A., 1965. The interpretation of genotypic ratios in domestic animal populations. Anim. Prod., 7: 319–324.
Robertson, A. and Asker, A.A., 1951a. The genetic history and breed structure of British Friesian cattle. Empire J. Exp. Agric., 19: 113–130.
Robertson, A. and Asker, A.A., 1951b. The expansion of a breed of dairy cattle. Empire J. Exp. Agric., 19: 191–201.
Robertson, F.W., 1972. Value and limitations of research in protein polymorphism. XIIth European Conference on Animal Blood Groups and Biochemical Polymorphism, Budapest, 1970, pp. 41–54.
Roe, F.G., 1972. The North American Buffalo. David and Charles, Newton Abbot.
Rognoni, G. and Finzi, A., 1984. Aspects of conservation of animal genetic resources — the Italian experiences. Livestock Prod. Sci., 11: 61–64.
Rouse, J.E., 1969. World Cattle, Vol. 1, Cattle of Europe, South America, Australia and New Zealand. University of Oklahoma Press, Norman.
Rouse, J.E., 1970. World Cattle, Vol. 2, Cattle of Africa and Asia. University of Oklahoma Press, Norman.
Rouse, J.E., 1973. World Cattle, Vol. 3, Cattle of North America. University of Oklahoma Press, Norman.
Rouse, J.E., 1977. The Criollo: Spanish Cattle in the Americas. University of Oklahoma Press, Norman.
Rowlands, I.W., 1964. Rare breeds of domesticated animals being preserved by the Zoological Society of London. Nature, 202: 131–132.
Rowlandson, T., 1853. Farming in Herefordshire. J. Royal Agric., Soc. England, 14: 433– 456.
Rudolph, W., Heine, C. and Sperlich, W., 1980. Zoologische gärten und die ausbildung von studenten in den grundlagen der tierproduktion. Zool. Gärten, 50: 393–400.
Rutman, G.L. and Werner, D.J., 1973. A test of the 'uneconomic culture' thesis: an economic rationale for the 'sacred cow'. Journal of Development Studies, 9: 566–580.
Ryder, M.L., 1970. Why preserve declining breeds of livestock? Animal Breeding Research Report, Agricultural Research Council, pp. 19–26.
Ryder, M.L., 1971. Keeping fossils alive. Nature, 233: 587.
Ryder, M.L., 1976. Why should rare breeds of livestock be saved. Int. Zoo Yearbook, 16: 244–249.
Ryder, M.L., 1980. Hair remains throw light on early British prehistoric cattle. J. Archaeol. Sci., 7: 389–392.
Saumande, J., Chupin, D., Mariana, J.C., Ortavant, R. and Mauleon, P., 1978. Factors affecting

the variability of ovulation rates after PMSG stimulation. In: J.R. Sreenan (Editor), Control of Reproduction in the Cow. Martinus Nijhoff, The Hague, pp. 195–224.
Schäper, W., 1936. Konstitutionsforschung und Krankheitsbekämpfung in der Tierzucht. Z. Tierz. Züchtungsbiol., 35: 1–88.
Scheifler, H., 1974. Durch kreuzung entstehen neue rinderrassen. Säugetierkund. Mitteil., 22: 104–108.
Schonewald-Cox, C.M., Chambers, S.M., MacBryde, B. and Thomas, W.L. (Editors), 1983. Genetics and Conservation. Benjamin/Cummings, Menlo Park, CA.
Schröffel, J., Glasnák, V., Fulka, J., Motlík, J., Pavlok, A., Riha, J. and Polášek, M., 1983. Blood types of twin cattle after embryo transfer to inseminated recipients. Vet. Rec., 22 January, pp. 77–79.
Schultze, H.E. and Heremans, J.F., 1966. Molecular Biology of Human Proteins with Special Reference to Plasma Proteins, Vol. 1. Elsevier, Amsterdam.
Schwabe, C.W., 1984. A unique surgical operation on the horns of African bulls in ancient and modern times. Agricultural History, 58: 138–156.
Scott, L. and Rivington, H., 1870. The agriculture of the Scilly Isles. J. Royal Agric. Soc. England, 2nd Series, 6: 374–392.
Scudder, G.G.E., 1974. Species concepts and speciation. Can. J. Zool., 52: 1121–1134.
Scudder, G.C.E. and Reveal, J.L. (Editors), 1981. Evolution Today. Hunt Institute for Botanical Documentation, Carnegie-Mellon University, Pittsburgh.
Seago, J.A., 1971. Problems of Extension in Traditional Cattle Societies. M.Sc. Thesis, University of Reading.
Seidel, G.E. and Seidel, S.M., 1981. The embryo transfer industry. In: B.G. Brackett, G.E. Seidel and S.M. Seidel (Editors), New Technologies in Animal Breeding. Academic Press, New York, pp. 41–80.
Senn, J., 1972. Das einheimische Koreanische rind (SüdKorea). Zeitschrift für Tierzüchtung und Züchtungsbiologie, 89: 312–322.
Shaw, C.R. and Koen, A.L., 1968. Starch gel zone electrophoresis of enzymes. In: I. Smith (Editor), Chromatographic and Electrophoretic Techniques, Vol. II (2nd Edition), Zone Electrophoresis. Heinemann, London, pp. 325–364.
Shrode, R.R. and Lush, J.L., 1947. The genetics of cattle. Adv. Genet., 1: 210–261.
Siegfried, W.R. and Hofmeyr, M.D., 1979. Cattle colours in Transkei. South African J. Sci., 75: 106–108.
Simmonds, N.W., 1962. Variability in crop plants, its use and conservation. Biol. Rev., 37: 442–465.
Simoons, F.J., 1979. Dairying, milk use and lactose malabsorption in Eurasia: a problem in culture history. Anthropos, 74: 61–80.
Simoons, F.J., 1984. Gayal or Mithan. In: I. Mason (Editor) Evolution of Domesticated Animals. Longman, London.
Simoons, F.J. and Simoons, E.S., 1968. A Ceremonial Ox of India. University of Wisconsin Press, Madison.
Sinclair, A.R.E., 1971. Wildlife as a resource. Outlook Agric., 6: 261–266.
Sinclair, A.R.E., 1977. The African Buffalo. University of Chicaco Press, Chicago.
Singh, H. and Bhat, P.N., 1980. Kinetics of the Friesian gene-flow in populations arising from their crosses with Indian cattle breeds. Ind. J. Anim. Sci., 50: 311–320.
Singh, H. and Bhat, P.N., 1981. Phylogenetic relationship between Indian cattle breeds. Ind. J. Anim. Sci., 51: 691–697.
Singh, H. Bhat, P.N. and Singh, R., 1981. Gene differentiation in Indian cattle. Ind. J. Anim. Sci., 51: 261–270.
Singh, H., Kumar, S. and Bhat, P.N., 1983. Genotypic plasticity of Friesian herds in India. Ind. J. Anim. Sci., 53: 1287–1291.
Slatis, H.M., 1960. An analysis of inbreeding in the European bison. Genetics, 45: 275–287.
Smith, C., 1984a. Major genes in animal breeding. Animal Breeding Research Organisation [U.K.] Report, pp. 23–27.
Smith, C., 1984b. Economic aspects of conserving animal genetic resources. Animal Genetic Resources Information, FAO–UNEP Food and Agriculture Organization, Rome.
Smith, C., 1984c. Estimated costs of genetic conservation in farm animals. In: Animal Genetic Resources Conservation by Management Data Banks and Training. Animal Production and Health Paper 44/1, Food and Agriculture Organization, Rome.
Smith, C.A.B., 1977. A note on genetic distance. Ann. Human Genet., 40: 463–479.
Smoliak, S. and Peters, H.F., 1955. Climatic effects on foraging performance of beef cows on winter range. Can. J. Agric. Sci., 35: 213–216.
Societé d'Ethnozootechnie, 1976. Le Yak. Ethnozootechnie, No. 15.
Sorokovoi, P.F., Bukarov, N.G. and Zagdsuren, E., 1982. [Blood groups in Mongolian cattle, yaks and their hybrids.] Genetika, 18: 306–312. (Russian, English Summary.)
Spooner, R.L., Oliver, R.A., Sales, D.I., McCoubrey, C.M., Millar, P., Morgan, A.P., Amorenca, B., Bailey, E., Bernoco, D., Brandon, M., Bull, R.W., Caldwell, J., Cwik, S., van Dam, R.H., Dodd, J., Gahne, B., Grosclaude, F., Hall, J.G., Hines, H., Leveziel, H., Newman, M.J., Stear, M.J.,

Stone, W.H. and Vaiman, M., 1979. Analysis of alloantisera against bovine lymphocytes. Joint Report of the First International Bovine Lymphocyte Antigen (BoLA) Workshop. Anim. Blood Groups Biochem. Genet., 10: 63–68.
Stallibrass, S., 1983. A bifid thoracic vertebral spine from a bovine in the Roman Fenland. J. Archaeol. Sci., 10: 265–266.
Stewart, J.L., 1938. The cattle of the Gold Coast. Empire J. Exp. Agric., 6: 85–94.
Stormont, C., 1977. Blood typing cattle and horses. In: Ensminger, M.E. (Editor), Beef Cattle Science Handbook, Vol. 14. Interstate Publishers, Danville, pp. 572–591.
Stormont, C.J., 1984. Genetic markers in the blood and their application in animal breeding. In: Proc. Second World Congress on Sheep and Beef Cattle Breeding, Pretoria, Vol. I, Paper No. 30, pp. 1–9.
Stufflebeam, C.E., 1983. Principles of Animal Agriculture. Prentice-Hall, Englewood Cliffs, NJ.
Sun, M., 1984. Use of antibiotics in animal feed challenged. Science, 226: 144–146.
Subandriyo, P.S., Zulbardi, M. and Roesyat, A., 1979. Performance of Bali Cattle as work animals and milk and beef producers. Indonesian Agricultural Research Development Journal, 1 (1&2): 9–10, 24.
Swaminathan, M.S., 1981. Keynote address. In: Animal Genetic Resources Conservation Managament. Animal Production and Health Paper 24, Food and Agriculture Organization, Rome, pp. 6–14.
Tajima, F. and Nei, M., 1982. Biases of the estimates of DNA divergence obtained by the restriction enzyme technique. J. Molec. Evolut., 18: 115–120.
Taneja, V.K., Bhat, P.N. and Garg, R.C., 1979. Genetic divergence in various Sahiwal x Holstein cross-bred grades. Theor. Appl. Genet., 54: 69–74.
Tanner, H., 1858. The cattle of the West of England. J. Bath and West of England Soc., n.s. 6: 178–220.
Taylor, St C.S., 1973. Genetic differences in milk production in relation to mature body weight. Proc. Br. Soc. Anim. Prod., 2: 15–26.
Templeton, A.R. and Read, B., 1983. The elimination of inbreeding depression in a captive herd of Speke's gazelle. In: C.M. Schonewald-Cox, S.M. Chambers, B. MacBryde and W.L. Thomas (Editors), Genetics and Conservation. Benjamin/Cummings, Menlo Park, CA, pp. 241–261.
Thenius, E., 1980. Grundzüge der Faunen — und Verbreitungsgeschichte der Säugetiere Ein historische Tiergeographie. Gustav Fischer Verlag, Stuttgart.
Thiele, O.W. and Urbaschek, B., 1966 (published 1967). Untersuchungen zur chemischen natur der J-Blutgruppe des rindes. Xth European Conference on Animal Blood Groups and Biochemical Polymorphism, Paris, 1966, pp. 97–100.
Thiele, O.W., Oulevey, J., Hennemuth, K. and Koch, J., 1979. Studies on the chemical nature of the lipidic J blood-group substance of cattle. Anim. Blood Groups Biochem. Genet., 10: 1–9.
Thomson, O., 1970. Buffalo steaks from Humpty Doo. The Australian, 5 October, p. 9.
Tisdell, C.A., 1982. Wild Pigs: Environmental Pest or Economic Resource. Pergamon Press, Oxford.
Todd, N.B., 1977. Cats and commerce. Sci. Am., 237: 100–107.
Topsell, E., 1607. The Historie of the Foure-Footed Beasts. William Jaggard, London. (Reprinted as No. 561 in The English Experience by Plenum Press, New York, 1973).
Touchberry, R.W., 1967. A Study of the N'Dama Cattle at the Musaia Animal Husbandry Station in Sierra Leone. Bulletin 724, University of Illinois Agricultural Experiment Station.
Trail, J.C.M., 1981. Work on conservation of animal genetic resources by the International Livestock Centre for Africa (ICLA). In: Animal Genetic Resources Conservation Management. Animal Production and Health Paper 24, Food and Agriculture Organization, Rome, pp. 29–41.
Train, J., 1845. An Historical and Statistical Account of the Isle of Man. 2 vols. Mary A. Quiggin, Douglas, Isle of Man.
Trela, E., Trela, J., Rychlik, T. and Kraszewska, D., 1979. Studies on the immunogenetic structure in a selected population of bulls. In: Proc. XVIth International Conference on Animal Blood Groups and Biochemical Polymorphism, Leningrad, 1978, Vol. 2, pp. 153–159.
Trow-Smith, R., 1959. A History of British Livestock Husbandry 1700–1900. Routledge and Kegan Paul, London.
Tucker, E.M., 1984. Applications of the hybridoma technique in studies of animal genetics. XIXth International Conference on Animal Blood Groups and Biochemical Polymorphisms, Göttingen, p. 121.
Turton, J.D., 1974. The collection, storage and dissemination of information on breeds of livestock. First World Congress on Genetics Applied to Livestock Production, Vol. 2, pp. 61–74.
Van Riper, W., 1932. Aesthetic notions in animal breeding. Q. Rev. Biol., 7: 84–92.
Van Zyl, J.G.E., Dreyer, C.J. and Venter, H.A.W., 1984. Comparative breed structure of Bonsmara and Drakensberger cattle. In: Proc. Second World Congress on Sheep and Beef Cattle Breeding, Pretoria, Vol. II, Paper No. P9, pp. 1–5.
Vasey, G., 1851. Delineations of the Ox Tribe. G. Biggs, London.
Vu Tien Khang, J., 1983. Méthodes d'analyse des données démographiques et généalogiques dans les populations d'animaux domestiques. Génét., Sélection Evolut., 15: 263–298.

Wahlund, S., 1928. Zusammensetzung von Populationen und Korrelationserscheinungen vom Standpunkt der Vererbungslehre aus betrachet. Hereditas, 11: 65–100.
Wallace, R., 1888. India in 1887. Oliver and Boyd, Edinburgh.
Wallace, R., 1896. Farming Industries of Cape Colony. King and Son, London.
Warriner, D., 1934. Economics of Peasant Farming. Frank Cass and Co., London.
Weinberg, A.M., 1967. Can technology replace social engineering? Am. Behav. Sci., 10(9): 7–10.
Wharton, C.H., 1957. An Ecological Study of the Kouprey, *Novibos sauveli* (Urbain). Philippines (Republic) Institute of Science and Technology, Monograph No. 5, Bureau of Printing, Manila.
Wharton, C.H., 1966. Man, fire and wild cattle in North Cambodia. In: Proc. Fifth Annual Tall Timbers Fire Ecology Conference, pp. 23–65.
Wharton, C.H., 1968. Man, fire and wild cattle in Southeast Asia. In: Proc. Annual Tall Timbers Fire Ecology Conference, Vol. 8, pp. 107–167.
Wharton, R.H., Utech, K.B.W. and Turner, H.G., 1970. Resistance to the cattle tick, *Boophilus microplus* in a herd of Australian Illawarra Shorthorn cattle: its assessment and heritability. Aust. J. Agric. Res., 21: 163–181.
White, W.T., Phillips, R.W. and Elting, E.C., 1946. Yaks and yak–cattle hybrids in Alaska. J. Heredity, 37: 355–358.
Whitlock, R., 1980. Rare Breeds. Prism Press, Dorchester.
Wiener, G., 1979. Review of genetic aspects of mineral metabolism with particular reference to copper in sheep. Livestock Prod. Sci., 6: 223–232.
Wiener, G. and Yao, T.S., 1952. Growth of the pedigree Ayrshire cattle population in Great Britain. Empire J. Exp. Agric., 20: 195–208.
Wilson, E.O., 1975. Sociobiology: The New Synthesis. Belknap Press, Cambridge, MA.
Wilson, J., 1909. The Evolution of British Cattle and the Fashioning of Breeds. Vinton and Co., London.
Winter, H., Mary, B., Schleger, W., Dworak, E., Krutzler, J. and Burger, B., 1984. Karyotyping, red blood cell and haemoglobin typing of the mithun (*Bos frontalis*), its wild ancestor and its hybrids. Res. Vet. Sci., 36: 276–283.
Wriedt, C., 1930. Heredity in Livestock. Macmillan, London.
Wright, C.M., 1984. Rare breeds hold their own in beef stakes. Ark, 11 (August): 101.
Wright, S., 1968. Evolution and Genetics of Populations, Vol. 1.1, Genetic and Biometric Foundations. University of Chicago Press, Chicago.
Wright, S., 1969. Evolution and the Genetics of Populations, Vol. 2. The Theory of Gene Frequencies, University of Chicago Press, Chicago.
Wright, S., 1977. Evolution and the Genetics of Populations, Vol. 3, Experimental Results and Evolutionary Deductions. University of Chicago Press, Chicago.
Wright, S., 1978. Evolution and the Genetics of Populations, Vol. 4, Variability Within and Among Natural Populations. University of Chicago Press, Chicago.
Wright, S., 1982. The shifting balance theory and macroevolution. Ann. Rev. Genet., 16: 1–19.
Yamane, J. and Kato, K., 1936. Über die abstammung der ostasiatischen hausrinder auf grund der vergleichenden morphologie der brustwirbel bei den boviden. Zoological Magazine, Tokyo, 48: 705–716 + 3 plates. (Japanese with German summary).
Young, A., 1771. The Farmers Tour Through the East of England. Strahan and Nicol, London.
Young, A., 1804. General View of the Agriculture of Hertfordshire. G. & W. Nicoll, Pall Mall.
Young, G.B., 1953. Population dynamics of the Dexter breed of cattle. J. Agric. Sci., 43: 369–374.
Youatt, W., 1934. Cattle. Their Breeds, Management and Diseases. Baldwin and Cradock, London.
Zeuner, F.E., 1963. A History of Domesticated Animals. Hutchinson, London.
Zeuner, F.E. and Mourant, A.E., 1963. Summary of the Symposium. In: A.E. Mourant, and F.E. Zeuner (Editors), Man and Cattle. Royal Anthropological Institute of Great Britain and Ireland, London, pp. 158–166.
Zhanchiv, T., 1978. Tipy gemoglobina i amilazy i ikh rol' v ekologo-geneticheskoi differentsiatsii populyatsii yaka i krupnogo rogatogo skota. Tsitologiya i Genetika, 12: 137–141.
Zuckerman, S., 1971. Preserving rare breeds. Nature, 234: 237.

List of Contributors

C.M. Ann BAKER, Chapter 10. Born in 1931, she obtained the degrees of B.Sc. (Dunelm.) in 1954 and M.Sc. (Dunelm.) in 1959. She was a Research Fellow in Zoology at the University of Adelaide until 1986; since then she has been engaged in research and consultancy. Her publications include (with C. Manwell) *Molecular Biology and the Origin of Species: Heterosis, Protein Polymorphism and Animal Breeding,* Sidgwick and Jackson, London and University of Washington Press, Seattle (1970); *Food Production: Good Husbandry or Agribusiness,* Friends of the Earth, Adelaide (1974); and (co-editor with B. Martin, C. Manwell and C. Pugh) *Intellectual Suppression,* Angus and Robertson, Sydney (1986).

Howard T. FREDEEN, B.S.A., M.Sc., Ph.D., Chapter 6. Born in 1921, he received his degrees in Biological Agriculture at the University of Saskatchewan, Ruminant Nutrition at the University of Alta. and Animal Breeding, Genetics and Statistics at Iowa State College, respectively. He was elected Fellow of the Agricultural Institute of Canada in 1967, awarded the Certificate of Merit, Canadian Society of Animal Science in 1976, given the Award of Excellence of the Canadian Society of Genetics and Cytology in 1978, and the Distinguished Alumni Award, University of Saskatchewan in 1981. He was Research Scientist in Animal Breeding at the Lacombe Research Station between 1947 and 1984 and Head of Animal Research from 1955 to 1980. He is author of 383 research and technical papers on meats, carcase evaluation and genetics of cattle, pigs and poultry. He has also written two books on the agricultural history of Alberta.

Philippe LHOSTE, Chapter 4. Born in 1941, he studied Agronomy and Animal Science at the Institut National Agronomie, Paris. He obtained his doctorate in Agronomic Sciences in Paris and worked as an animal scientist in the tropics (Cameroon, Ivory Coast, Senegal and Mexico) for about 20 years. Now based in France he works as an Animal Scientist at the Institut d'Elevage et de Médecine Vétérinaire des Pays Tropicaux in charge of research programmes on livestock production, systems analysis and integration of agriculture and animal husbandry in the tropics. From 1977 to 1978 he was the main consultant for the FAO/ILCA study 'Trypanotolerant livestock in West and Central Africa' (ILCA, 1979 and FAO, 1980).

J. Douglas MACKECHNIE, B. Sc. (Agr.) P.Ag., Chapter 9. Born in 1927 he studied Animal Science at Macdonald College, McGill University, Montreal, where he was awarded the Stern Cup for livestock judging. For the last ten years he has been Program Manager for Dairy Cattle Production at Agriculture Canada, with responsibilities that include the administration of a national milk recording program. He served as Acting Director of the Department's Animal Production Division for a two year period and was a recipient of the Department's Agcellence Award in 1989. He has written a number of articles for the national breed magazines in Canada and has served as President, Ottawa Valley Branch, Agriculture Institute of Canada and a Director of the Ontario Institute of Agrologists.

Clyde MANWELL, Chapter 10. Born in 1930, he obtained the degrees of B.A. at Stanford in 1952, M.S. at University of Washington in 1955, and Ph.D. at Stanford in 1957. He was elected a Fellow of the American Association for the Advancement of Science in 1978. From 1969 until his retirement in 1986 he was Professor of Zoology at the University of Adelaide; since then he has been engaged in research and consultancy. His publications include (with C.M.A. Baker) *Molecular Biology and the Origin of Species: Heterosis, Protein Polymorphism and Animal Breeding,* Sidgwick and Jackson, London and University of Washinton Press, Seattle (1970); and (co-editor with B. Martin, C.M.A. Baker and C. Pugh) *Intellectual Suppression,* Angus and Robertson, Sydney (1986).

Truman G. MARTIN, B.S., M.S., Ph.D., Chapter 7. Born in 1928, he studied Agriculture Education at Texas A&M University, College Station, Texas, and earned the M.S. and Ph.D. degrees at Iowa State University, Ames, Iowa. He has been Professor of Animal Sciences, Purdue University, West Lafayette, Indiana, since 1963. He has authored or co-authored 75 research papers and 43 research abstracts. He was visiting scientist at Animal Breeding Research Organisation, Edinburgh, Scotland (1978–79) and at Instituto Nacional Investigaciones Agrarias, Madrid, Spain (1985–86).

Klaus MEYN. Dr. Sc. Agr., Chapter 9. A graduate of Göttingen university West Germany, he read his degree in general agriculture and later took his doctorate in animal breeding.

His experience includes international livestock development, both as a researcher in Kenya and as a livestock specialist with the World Bank. Since 1981 he has directed the Animal Breeders' Federation in West Germany with responsibilities also at the European level. Since 1986 he has been vice-President of ICRPMA.

W.J.A. PAYNE, Chapter 3. Born in 1918, he studied physiology at Cambrige and gained a Ph.D. at Glasgow University. Further studies in Climate Physiology were made at Louisiana State University. After conducting animal husbandry research in the tropics for 20 years he became an international consultant on livestock development and research in the tropics. He is the author of two major textbooks *An Introduction to Animal Husbandry in the Tropics* and *Cattle Production in the Tropics.*

Ralph W. PHILLIPS, Chapter 1. Born in 1909, he received a B.S. (Agric.) degree from Berea College and M.A. and Ph.D. degrees from the University of Missouri. He also holds Honorary D.Sc. degrees from Berea College and West Virginia University. His posts have included Executive Director, International Organization Affairs, U.S. Department of Agriculture; Deputy Director, Agriculture Division, FAO; Chief, Animal Production Branch, FAO; In Charge Genetics Investigations, U.S. Department of Agriculture; Head, Animal Husbandry Department, Utah State University. For four years until his retirement in 1981 he served as Deputy Director General of FAO in Rome.

Paul STARKEY, M.A., M.Sc., P.G.C.E., Chapter 8. Born in 1949, he qualified in Natural Science at Oxford University and in Education at Cambridge University. Having worked in Malawi, he gained a Distinction in his M.Sc. in Tropical Agricultural Development at Reading University. He worked for 7 years in Sierra Leone, where he initiated a national animal traction programme. Since 1986 he has worked as a consultant involved in stimulating international liaison relating to animal traction, notably in his role as Technical Adviser to the West Africa Animal Traction Network. In 1987 he was appointed an Honorary Research Fellow at the Centre for Agricultural Strategy of the University of Reading. He has had 20 papers published in international journals. His first book *Farming with Work Oxen in Sierra Leone* was published in 1981. His most recent books *Animal-drawn Wheeled Toolcarriers: Perfected Yet Rejected, Animal Traction Directory: Africa, Animal Power in Farming Systems* (the proceedings of an international workshop for which he was Chief Editor) and *Harnessing and Equipment for Animal Traction* have been published by Vieweg, Braunschweig, in cooperation with the German Appropriate Technology Exchange, GATE.

J.D. TURTON, B.Sc., M.R.C.V.S., D.T.V.M., Chapter 2. Born in 1928, he graduated in Veterinary Medicine and Science from the Royal (Dick) Veterinary College and Edinburgh University in 1950, returning in 1957 to study Tropical Veterinary Medicine. After general agricultural practice in the U.K., he worked in the Animal Health Department, Ghana, from 1952 to 1962, becoming Deputy Chief Veterinary Officer. In 1962 he joined the Commonwealth Bureau of Animal Breeding and Genetics as Assistant Director, becoming Director in 1972. He also lectures on animal breeding to postgraduate courses at Edinburgh University's Centre for Tropical Veterinary Medicine, and is currently a member of the FAO Expert Panel on the Conservation of Animal Genetic Resources.

John Vernon WILKINS, N.D.A., M.Sc., M.I. Biol., C. Biol., Chapter 5. Born in 1934, he graduated from the University of Reading. He worked in Kenya for 15 years where he directed the National Sahiwal Stud and planned and initiated the national beef recording scheme. He has worked in Latin America for 12 years and has been team leader of the British Tropical Agricultural Mission in Santa Cruz, Bolivia, since 1983. This is a multi-disciplinary team studying agricultural problems in the lowlands of that country.

Subject Index